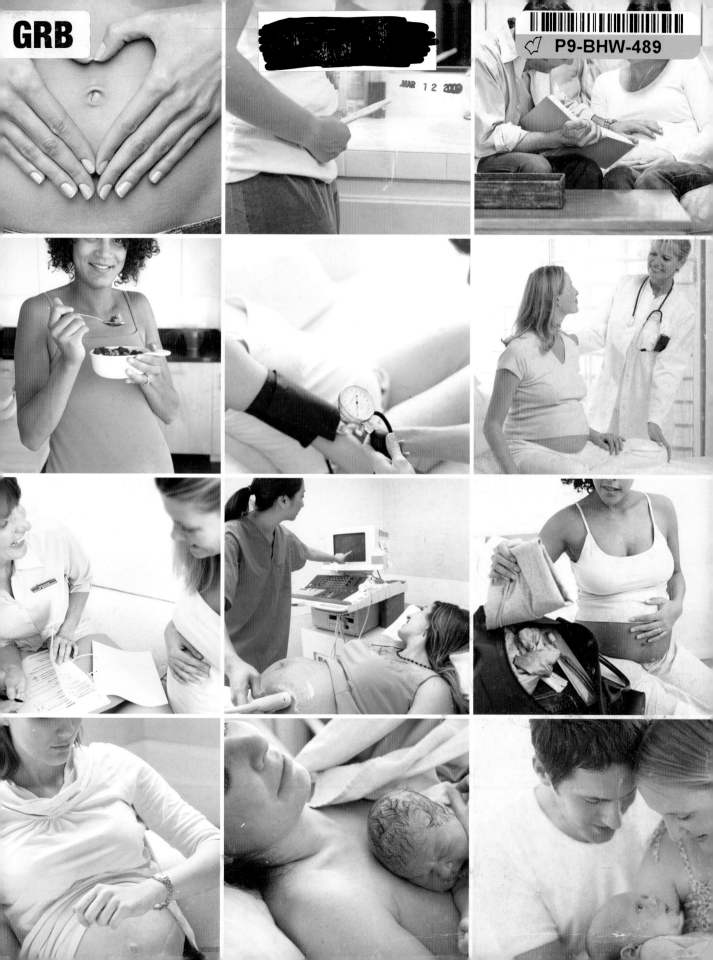

GRB

MAR 1 2 2009

P9-BHW-489

*For my family—each and every one
of you is a blessing in my life.*

*—Robin*

*To my wife Tammy whose constant
support and encouragement made
this book possible for other mothers.*

*—Marcello*

Text © 2009 by Robin Elise Weiss
and Marcello Pietrantoni, M.D.

First published in the USA in 2009 by
Fair Winds Press, a member of
Quayside Publishing Group
100 Cummings Center
Suite 406-L
Beverly, MA 01915-6101
www.fairwindspress.com

13 12 11 10 09          1 2 3 4 5

ISBN-13: 978-1-59233-358-5
ISBN-10: 1-59233-358-3

Library of Congress Cataloging-in-Publication Data available

Cover and book design: HOLTZ DESIGN
Photography: **www.alamy.com:** p. 4 (top), 64, 95, 98 (bottom), 118 (bottom), 120, 141, 142, 143, 148,
156, 161, 168, 176, 200 (bottom), 237, 244, 246, 248 (bottom), 249, 257, 260 (bottom), 282, 288, 303
(left); **www.apimages.com:** p. 26, 86; **www.gettyimages.com:** p. 8, 10 (top), 14, 16, 17, 20, 22, 24,
31, 35, 40, 42, 47, 48, 53, 73, 74, 78, 79, 94, 100, 106, 113, 116, 124 (bottom), 135, 139, 149, 154, 157, 164,
167, 170, 174, 175, 178, 183, 186 (bottom), 194, 195, 200 (top), 208, 209, 218 (bottom), 222, 226, 231,
255, 258, 263, 264, 285, 303 (right), 305; **www.istockphoto.com:** p. 4 (bottom), 10 (bottom), 13, 25,
29, 30, 32, 36, 38, 44, 50, 54, 56, 58, 76, 82, 84 (bottom), 87, 88, 91, 96, 102, 105, 110, 112 (bottom), 122,
126, 128, 136, 144, 150, 152, 153, 158, 190, 204, 210, 213, 216, 218 (top), 234, 252, 254 (bottom), 262;
**www.photoresearchers.com:** p. 4 (bottom), 5 (top), 7, 19, 28, 34, 37, 46, 52, 60, 62, 66, 70, 72, 80, 84
(top), 90, 92, 98 (top), 104, 109, 112 (top), 118 (top), 124 (top), 130, 131, 132, 138, 146, 160, 162, 163, 166,
172, 180, 184, 186 (top), 192, 198, 202, 206, 212, 224, 228, 230, 236, 240, 242, 248 (top), 251, 254 (top),
260 (top), 266, 276, 281

Courtesy of Medela Inc., p. 201; courtesy of www.ababy.com, p. 215; courtesy of Motherwear Int'l,
p. 219.

Printed and bound in Singapore

The information in this book is for educational purposes only.
It is not intended to replace the advice of a physician or medical practitioner.
Please see your health care provider before beginning any new health program.

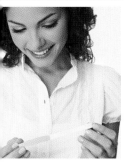
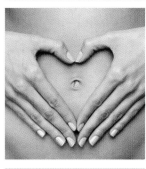
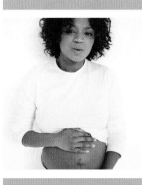
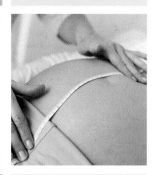
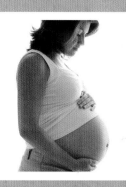

# the complete illustrated
# pregnancy
## companion

*OVER 200 COLOR PHOTOS SHOW YOU WHAT TO EXPECT IN EACH OF YOUR 40 WEEKS*

## A Week-by-Week Guide to Everything You Need to Do for a Healthy Pregnancy

Robin Elise Weiss, L.C.C.E., C.D. (DONA)
with Dr. Marcello Pietrantoni, M.D., F.A.C.O.G.

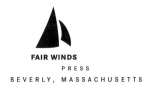

FAIR WINDS
PRESS
BEVERLY, MASSACHUSETTS

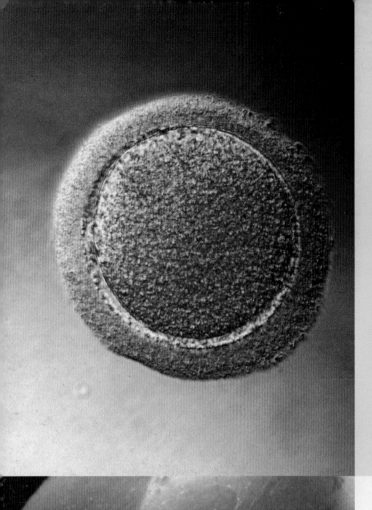

# contents

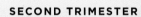

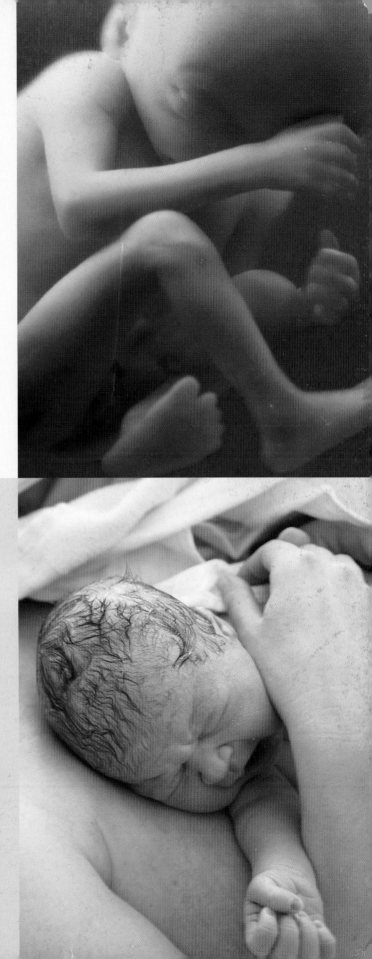

## THIRD TRIMESTER

# HOW TO USE
# THIS BOOK

WELCOME TO YOUR PREGNANCY companion and instruction guide! This book is your week-by-week reference to forty of the most fascinating weeks of your life.

Each chapter of this book is dedicated to a week of your pregnancy. And each chapter kicks off with a handy Checklist, Baby Data about how your baby is growing, and Body Basics about how your body may be changing. Consider this section your crash course in pregnancy for the week. You can use it to sit down with your partner to review the week while you spend time talking and dreaming about the baby, or you might consider using it to update loved ones and friends on what's going on inside your body at this stage of development. Here you will also find a What to Watch For reference section to let you know things to watch out for each week.

After the crash course, you'll find in-depth discussions about what matters most during each week: Pregnancy Particulars. In this section, you'll read about issues that you're likely to discuss with your doctor or midwife that week and questions you should be asking about your prenatal care. This gives you a chance to look at all of your options and entertain various thoughts about them before deciding what will work best for you and your family.

In each chapter, you'll also find Hot Mama tips to help you stay looking and feeling great during

your pregnancy and after. From the maternity fashion scene to building a safe and comfortable nursery, you're covered here. Take a look at the latest and greatest maternity clothes, baby products, and must-have items for your pregnancy, baby, and nursery.

Some chapters also offer a Memorable Moment. These quotes came from women who have been there before you and wanted to share their wisdom and what they learned along to way.

You have probably been told that pregnancy is all about the beautiful process of growing a baby and how wonderful that process can be, only to have that followed with a lengthy list of what can go wrong. This can lead to a very frightening experience for many pregnant women and their families. That's why each chapter of this book includes an affirmation or positive thought. This is meant to reassure you that millions of women have successfully come before you and that you too will get through this process—fully prepared to welcome a healthy, gorgeous baby into your life. Try to incorporate these affirmations into your everyday life because they really can help soothe you and focus your attention. Each week, you may want to tape the new affirmation someplace you will see it every day, such as on your bathroom mirror. Say the affirmation aloud and quietly to yourself throughout the day to help ingrain its message.

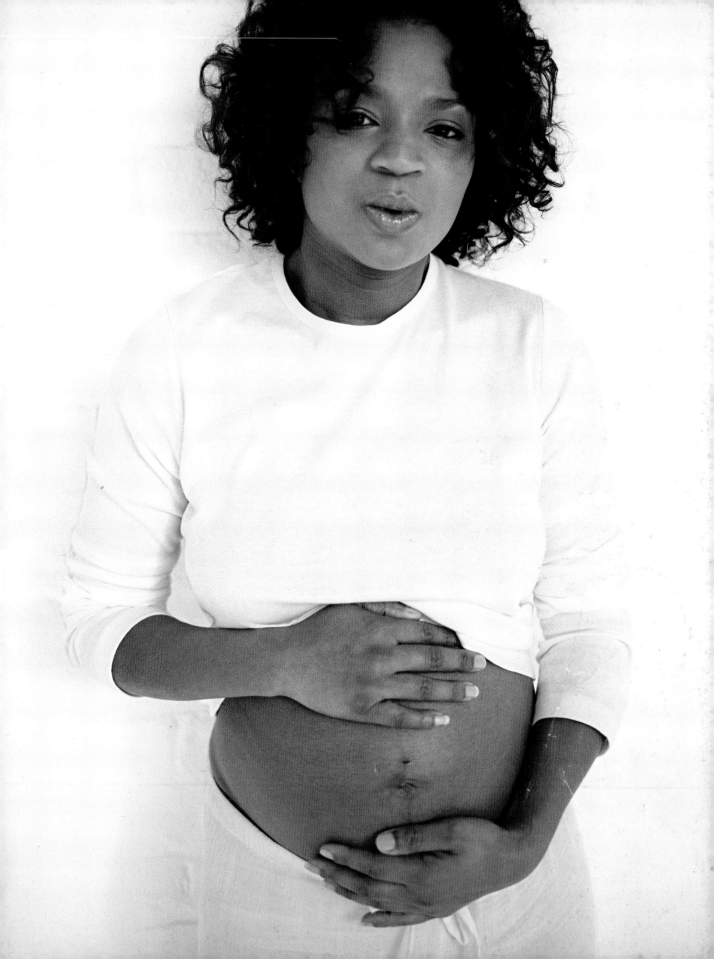

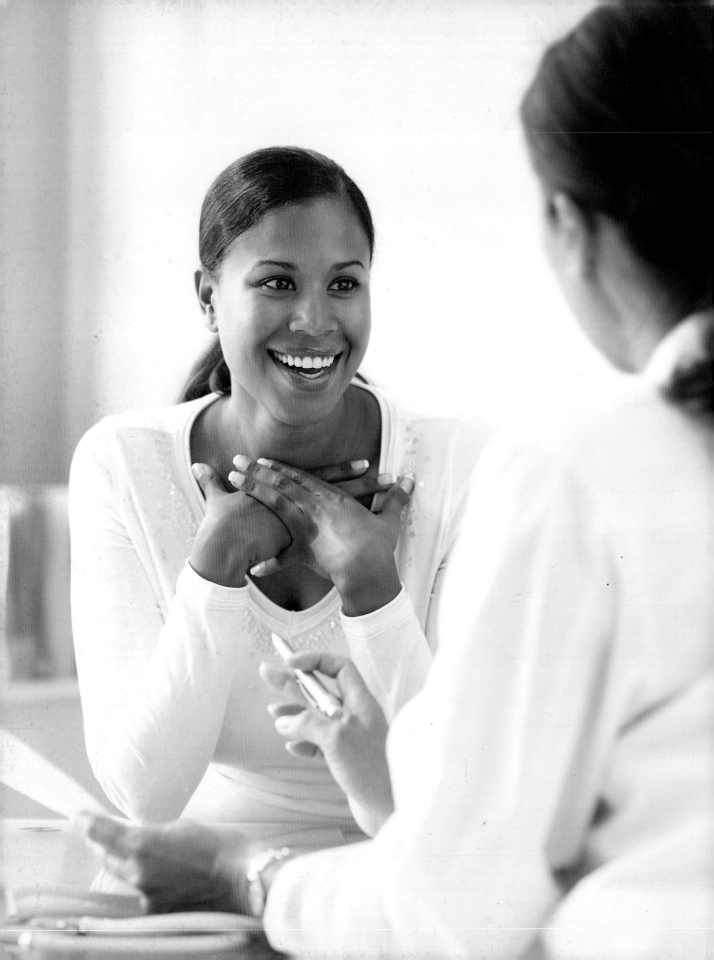

# WEEK 1

## ✎ CHECKLIST FOR WEEK 1

[ ]  Select a prenatal vitamin.
[ ]  Plan your preconceptional health visit.
[ ]  Decide if you need genetic counseling.
[ ]  Define your philosophy of prenatal care.
[ ]  Start developing a comprehensive list
     of your family medical history.

## ○ WHAT TO WATCH FOR THIS WEEK

**Bleeding or spotting:** Red or brown bleeding or spotting when
it is not expected could be a sign of problems with your menstrual
cycle. When reported to your practitioner early, any potential
problems can be addressed.

**One-sided pain:** One-sided pain in your abdomen can indicate
the presence of an ovarian cyst, which might interfere with
conception attempts, or it could simply be an indication of
ovulation.

**Irregular menstrual cycles:** Menstrual irregularities can be long
or short cycles or cycles where you experience breakthrough
bleeding or bleeding at any point other than when your period is
expected. Because these can impede your ability to get pregnant,
you should see your midwife or doctor for further information.

*Report any strange or troublesome symptoms to your practitioner
immediately.*

##  BODY BASICS

Every menstrual cycle, your body goes through a complex dance
of hormones and timing that sets into motion the process of
ovulation—where an egg is released and available to be fertilized.
From there, if you are trying to get pregnant, the goal is for the egg
to be implanted inside your uterus, where it will nestle and grow for
the next 266 days or so until your baby is ready to be born.

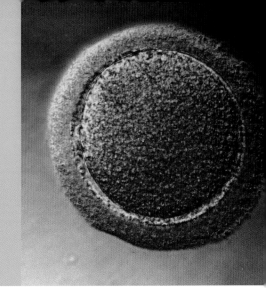

## 🛒 BABY DATA

There isn't a baby to speak of this week. However, your body is shedding its uterine lining in preparation for a new cycle. An egg is finishing up the process of ripening this week, but it won't be released from its home in your ovary until ovulation occurs more than a week from now.

## Select a Prenatal Vitamin

Taking a multivitamin before you get pregnant is a quick and easy way to increase your chances of a healthy pregnancy and to prevent problems with your baby due to a lack of certain vitamins and minerals. Many women, even before they get pregnant, have heard that taking 400 micrograms of folic acid prior to pregnancy can substantially decrease a baby's risk of neural tube defects. This is where the neural tube (spinal cord precursor) does not close properly, leaving your baby with a birth defect such as spina bifida or anencephaly.

When choosing the right multivitamin for you, there are a number of things to take into consideration. Ask yourself the following questions:

- Does this contain the right vitamins and minerals?
- Is it safe to take during pregnancy?
- How much does it cost?
- Will my insurance cover it?
- Does it agree with my digestive tract?
- How easily available is it?
- In what form does it come?
- Does it contain DHA or Omega Fatty acids?
- How many times a day should I take it?
- How many capsules are in a dose?

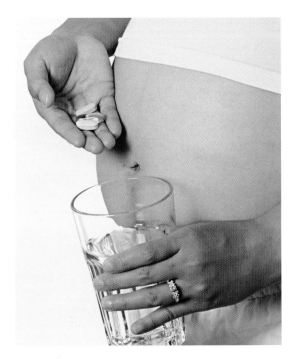

*Taking prenatal vitamins is a must. Try to find a time that works in your schedule to help you to remember to take the vitamins that you have chosen.*

Many women are surprised to note that it is not necessary to take a prescription vitamin when trying to get pregnant or during pregnancy. While there are vitamins available under prescriptive labels, the majority do not differ substantially from the over-the-counter products available at nearly any store, including the generic brands.

If you are already taking a multivitamin, you might simply want to bring the bottle to your midwife or doctor and ask if it is fine to continue. The primary concerns are that a regular multivitamin might not contain enough folic acid and too much vitamin A. If you are consuming the proper levels, your practitioner will most likely say to stick with what works!

## Plan Your Preconceptional Health Visit

A preconceptional health visit is not a new idea, but it is an idea that has been underused until fairly recently. Experts now recognize that there are huge advantages to having a health screening prior to pregnancy, and more and more women take this healthy step to protect their future babies.

During a preconceptional health visit, you will discuss many issues pertaining to your past and current health history. Your responses will be used to predict how your pregnancy should proceed health wise. You and your practitioner can then discuss what changes, if any, you should make to have the healthiest body possible for pregnancy.

The discussion may include the following:

- Should you change your current medications or stay on them?
- At what point should you stop your birth control method?
- Do you have any chronic health issues, such as a thyroid condition, diabetes, or high blood pressure?
- What is your health history?
- What is your age, weight, and general current health picture?
- Do you have any fertility issues, such as past problems getting pregnant or cycle problems?
- Any other questions you may have

PREGNANCY AFFIRMATION
FOR WEEK 1

# I am preparing my body to welcome a baby.

## Decide If You Need Genetic Counseling

The decision about whether or not to undergo genetic counseling may or may not be an easy task for you and your family. One of the best things you can do before making the decision is to have a genetic counselor help you sort through your medical histories and familial histories. This may give you a much clearer picture of the real risks associated with genetic factors and pregnancy for your specific situation. For example, if the risk of a certain genetic disease is 1 in 1,000 given your age group, but when you factor in personal issues the risk then drops to 1 in 5,000, the last number is more customized and specific to you.

People choose to have genetic counseling for the following reasons:

- Family history of genetic disorders
- Prenatal testing that places them in a higher risk category
- Age or other predetermining factor

Many people know ahead of pregnancy that they will or will not have genetic testing. What you may not expect is for those feelings or decisions, even deep-seated ones, to change once you become pregnant. Your reasons or beliefs may change for a variety of reasons, including:

- Screening tests indicating a potential problem
- Further discussion with your care provider or genetic counselor
- Change of heart for either you or your partner

If you are struggling with the decision concerning genetic testing, you should know the following things before making up your mind:

- Which tests are available
- What risks each test presents
- How and when each test is done
- How the results will be delivered
- How likely it is that the results are correct

In the end, the central question is how will you and your partner react to the test results. For example, if you know that you will not make any changes in your pregnancy, birth, or parenting plans because of the genetic test results, are you willing to accept the risks to the pregnancy just to find out?

This question is not one that is easily answered, nor is it a question that many people feel that they can discuss openly. Be sure to talk to as many people as you can, including your family, religious leaders, medical practitioners, and genetic counselors to help you make these decisions.

## Define Your Philosophy of Prenatal Care

The choice of practitioner is a huge decision, and the sooner you make it, the more time you have to get to know this person. For some women, the obvious choice is whoever they have been seeing for their well-woman care such as birth control and Pap smears. The doctor or midwife who cares for you on an annual basis should definitely be a candidate for the position of baby catcher, but it is also wise to look around because many women find, often later in pregnancy, that what they need for prenatal care is often very different from what they need for yearly checkups.

One of the best methods for figuring out if a midwife or doctor is right for you is to formulate your philosophy of prenatal care. Ask yourself the following questions:

- How much do I already know about pregnancy and birth?
- Do I have strong opinions?
- Would I prefer to define my practitioner as a partner in my health care or as a director?
- Do I have any special needs for my pregnancy?
- What do I know about informed consent and informed refusal?
- How much emotional support do I need from my medical care provider?
- Do I need someone to hold my hand?

The answers to these questions should give you a basic sense of your requirements and preferences for a practitioner for pregnancy and birth. Some women will know right away the qualities they want in a practitioner. Others aren't so sure, even after answering the questions.

It is okay to be unsure. You are simply trying to get a step ahead of pregnancy by figuring out where to start. The good news is that most women have a number of choices when it comes to practitioners. You should look for the person with the medical skills and the personality that best suits you for one of the most amazing, at times frightening, and intense journeys of your life.

## Start Developing a Comprehensive List of Your Family Medical History

Your family medical history may be something about which you have a vague understanding. You know the major things, right? But do you, really? Most people are confident that they know who had what and when, but in a medical office, when pressed for details, most people come up short.

Now that you are thinking about becoming pregnant, it's a great time to sit down and find a way to collect that history and also to find a way to preserve that information so you can pass it along

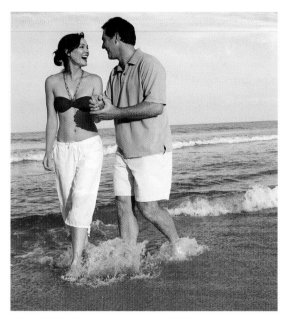

*Spending time with your partner is a great way to discuss your future plans, as well as any concerns either of you may have about being parents.*

- Learning disabilities
- Birth defects

Put all of the information in a binder or save it on your computer. When you update the information, be sure to print a new copy for your practitioner and for keeping in your wallet. This information will eventually expand to include future data on your children.

**HOT MAMA**

Starting a fitness program before you get pregnant can help in many ways. Although the health benefits may be obvious, you may not know about the added benefits for your post-baby body. For example, women who are fit prior to becoming pregnant tend to gain less weight in pregnancy, which usually means they are able to lose their pregnancy weight faster once their babies are born.

to your children and subsequent generations. This means that you will need a system of recording and updating information.

The information that you obtain is important because the history of your family's health and that of your partner will strongly influence your health and that of your children. Relying on these clues from the past helps shape your future by encouraging you to make healthy choices and schedule appropriate medical screenings, including genetic counseling.

First, find out if your parents, siblings, and grandparents had the following:

- Cardiac problems
- Diabetes
- Cancer
- Genetic diseases
- Hearing loss
- Vision problems, including wearing eyeglasses or contact lenses
- High blood pressure

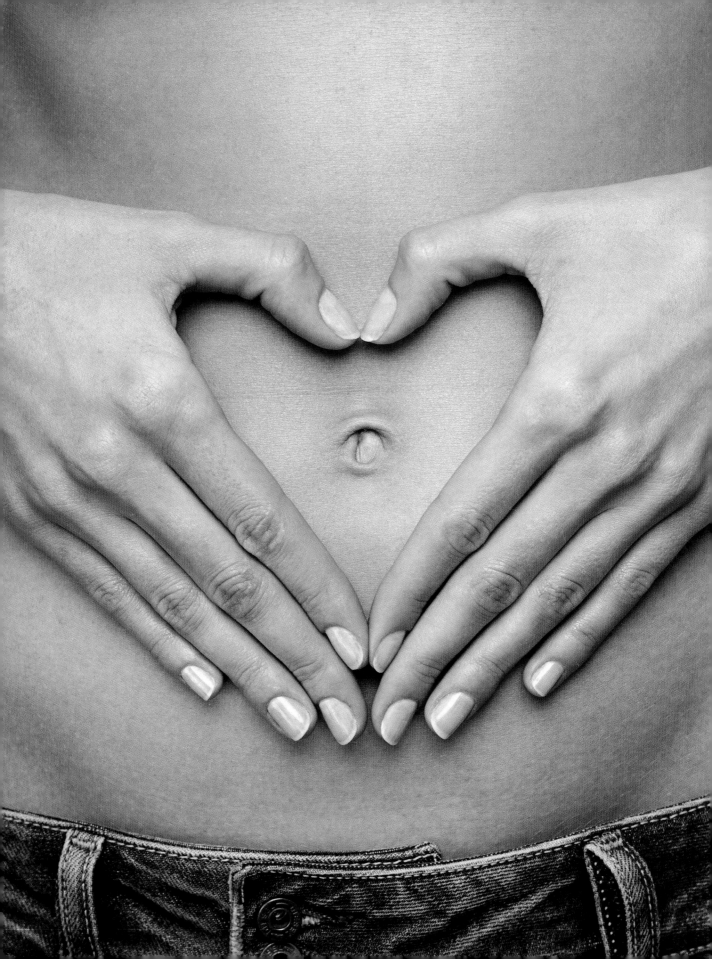

# WEEK 2

## ✏ CHECKLIST FOR WEEK 2

[ ]  Know your body's signs of ovulation.
[ ]  Plan a healthy lifestyle.
[ ]  Clean out your medicine cabinet.
[ ]  Choose questions to ask your practitioner.
[ ]  Select an ovulation prediction kit.

## ⌕ WHAT TO WATCH FOR THIS WEEK

### Double Check

**One-sided pain:** One-sided pain in your abdomen that doesn't go away may be a sign that you have an ovarian cyst. Some ovarian cysts are considered functional and not problematic. But knowing this will likely ease your mind even if it doesn't abate the pain.

**Bleeding or spotting:** Bleeding or spotting can be normal at this stage of your menstrual cycle. However, be sure to talk to your practitioner about potential problems with your cycle if you experience frequent or prolonged bleeding or spotting.

*Report any strange or troublesome symptoms to your practitioner immediately.*

##  BODY BASICS

As you get closer to releasing the egg in your ovary via ovulation, you may notice some changes in your body. These subtle and not-so-subtle changes, which are listed below, indicate that you are about to ovulate. By tuning in to these changes, you can increase your chances of conceiving.

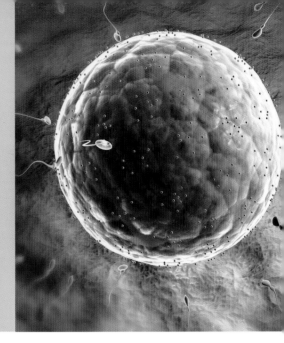

## 🛒 BABY DATA

At this point in your cycle, your baby is still not formed. However, you have a follicle with a ripening egg that is getting ready to be released. Once the egg is released, you have ovulated! During ovulation, the egg has approximately twenty-four hours in which to be fertilized by sperm. This makes knowing when you ovulate crucial to getting pregnant. It goes without saying that having sex this week is optimal for conception.

**PREGNANCY PARTICULARS**

# Know Your Body's Signs of Ovulation

Your body's process of releasing an egg is known as ovulation. It's important to know when you're ovulating because the released egg is only viable for about twenty-four hours. Talk about your pressure to get pregnant! The good news is that while the egg may only be viable for a short time, a man's sperm lasts longer, which widens the period during which you have to get pregnant.

Generally speaking, you will ovulate once every cycle. The average cycle lasts about twenty-eight days, though it is quite normal to be above or below this number. The first day of your cycle is the day you start your period. A basic rule is that you will ovulate fourteen days before the *end* of your cycle. So if your cycle is thirty days long, you will typically ovulate on day sixteen. This is a good estimate to use if you are new to trying to get pregnant and don't have a specific need to pinpoint your exact day of ovulation. And then when you look for some of the more obvious body signals that you are ovulating, you increase the chances that you be able to tell when you are ovulating.

Your body actually gives you lots of little clues and signals that you are about to ovulate. These include the following:

- Increase in vaginal discharge
- Brief, one-sided ache in your ovary near your lower pelvis
- Changes in consistency of vagina secretions
- Cervical changes
- Temperature fluctuations

Some of these changes are obvious, such as the increase in vaginal discharge. This is your body's natural lubricant that helps you enjoy sex and acts as a medium between the sperm and your reproductive tract. Many women notice this discharge but haven't really focused on it until now.

You may also experience a slight cramping on one side in the middle of every monthly cycle. This mild pain is known as mittelschmerz, and it lets you know that you've ovulated.

The other signs take a bit of work to interpret. For example, there is a change in the consistency of the vaginal discharge as you near ovulation. Fertile mucous, as it is called, is very slippery and can be easily stretched between your fingers. Mucous that appears during the rest of your cycle is a bit more tacky and doesn't stretch.

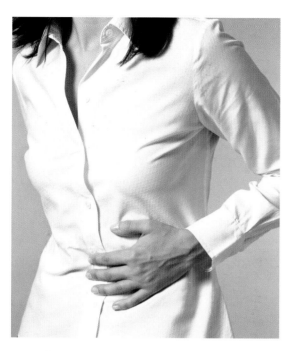

*Signs of ovulation can be as simple as a cramping feeling mid-month, or you may have to do a bit more investigating to pinpoint ovulation.*

You can also do a quick check of your cervix to see where it is and if it is open. When you are not ovulating, your cervix is rather difficult to feel, and if you can feel it, it would be closed. During ovulation, it is easier to feel, and you may be able to feel that it is slightly open and receptive to semen.

Looking for minute fluctuations in body temperature can be tracked using a thermometer that measures in tenths of degrees. Take your temperature once a day, ideally first thing in the morning. You then chart this information and look for a drop and then spike in your temperature. This is a graphical representation of your hormones at work that cause you to ovulate. The chart is also valuable to bring to future appointments with your practitioner and can help if you have questions concerning possible infertility.

# PREGNANCY AFFIRMATION FOR WEEK 2

## My body is strong and healthy.

### Plan a Healthy Lifestyle

Just as an unhealthy lifestyle takes practice and reinforcement, being healthy may take you a while to get the hang of before it becomes routine. For example, if you're used to grabbing a bite to eat from the snack machine during the day, trying to get pregnant or being pregnant won't automatically change that habit. Instead you need to consciously make an effort every day to pack healthy snacks or to bypass the vending machine and opt for healthier options.

Eat a variety of foods from all the food groups, focusing on healthy alternatives to processed snack foods. Be sure to include green and orange vegetables, whole grains, and protein. It is perfectly acceptable to eat sweets and fats, just do so in moderation.

Try to sleep seven to eight hours every night, and nap when you need to without overdoing it. Avoid alcohol, cigarettes, nicotine, recreational drugs, and medications that can be harmful to you or your baby in pregnancy. And if possible, you should incorporate thirty to sixty minutes of exercise into your daily routine—even if that means going for a walk after dinner.

## Clean Out Your Medicine Cabinet

As you plan for pregnancy, it's time to reevaluate your medicine cabinet and its contents. Going through your medicine cabinet can help you plan for pregnancy because it may remind you of little things you quite possibly have forgotten, such as the allergies that you experience every spring or the fact that you like to take a pain reliever at the first sign of a headache. These seemingly minor issues are easily overlooked simply because you aren't currently suffering from them.

A glance in your medicine cabinet can also show you just how many medications you take, including over-the-counter medications. When you aren't pregnant, the risks from medication are small, and you probably don't think about them every time you open the cabinet door. But during pregnancy, something as simple as a pain killer can cause grave problems, such as bleeding difficulties for the baby or bleeding issues for both the baby and Mom. Now is the time to conduct a thorough evaluation. Then, consider what you can do for chronic issues such as headaches and allergies that do not involve medication.

If you can't avoid medications, which is sometimes the case, you need to find a suitable alternative during pregnancy. Finding replacements now, before you get pregnant, avoids a 3 A.M. call to your practitioner because your head is pounding and you can't sleep but don't want to reach for a pain reliever. A review of your medicine cabinet also helps you with the following:

- Remove medicine that is out-of-date
- Remind yourself what you have and what you need
- Jog your memory to ask your practitioner about common medications, such as those for pain relief, fever reduction, allergies, and heartburn

## Choose Questions to Ask Your Practitioner

If you visit your practitioner around this point in your menstrual cycle, you might want to talk about your ovulatory cycle. Your doctor or midwife may be able to help you identify some of the finer details that you may have missed when trying to chart your cycle. For example, perhaps you have a slightly longer cycle and missed some of the earlier cues that you were ovulating.

The insight that you gain from a medical professional may also include ways to make your body more baby friendly, such as nutrients that can help with conception or provide a healthy space for your baby. You may gain knowledge of sex positions that can enhance or hinder conception. For example, having sex standing up goes against gravity and makes the sperm work harder than they need to.

## Select an Ovulation Prediction Kit

Ovulation prediction kits, also know as OPKs, are used to help you pinpoint ovulation. These test kits work by screening your urine for luteinizing hormone (LH), which is only produced for a short period of time when you ovulate. Typically you start using a kit around the eighth or ninth day of your cycle, depending on your cycle length. You use the tests daily until you receive a positive sign of ovulation.

Ovulation kits can be quite costly; you might even spend $35 or more per cycle. This normally includes seven kits with which to test. If your cycle is longer, you will need to purchase additional test kits. You can buy less expensive strips that test for LH and sell for as little as $1 per test. On the other hand, you can also use more technically advanced equipment that costs hundreds of dollars up front and then about $35 per cycle.

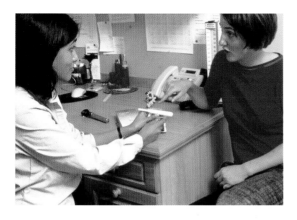

*Finding a midwife or doctor that you feel comfortable with is the most important decision you will make. Don't shy away from interviews.*

If none of these options suits you or factors into your budget, you have other choices. There are ovulation predicting microscope kits that use saliva or vaginal secretions to detect ovulation. For a $35 initial investment, you can use this type of kit for years. Another advantage is that it allows you to test every few hours. You simply place saliva on the slide and view it through a microscope, which lets you know if you are ovulating or not.

By knowing when you ovulate, you can pinpoint the right time to have sex in order to maximize your chances of conception.

**HOT MAMA**

It's said that fertile women are more attractive to the opposite sex. If so, then this is your week to shine! Your might find that your skin looks better than ever and that you feel sexier than ever. This is part of your body's attempt to help you get pregnant. Use it to your advantage. Take a few extra minutes in the shower and use some of the salts or scrubs you've been saving for a special day. You might also consider a special outfit and a date night out with your spouse.

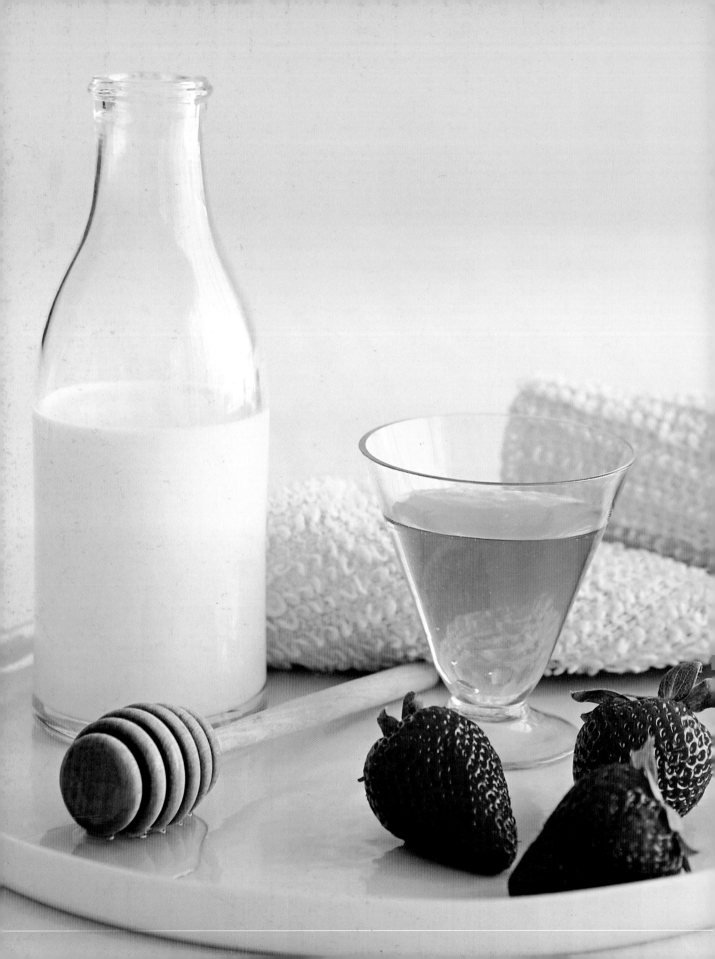

# WEEK 3

## ✏ CHECKLIST FOR WEEK 3

[ ]  Enjoy the two-week wait.
[ ]  Make a list of medications that you take currently or seasonally.
[ ]  See a fertility specialist if necessary.
[ ]  Recognize early pregnancy symptoms.
[ ]  Be prepared emotionally.
[ ]  Avoid the litter box.
[ ]  Assess your intake of sugar substitutes.

## ♀ WHAT TO WATCH FOR THIS WEEK

*Double Check*

**One-sided pain:** One-sided pain in your abdomen that doesn't go away may be an ovarian cyst.

**Bleeding or spotting:** Bleeding or spotting during this week can mean that you are having implantation bleeding—brief bleeding from where the egg implants into the uterus—or that you have menstrual cycle irregularities.

*Report any strange or troublesome symptoms to your practitioner immediately.*

##  BODY BASICS

The blastocyst is now making its way down your Fallopian tube. This journey will take three to seven days. However, while the journey is taking place, the cells continue their work. They are ready to embed into the uterine lining that has been built up over the past few weeks. Once the blastocyst has landed in the uterus and made that connection, it will send out signals to alert your body to its presence. You do not yet have any symptoms of pregnancy.

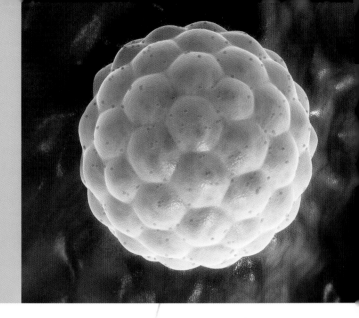

## BABY DATA

After a long arduous journey, the egg and sperm have joined. As the cells that are your baby begin to divide, you are blissfully unaware of what is going on in your body. While you may be hoping that these cells are rapidly dividing and heading toward your uterus, you have no way of knowing.

**PREGNANCY PARTICULARS**

## Enjoy the Two-Week Wait

The time between ovulation and when the results of a pregnancy test would be positive or when your next period is due is known as the two-week wait. During this time, you may be pregnant but not know or feel it yet. This is because of the time it takes the egg and sperm to take their journey down the Fallopian tube.

This period of time tends to be very frustrating for most women. You're probably anxious to know if you've conceived or if it's back to the drawing board. Many women spend this time analyzing their cycles and trying to guess—or second-guess—at the chances of conception. When you look at the fact that so many things have to be just right for pregnancy to occur, you may begin to wonder how anyone ever gets pregnant.

Rather than spend this time in constant wonder about your pregnancy status, try to focus on some of the positive aspects that you have some control over. First of all, you're probably already acting pregnant to avoid issues with alcohol and other substances that are frowned upon in pregnancy. Secondly, you can be sure that you are providing a positive and appropriate body for your baby to grow in. Part of this has to do with health and nutrition, but another part is building a positive mental attitude and emotional outlook as you prepare for pregnancy.

Consider this time period a break. You no longer need to worry about whether or not you've correctly identified ovulation. Sexual relations can be spontaneous without either party worrying about whether the timing is right or not. If you or your partner were tense or stressed about the conception process, now is the time to put that behind you. Try to take some time to be alone as a couple. You have the right to declare this as baby-talk free time or time in which to focus on your expectant miracle.

So devote some energy this week to planning ahead. If you are pregnant, how will you react? Have you thought beyond the pregnancy test? This is probably where most women spend their time planning. However, there is also the possibility that your period will start. As your cycle resets itself to begin again, what will you do to comfort yourself?

## Make a List of Medications That You Take Currently or Seasonally

When you're planning a pregnancy, it's helpful to sit down and have a date with your medicine cabinet. While many medications may be safe to continue taking during your pregnancy, there may be special rules to taking them. For instance, it may be that a certain medication should be avoided in the first trimester but fine to take later in the pregnancy. It may also be smart to find substitutes for certain medications that are safer during pregnancy. Your doctor or midwife will be able to help you in this assessment.

Some medications you are currently taking may need to be switched. If you haven't already reviewed your list of medications with your practitioner to determine whether they are safe to take during pregnancy, call as soon as you find out that you are pregnant to discuss the matter. You will want to ask about seasonal medication such as allergy medications and occasional medications such as inhalers or pain medications. Informing yourself now on how to safely stock your medicine cabinet will prevent some potentially sleepless nights later when you develop a cold and wonder what you can take before your practitioner's office opens up in the morning.

## Recognize Early Pregnancy Symptoms

Early pregnancy symptoms are typically described as resembling premenstrual symptoms. As a result, many women feel upset when they start to notice what they think are symptoms of premenstrual syndrome (PMS). Some women find that ignoring every little symptom and waiting for their period is the most helpful way to approach it while others swear that they can tell the difference between PMS and early pregnancy.

Some common early pregnancy symptoms include:

- Sore breasts
- Feeling bloated
- Fatigue
- Crankiness
- Sensitivity to certain smells
- Aversions to certain foods

If you have suffered from bad bouts of PMS prior to trying to conceive, you may have kept journals or logs of symptoms prior to your period. This information may be handy in working out whether these symptoms are different.

PREGNANCY AFFIRMATION
FOR WEEK 3

## My mind and body are open to pregnancy.

### Be Prepared Emotionally

You can expect to experience emotional as well as physical symptoms in early pregnancy. For one, what seemed like the best plan in the world—having a baby—now may seem like a really bad idea. You may find that you go back and forth between being insanely excited and incredibly worried. Emotional acceptance of pregnancy will come in time, though how long it takes varies from woman to woman.

This feeling can be worrisome for you. Do not panic. It doesn't mean that you will be a bad mother or that you don't care. In fact, it means quite the opposite: that you are putting a great deal of thought into your pregnancy. Even women who have been trying to get pregnant for years and those who have been given fertility treatments to aid in conception may have these feelings. They are completely normal. You shouldn't ignore them, but you should realize that they will, for the most part, work themselves out during pregnancy. If these feelings persist well into the pregnancy and you are truly concerned, consider speaking to a counselor about your fears.

**MEMORABLE MOMENTS**

"The first half of my cycle we had stuff to do. You know, taking temperatures, planning romantic trysts, so that we would always remember 'the night.' But the second half was pretty much hurry up and wait. It was a real drag, and we were so anxious. We even got a bit snippy at each other toward the end. But it was all worth it."

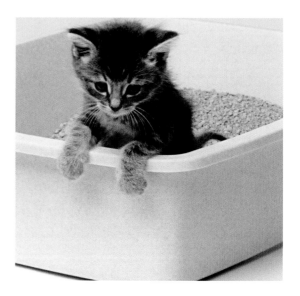

*Changing the cat litter is someone else's job for the duration of pregnancy. This helps prevent you from contracting toxoplasmosis.*

## Avoid the Litter Box

In pregnancy, one of the things you will have to get used to is avoiding the litter box because cat feces can carry toxoplasmosis, which is a disease caused by a parasite. While the disease will have very little effect on you, it can cause problems in your pregnancy and with your baby. It is usually recommended that you avoid changing the litter box at all costs and that you leave the room to avoid flying particles when someone else changes it.

If you have had a cat for awhile, you have probably already been exposed to toxoplasmosis and did not even realize it. Your practitioner can do a blood test to see if you have the lifelong immunity if you are concerned that you have contracted toxoplasmosis or if you are just concerned about it. However, it is still a good idea to avoid the litter box for the duration of your pregnancy.

You can still cuddle with your cat because your cat cannot give you toxoplasmosis. So do not fear being around your cat or playing with your cat as usual. This will not pose a problem.

You should also avoid uncooked or under-cooked meats and sushi for the same reason; they can contain toxoplasmosis. If you have a garden, make sure that you wear gloves while gardening to avoid exposure from contaminated soil. You may also wish to wear gloves while handling raw meats.

## Assess Your Intake of Sugar Substitutes

Many women try to give up sugar before or during pregnancy. What they may not realize is that switching to diet or sugar-free foods introduces artificial sweeteners or sugar substitutes into their system. These chemicals, designed to sweeten food without calories, may not be safe to consume in pregnancy. The following products should not be used in pregnancy:

- Stevia (a natural sweetener)
- Saccharine (Brand name: Sweet'N Low)

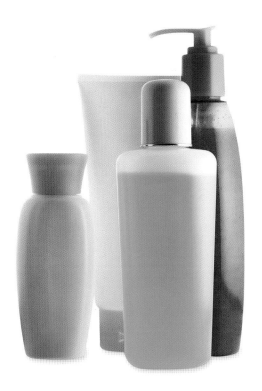

*Just like your medicine cabinet, check your makeup and lotions for harmful chemicals that aren't pregnancy friendly.*

**HOT MAMA**

You might want to look through your makeup and toiletries as you prepare for pregnancy. Do you have any lotions that contain things that might be harmful to your growing baby, such as petroleum, retin-A, salicylic acid, retinol, oxybenzone, and vitamin A? Chemicals are absorbed through your skin and can be passed onto your baby. Look for products containing all-natural ingredients and fewer chemicals, although even some all-natural ingredients are not safe for your baby. Bottom line: Ask your practitioner if you have questions.

Some artificial sweeteners are considered by the FDA to be safe to consume during pregnancy. These include the following:

- Aspartame (Brand names: Equal and Nutra-Sweet)
- Sucralose (Brand name: Splenda)
- Acesulfame (Brand name: Sunett)

In addition, you can always choose to use sugar or honey to sweeten your foods and drinks

Your doctor or midwife may ask you to limit artificial sweeteners, even if they are considered safe, for a variety of reasons. Some practitioners ask that you have no more than one serving of a food or drink item per day that contains these chemicals.

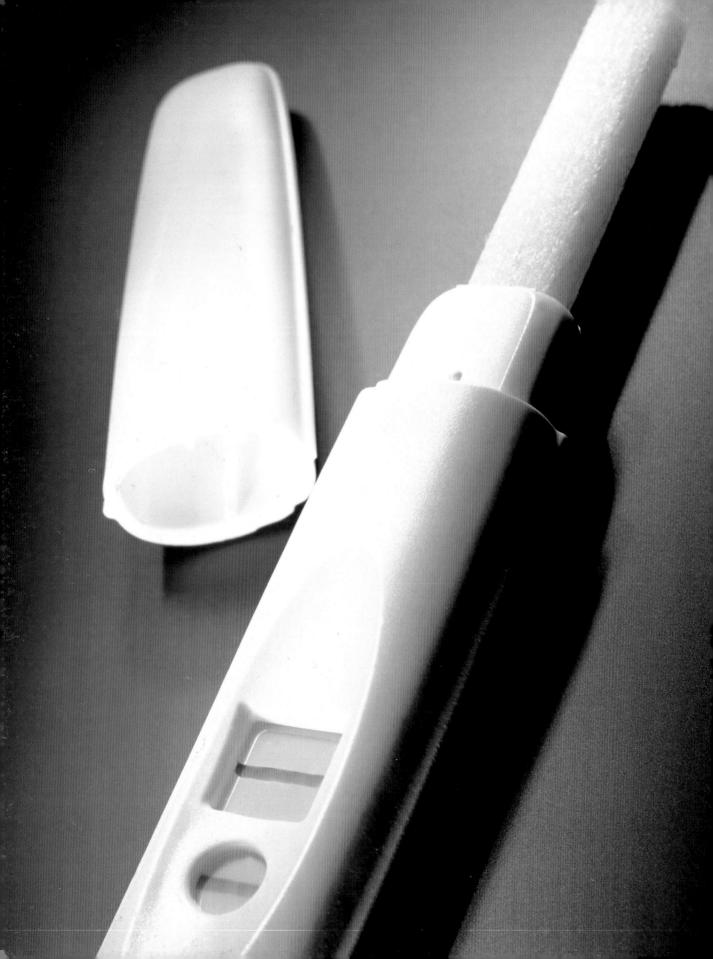

# WEEK 4

✎ **CHECKLIST FOR WEEK 4**

[ ] Take a pregnancy test.
[ ] Choose a practitioner.
[ ] Watch for signs of pregnancy.
[ ] Cope with morning sickness.
[ ] Have sex.
[ ] Find out how twins come to be.

🔎 **WHAT TO WATCH FOR THIS WEEK**

*Double Check*

**One-sided pain:** One-sided pain in your abdomen that doesn't go away may indicate an ovarian cyst or an ectopic pregnancy.

**Bleeding or spotting:** Bleeding or spotting can be a normal part of the pregnancy at this stage. It may actually be implantation bleeding. But if you are concerned, mention it to your practitioner and keep a record of abnormal bleeding.

*Report any strange or troublesome symptoms to your practitioner immediately.*

 **BODY BASICS**

Congratulations! You're pregnant! Your period is most likely tardy at this point, which may be what clued you in to your new pregnancy. Other than that, however, you may not have any symptoms of pregnancy. Typically the first signs of pregnancy to emerge are sore breasts, exhaustion, and frequent urination. These are the result of the hormone levels, namely progesterone, increasing in your body. Occasionally moms will report feelings of morning sickness or nausea this week.

## 🍼 BABY DATA

This is the first week that you are sure that your baby is in there! Though what is going on is still very hard to see. Even with high-tech ultrasound equipment, you would be lucky to see the gestational sac—the small bubble where your baby is busy forming and growing—this week. Using a transvaginal ultrasound, which is an ultrasound done from inside your vagina, is your only hope of seeing it at this point in pregnancy. In that gestational sac, you will also have a yolk sac forming. This will help feed your baby until the placenta has fully formed around the end of the first trimester. At the end of week 4, the chorionic villi are completely formed.

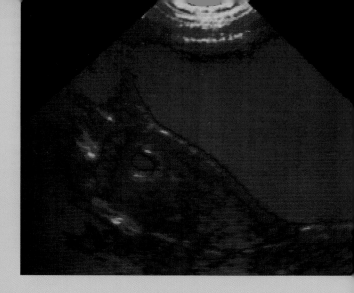

These are finger-like projections of placental tissue. They contain the same genetic material as your baby and can be helpful later for genetic testing.

### PREGNANCY PARTICULARS

## Take a Pregnancy Test

At this stage of pregnancy, your body is secreting human chorionic gonadotropin (hCG), the pregnancy hormone, at levels that can be detected in the urine as well as in the blood. This means that a urine or blood test should be positive for you, depending on the specific limits of the individual test. Everyone's hormones are slightly different, as shown by the wide range of normal in the early weeks of pregnancy.

BLOOD TESTS: Blood tests work by measuring the amount of hCG in your blood. Typically a result of more than 5 mIU is considered a positive test. The type of blood test that tells you the exact amount of hCG is called a quantitative hCG. Sometimes a midwife or doctor may simply order a qualitative hCG, which will detect whether hCG is present in your blood without providing an exact measurement.

Blood work would be the optimal route if you need to know the exact amount of hCG. By repeating the test forty-eight hours later, you can get a good picture of the health of the pregnancy, even before an ultrasound could detect anything. That's because generally in early pregnancy, hCG levels should double every forty-eight to seventy-two hours. A blood test is particularly important for women who are having issues with their pregnancy such as bleeding, spotting, or cramping or other potential problems such as a history of ectopic (tubal) pregnancies. A blood test is also a way to approximate the start of the pregnancy—to figure out how far along you are if you are unsure.

URINE TESTS: Urine tests function much in the way that the qualitative hCG works: They will say yes or no to the presence of hCG, depending on the threshold of the specific test. Some home pregnancy tests measure very small amounts of hCG in the urine, as low as 10 to 15 mIU. Other home tests are not as sensitive and detect hCG at higher levels, such as 200 mIU. To find out the hCG level detected by a particular brand, you might have to call the manufacturer because the information is rarely printed on the package.

When you are testing urine, the concentration of hCG varies throughout the day, depending on when you last urinated and how many fluids you've consumed. While hCG is said to nearly double every forty-eight hours, the numbers can still be very small and the difference that a day makes can be very large. This is why pregnancy test manufacturers often suggest that you use first morning urine. This is because you've been asleep and not going to the bathroom all night, nor have you been drinking. Your hCG levels will be higher and, thus, more likely to be detected by the test.

If you have a negative urine test and your period still doesn't come, you should retest. In early pregnancy, if your hCG is 2 mIU on Monday, doubling makes it only 4 mIU on Wednesday, which with a urine test would still produce a negative result. When you choose to retest depends on many factors, including your degree of patience. Some women choose to test daily until they get a positive result or their period starts, or even after they have a positive test. The product instructions usually recommend that you wait several days to a week before retesting.

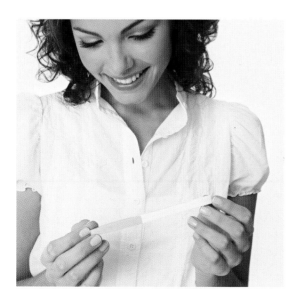

# PREGNANCY AFFIRMATION FOR WEEK 4

## My body is a healthy place to grow my baby.

It's important to take home pregnancy tests according to the instructions on the box. Many women wait too long to read the results, which can fade or darken, leading to a false positive reading. With the newer digital pregnancy tests, you don't have to sweat over how dark or faint the line is; the answer is spelled out in LCD letters.

### Choose a Practitioner

One of the first things you'll do when the pregnancy test turns positive is to run for the phone to make your first prenatal appointment. Your choice of practitioner is extremely important. Practitioners fall into the following two categories:

MIDWIVES: There are many types of midwives who care for low-risk pregnant women and their families. Where you live will determine what types of midwives are available and where they practice: in homes, birth centers, or hospitals. Some midwives are certified by various national organizations such as the North American Registry of Midwives or the American College of Nurse Midwives, which certifies both nurse and nonnurse midwives.

*Choose a pregnancy test that you have confidence in to avoid the desire to spend lots of time and money with additional pregnancy tests.*

DOCTORS: Doctors have a variety of specialties. Some are family practitioners, trained to take care of families in all stages of life; others are obstetricians who specialize in pregnancy and women's gynecological issues; and still others are maternal fetal medicine specialists who specialize in high-risk pregnancies. Doctors usually practice in a hospitals or birth centers, but they do occasionally attend home births.

Your decision on which type of practitioner is right for you might be simple if you've already decided on your birth philosophy. It may also make sense for you to find a middle ground, such as a doctor and midwife team, that allows you to make a final choice later down the road.

Don't fret over your decision too much because you can always make a change later if you find that your relationship with your practitioner isn't what you had hoped for during the early stage of your pregnancy.

## Watch for Signs of Pregnancy

Perhaps you already know that you're pregnant from a pregnancy test or you strongly suspect it based on your body's signs and symptoms, but having a list of things to look for can be oddly comforting. Here is a list of the most common signs of early pregnancy:

SORE BREASTS: This is caused by changes in your hormone levels. If you normally have sore breasts before your menstrual cycle starts, this may not be a noticeable difference; for other women it is very noticeable.

FREQUENT URINATION: Needing to know the location of the nearest restroom or having to get up during the night to go to the bathroom can be a common first sign of pregnancy. This is caused more by hormones than changes in the uterus at this point.

NAUSEA AND VOMITING: Yet another symptom to chalk up to hormones, this one can take many shapes and degrees of intensity.

EXHAUSTION: The need to sleep more or feeling tired or lethargic is a very common sign of pregnancy.

HEADACHES: They can be caused by hormones, dehydration, and even caffeine withdrawal.

ODD BEHAVIOR: Many women complain of an assortment of symptoms that range from dropping things to being hyper-emotional that they can't quite explain.

## Cope with Morning Sickness

Morning sickness is a misnomer, because it can happen at any time of the day or night. That said, many women find that they have a particular time of day when the problem tends to bother them more than at other times. Other women simply feel nauseated all day without ever progressing to the point of vomiting. Whether or when you experience morning sickness is impossible to predict and which form of nausea you suffer from can vary from day to day.

Here are some tips that have proven helpful in alleviating morning sickness:

- Eating something before getting out of bed
- Snacking throughout the day

*Morning sickness can happen at any time of the day or night. Be prepared to deal with it as best you can. This can take some trial and error.*

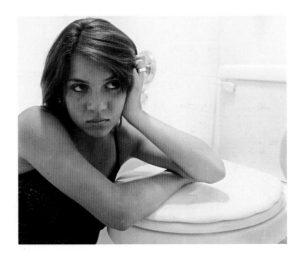

- Wearing bands around the wrists that hit acupressure points
- Sucking on sour candies
- Drinking special teas or treats designed to promote nausea relief

## Have Sex

Early pregnancy is typically a time when couples start altering their normal activities, and this can extend to sexual relations. Couples can become apprehensive, believing that sex will somehow harm the baby. The truth is that sex in pregnancy is natural and healthy. Sometimes it's harder to enjoy sex in the first trimester because of the exhaustion, sore breasts, and nausea. But it is perfectly fine to have sex and orgasms during pregnancy, even in the first trimester, because the baby is well protected. You should only avoid sex in the following circumstances:

- You are or have been bleeding.
- You have a history of preterm labor.
- You or your partner has an active sexually transmitted infection (STI).
- Your water has broken.
- You have placenta previa, which is a condition where the placenta covers or is near the cervix.

Sex can be a wonderful way to connect with your partner and relieve stress throughout pregnancy. If you heed the cautions above, you can enjoy sex right up until you go into labor. Communication is key. ("I feel too nauseous to have sex now." "Will you be attracted to me even when I have a huge belly?") Certain positions may be better than others. Even early on some women find some positions make them feel light-headed or nauseated.

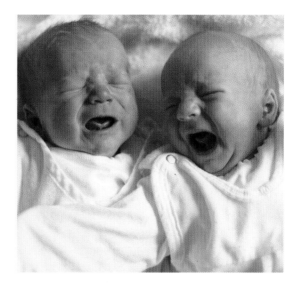

*Twin births are on the rise. Certain things can put you at a higher risk of having twins and other multiples, including your age, family history, and medications.*

## Find Out How Twins Come to Be

About one in ninety births is a twin birth. Twins can come from one egg or from two eggs. Twins resulting from a single egg splitting are known as monozygotic, or identical, twins. This can occur spontaneously or as the result of fertility treatments.

Twins from two eggs are called dizygotic, or fraternal, twins. This can happen because a mother ovulates more than once in a cycle, either naturally or because of medications used to aid fertility, or it can happen because multiple embryos were placed in the uterus during in vitro fertilization treatments.

The rate for twins and multiple births has risen in the past decade due to fertility treatments, including the use of ovulatory medications such as Clomid.

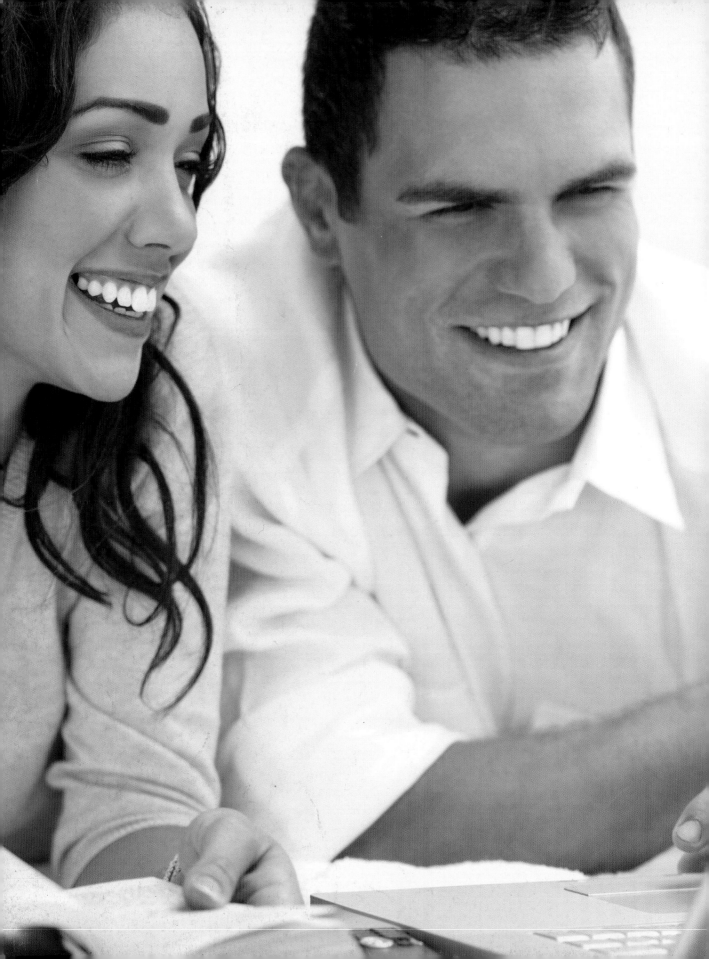

# WEEK 5

## ✏ CHECKLIST FOR WEEK 5

[ ] Make your first prenatal appointment.

[ ] Learn to cope with exhaustion.

[ ] Understand why you have to go to the bathroom all the time.

[ ] Consider telling your family.

[ ] Learn what an early ultrasound can tell you.

[ ] Calculate your due date.

## 🔍 WHAT TO WATCH FOR THIS WEEK

**Back pain:** Pain in your back can be a sign of uterine cramping and potential miscarriage. It may also be a sign of infection or of your uterus stretching. Report severe pain and pain that does not abate to your midwife or doctor.

**Sudden disappearance of pregnancy symptoms:** If you've been having a lot of pregnancy symptoms, such as sore breasts, nausea and/ or vomiting, and sensitivities to smell, that suddenly disappear, you should report this to your doctor or midwife. These things can come in waves, but a complete loss may indicate a hormonal issue, and you should have your levels checked.

**Inability to keep food or liquid down:** You may have expected to throw up during your pregnancy, but the risk of dehydration can be real for many pregnant women. You need to report this to your practitioner.

### Double Check

**One-sided pain:** One-sided pain in your abdomen that doesn't go away can be a potential sign of an ovarian cyst or ectopic pregnancy.

**Bleeding or spotting:** While bleeding is rarely considered a good thing, it may still be implantation bleeding or other "normal" sign. Either way you should alert your practitioner because the possibility of miscarriage, ectopic pregnancy, or blighted ovum (where a fertilized egg fails to grow) is present. *Report any strange or troublesome symptoms to your practitioner immediately.*

##  BODY BASICS

You have probably joined one of two camps: the not-feeling-so-well camp or the can't-tell-I'm-pregnant camp. If you're not feeling so well, you may have predicted or expected it—just not so soon. Symptoms you might be grappling with include:

- Headaches
- Frequent urination
- Exhaustion
- Nausea or vomiting

But on the other hand, plenty of women experience no symptoms of early pregnancy. If this applies to you, don't worry; it does not mean that anything is wrong. You should only worry if you start your pregnancy with really bad or strong symptoms that suddenly disappear. If this happens, it could mean that your hormone levels are falling, and you should call your doctor or midwife to investigate further.

## 👶 BABY DATA

One way to measure a baby this size is called crown to rump length (CRL). From the crown, or top of your baby's head, to the bottom (rump), your baby measures about 1.5 to 2.5 millimeters by the end of this week. Very small, but very busy. A couple of major milestones happen this week: Your baby's heart begins to beat, and the neural folds (the folds of tissue that become the brain and spinal cord) are fusing. This means that you can almost begin to differentiate the head from the tail (a vestige that reabsorbs into the body as the baby becomes a fetus). But even with ultrasound, you still may not see as much as you'd like.

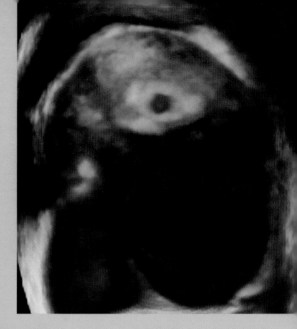

## Make Your First Prenatal Appointment

Once you have a positive pregnancy test result, you will be anxious to make your first prenatal appointment. Be prepared when you call to spend about fifteen to twenty minutes talking to the receptionist.

The office will record some basic information, including your name, address, phone number, insurance information, and possibly your health history. What surprises most pregnant women is how far off that first appointment is scheduled.

There are many reasons why your appointment may not be soon after you call. It may depend on your practitioner's preference or how busy the practice is. Many doctors prefer that you wait until you have missed your second period before coming in to be seen. This helps ensure that the pregnancy is viable. If you have problems with your pregnancy before the appointment, you are always welcome to call and come in earlier.

You may wish to make this first appointment for a time when your husband or partner can go with you. This ensures that you both get a sense of the practice and the practitioner.

## Learn to Cope with Exhaustion

Being super tired is hard to live with when you have other things to do. The exhaustion that comes with pregnancy tends to differ from any other tired you have felt before. And when you're not expecting it, the feeling can be particularly debilitating.

The best way to deal with exhaustion is to combat it head on. Try to go to bed earlier when you can and sleep in whenever possible. Naps, while tempting, may not be a great solution, particularly if you end up napping for long periods of time. You don't want to interfere with a good night's sleep, nor do you want to sleep away a good chunk of the day. Quick naps of thirty minutes or less can be very refreshing and are easier to recover from and get on with your day.

Other tips for getting better sleep at night include:

- Exercise during the day to help you sleep better at night.
- But avoid exercise several hours before going to bed.
- Avoid caffeine past 4 p.m.
- Don't eat for several hours before going to bed.

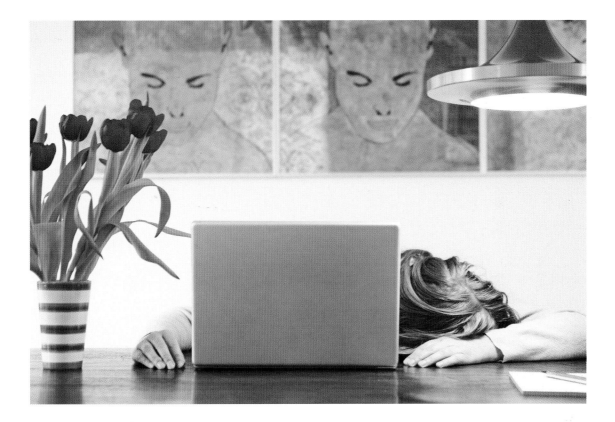

- Avoid lengthy naps.
- Try to establish regular bedtimes and times to get up.

## Understand Why You Have to Go to the Bathroom All the Time

Urinary frequency is something many women experience at the start of their pregnancies, even though they may not notice it right away. While it tends to be a symptom associated with late-term pregnancies, many women find that they have to get up to urinate in the middle of the night even before their pregnancy tests are positive.

The need to urinate more often is not from the size of your baby but rather your lovely hormones. Remember that the purpose of urination is to help excrete waste products from your body. Your internal construction zone is busy building away, even though it's on a microscopic level.

PREGNANCY AFFIRMATION
FOR WEEK 5

## Changes in my body are healthy for my baby.

It will be a long nine months of trips to the bathroom, although some women get a brief reprieve during the second trimester. Try the following tips to help address this issue:

- Plan ahead and know where the restrooms are located.
- Limit your intake of fluids before bedtime.
- Avoid caffeine, which is a diuretic.

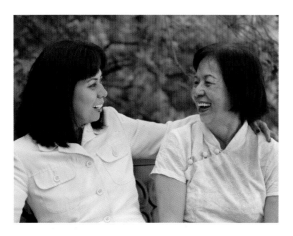

*Telling your family will hopefully be a joyous occasion. Just as you wanted to remember the moment fondly, they do too.*

## Consider Telling Your Family

Knowing when and how to tell your family that you're pregnant can be a tough decision. There tend to be two schools of thought on the matter: telling early or waiting until the end of the first trimester. Both approaches are valid, but only you can decide which is right for your family.

Sharing the news early gives you a chance to spread your cheer sooner. It also earns you a lot of support for those days when you aren't feeling very well. Some women have a hard time hiding pregnancy symptoms or changes in their behavior, such as cutting out alcoholic beverages. The critics of the tell-early side are concerned what should happen if you have a miscarriage and have to take the good news back. The upside here again is that you have people to support you during a difficult time.

Some families try to take a middle ground in the pregnancy announcement arena. They tell only close family and friends in the beginning and wait till later to tell others. Again, it's completely up to you who you tell when and how.

## Learn What an Early Ultrasound Can Tell You

Early ultrasounds are limited to a few uses. These include confirming that a pregnancy exists and where the pregnancy is growing to rule out an ectopic pregnancy. This surprises people who are used to seeing ultrasound images everywhere.

Most people are familiar with the ultrasound that is used externally on a woman's abdomen, but in early pregnancy, the test needs to be even closer and therefore involves internal or transvaginal ultrasound to get the best images. During an early ultrasound, you're hoping to see the gestational sac, where your baby is developing. You may also see the yolk sac, which is helping to feed your baby. You can also look at the uterus, cervix, and ovaries for potential problems—such as subchorionic hemorrhages, ectopic pregnancy, cysts, and improper development—or a lesson in simply anatomy.

Early ultrasounds are generally reserved for women who are having problems in their pregnancies or who have a history of ectopic pregnancies. You may have an ultrasound if you are bleeding; unsure of your dates of conception, period, or ovulation; or if you are experiencing a complication such as unexplained pain. Because so little can be seen at this stage, many women are more concerned than relieved following an early ultrasound.

As the weeks pass, more can be seen, including a fetal pole (your baby) and a heartbeat. Your practitioner may schedule you for an ultrasound if you are having complications or if an earlier ultrasound failed to provide all of the necessary information.

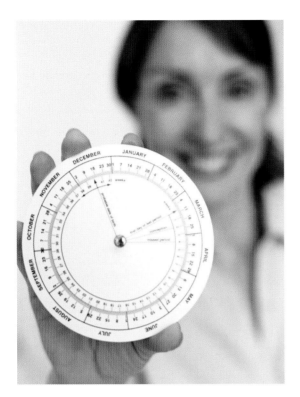

*Your due date is simply a guess. You can expect your baby up to two weeks after your anticipated due date or two weeks before.*

## Calculate Your Due Date

One of the first question people ask a pregnant woman is her due date. It is typically calculated from the first day of your last normal period. (Sometimes women have a light period and then skip a period and are really more pregnant than they believe. The light period could have been implantation bleeding.) Pregnancy usually lasts 280 days from the first day of your last normal period (if you have twenty-eight day cycles), or 266 days from conception.

If you have cycles of differing lengths or consistent cycles that are shorter or longer than twenty-eight days, it is easier to calculate your due date from when you ovulated. Not everyone will know this date, but your practitioner can help you with the calculation. There are other tools by which to measure your baby's growth, including when you first feel movements, when your uterus reaches certain stages, and ultrasound dating.

The most important thing to remember about your due date is that it is at best an estimate. Only 4 to 5 percent of babies are born on their due dates. Birth without intervention occurs at a range of normal. That range runs from week 37 through week 42 of gestation. Before 37 weeks, a baby is considered premature. And after 42 weeks, the American College of Obstetricians suggests that labor be induced, meaning that labor is started using artificial means.

Once you're told your due date, try to think of it as an estimate. Some practitioners advocate that women be given due months. In that case you'd be told, for example, that you are due at the end of August or early September, rather than an exact date such as August 23.

### HOT MAMA

If you're feeling sluggish and sick, you might not have that glow you were hoping for as a pregnant woman. For now, get your glow from a bottle or brush by applying blush to your cheeks. You'll look the part of a healthy mother-to-be, even if you're feeling less than radiant.

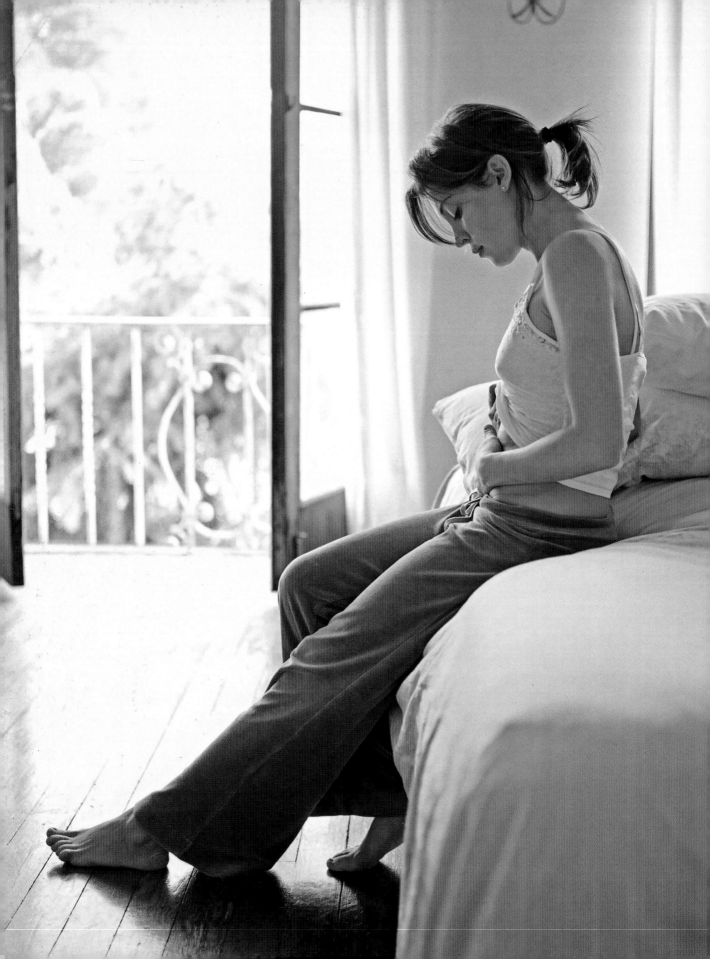

# WEEK 6

## ✎ CHECKLIST FOR WEEK 6

[ ]  Learn about prenatal visit schedules.
[ ]  Check your breasts.
[ ]  Consider chorionic villus sampling.
[ ]  Understand what an ectopic pregnancy is.
[ ]  Deal with constipation.
[ ]  Don't panic over vaginal discharge.

## ⌕ WHAT TO WATCH FOR THIS WEEK

### Double Check

**One-sided pain:** One-sided pain in your abdomen that doesn't go away can be evidence of an ovarian cyst or ectopic pregnancy.

**Bleeding or spotting:** While bleeding is rarely considered a good thing, it may still be implantation bleeding or another "normal" sign. Either way you should alert your practitioner because the possibility of miscarriage, ectopic pregnancy, or blighted ovum (where a fertilized egg fails to grow) is present.

**Back pain:** Pain in your lower back can be a sign of many things: uterine cramping, potential miscarriage, infection, or the uterus stretching. Make sure to report severe pain and pain that does not abate to your midwife or doctor.

**Sudden disappearance of pregnancy symptoms:** If the start of your pregnancy involved strong symptoms such as sore breasts, nausea and/or vomiting, and certain sensitivities, and some or all of these suddenly disappear, you should alert your doctor or midwife. Symptoms can come and go, but when they disappear entirely, there may be a hormonal issue worth investigating.

**Inability to keep food or liquid down:** Throwing up during pregnancy is normal for many women, but you don't want to risk becoming dehydrated. Talk to your practitioner if you simply can't keep any solids or liquids down.

*Report any strange or troublesome symptoms to your practitioner immediately.*

##  BODY BASICS

You may be experiencing more pregnancy symptoms in addition to those you had last week. There is no particular order for pregnancy symptoms to appear or disappear.

This week you may be experiencing changes in your breasts. Perhaps your breasts are sore to the touch or simply sensitive to movement. Some women will also start to notice an increase in breast size as well as changes to the areola (the dark skin encircling the nipple). The areola may become larger or grow darker. These are small changes that occur as your body begins preparations for breastfeeding once your baby is born.

## 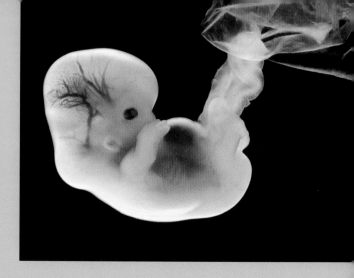 BABY DATA

From the crown, or top of your baby's head, to the bottom (rump), your baby measures about ⅕ inch (4 to 6 millimeters) or about half of a centimeter. Still very small, but working very hard, including a beating heart!

Your baby's heart is circulating blood through its tiny body, though the heart is still a bulge in the front of the body. (It will eventually move into the chest cavity.) The cells that will become your baby's stomach, liver, lungs, and pancreas are also present. In other big news, at the end of this week, upper and lower limb buds will appear. Your baby is also working on developing its inner ear and larynx.

The placenta is working too. It is getting ready to take over the production of hormones from the corpus luteum, which is spot on the ovary where you ovulated. Though this won't happen for about another six weeks, plans are in place now.

An ultrasound at this point would reveal a fetal pole with a heartbeat in 86 percent of the cases, and 100 percent should see a yolk sac. If your midwife or doctor doesn't see what they think they should, you may not be as far along in your pregnancy as you had believed. You will most likely be asked to repeat the transvaginal ultrasound in a few weeks.

## Learn about Prenatal Visit Schedules

Prenatal visits have a rhythm. During the first and second trimester, you will see your practitioner about every four weeks or once a month. Around the 28-3week mark, you will begin to see your midwife or doctor every other week, or once every two weeks. After 36 weeks, you will see him or her every week until your baby is born.

If you are experiencing problems, have a high-risk pregnancy, or are expecting twins or multiple babies, you will be seen more frequently. You will decide this schedule based on what's going on with your doctor or midwife. If you have questions in between your regularly scheduled visits that can't or shouldn't wait, you should vcall your practitioner and request an appointment.

When calling to schedule an appointment, be prepared to give your name, due date, how many weeks pregnant you are, and which practitioner you are seeing. You may talk to a nurse or a medical assistant when you call, or you may have to leave a voice message with your question or concern. If you have not received an answer within twenty-four hours during the normal work week, feel free to call again. In case of an emergency, page the doctor or midwife on call.

## Check Your Breasts

During pregnancy, your breasts begin to change fairly quickly. There are numerous changes that can occur, including:

- Increase in size
- Increase in sensitivity
- More pronounced veins
- Darkening of areola and development of tiny bumps

These changes in your breasts are your body's way of preparing for breastfeeding. You may also notice that in the early weeks of pregnancy your nipples or breasts are incredibly sore or sensitive. This will usually decrease as the pregnancy continues. Wearing a well-fitting bra, even at night, can help decrease painful sensations. These changes are quite common and are not a cause for concern.

Some women do not notice drastic changes in their breasts at the start of their pregnancy. It may happen slowly until one day you or your partner notices the change. If you are concerned about this or any other change, you should discuss it with your practitioner.

## Consider Chorionic Villus Sampling

Chorionic villus sampling (CVS) is a type of genetic testing. A small straw is inserted into the uterus inside the vagina or via a hollow needle through the abdomen to extract chorionic villi, which are finger-like projections of placental tissue. These cells are analyzed for chromosomal abnormalities, and the results are available within a couple of weeks.

In recent years, studies have shown that CVS causes miscarriage in roughly 1 to 2 percent of the pregnancies, regardless of the health of your baby. This number is very close to the rates of pregnancy

PREGNANCY AFFIRMATION FOR WEEK 6

# My baby is growing steadily.

complications that result from amniocentesis, which is a procedure that was previously thought to be less risky than CVS.

CVS can be done earlier in pregnancy than any screening, including amniocentesis and ultrasound screenings for birth defects, although exactly how early depends on your practitioner. In addition, compared to other forms of screening, it takes less time to receive results, including the sex of your baby.

If you are unsure whether or not you need genetic testing, speak to your practitioner. Genetic counseling can provide specific information bearing on your particular risks related to your age, the age of your partner, and your familys' medical histories.

Not all practitioners offer CVS. Talk to yours about whether or not they offer it, and if they don't ask where you can go to have the test. Most major cities have someone who does the test. The more tests they do, the more skilled they should be at doing the test. Having this procedure performed by a more practiced professional can lead to a less risky—and less painful—procedure.

After having the CVS test, you will generally be asked to take it easy for a day or two. After having a CVS, whether vaginally or abdominally, many women have some pain and cramping. An abdominal CVS is more like amniocentesis. If the placenta is in the way of the cervix, as is the case with placenta previa, it is necessary to go through the

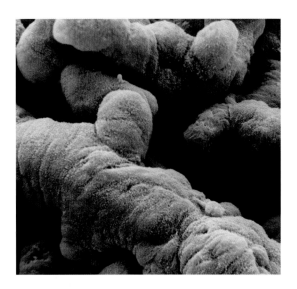

*The fallopian tube is where your baby, as a fertilized egg, travels toward your uterus. Sometimes a baby implants here accidentally, known as a tubal pregnancy.*

abdominal wall to collect the villi. This test is still performed earlier than amnio or ultrasound, and it doesn't use the amniotic fluid.

## Understand What an Ectopic Pregnancy Is

An ectopic pregnancy is a generic term used for a pregnancy that develops in the wrong location. The most common place for an ectopic pregnancy is in the fallopian tube, and it is known as a tubal pregnancy. Ectopic pregnancies can also develop in the abdomen, the cervix, or the ovary, among other places.

Ectopics are more common in certain women, including those with:

- Prior ectopic pregnancies
- History of pelvic inflammatory disease
- Endometriosis
- Tubal ligation
- Currently using an intrauterine device (IUD)
- Previous pelvic surgery

Signs of an ectopic pregnancy can include sharp, one-sided pain and shoulder pain (from internal bleeding). If you experience severe, one-sided pain, it is best to talk to your midwife or doctor. It may be something as simple as a benign ovarian cyst, but it is necessary to rule out an ectopic pregnancy.

Because ectopic pregnancies are the number one reason women die in the first trimester, they should not be taken lightly. One treatment option is medication therapy to help the pregnancy resolve itself without surgery. The medication used is called methotrexate, and it is extremely effective. Sometimes, however, surgery to remove the pregnancy is the best option. Which approach is right for you is a decision that you and your practitioner will make together.

**HOT MAMA**

Find ways to freshen your breath if you've been feeling ill or throwing up. Carry a travel-sized toothbrush or a packet of breath freshener wherever you go. This will help you feel better about your breath and how your mouth feels.

## Deal with Constipation

Constipation (having infrequent or hard-to-pass stools) is fairly common in pregnancy. In early pregnancy, it is due to the influx of progesterone in your system. This causes the lining of the intestines to move more slowly. Constipation can be miserable to deal with, and it can lead to other problems including hemorrhoids, which are varicose veins in the rectum.

Prevention is the best approach. To try to prevent constipation, you should do the following:

- Drink plenty of water every day (64 ounces).
- Exercise fifteen to thirty minutes every day.
- Eat lots of fresh fruits and vegetables.
- Consume foods that are high in fiber, such as sweet potatoes, some grains, etc.
- Take fiber supplements if necessary.

If constipation is a problem for you, it's worth examining the amount of iron in your prenatal vitamin. The higher the iron content, the greater chances of constipation and gastrointestinal upset. Your midwife or doctor might recommend that you switch brands or take your iron in a liquid form that is more readily absorbed.

Your practitioner can help you determine the best route if you're suffering from constipation in your pregnancy.

## Don't Panic over Vaginal Discharge

It is normal to have an increased vaginal discharge (called leukorrhea) during pregnancy. The discharge is the result of more blood flow to the vaginal area as well as more estrogen in your body. The discharge consists of normal secretions from the vagina and the cervix. It is a clear to milky white fluid that is neither foul smelling nor harmful. Some women choose to wear panty liners to absorb the discharge.

You should speak with your doctor or midwife if you experience the following:

- You have a drastic increase in discharge.
- The discharge is painful.
- You experience burning or itching.
- You notice a foul odor.
- You are concerned.

**MEMORABLE MOMENTS**

"Six weeks was a big milestone for me. I felt more pregnant every day my period didn't show up. I was able to get more into being pregnant by eating better and actually trying to stop and enjoy the symptoms I was having. We hadn't told anyone, so it was something for me to focus on."

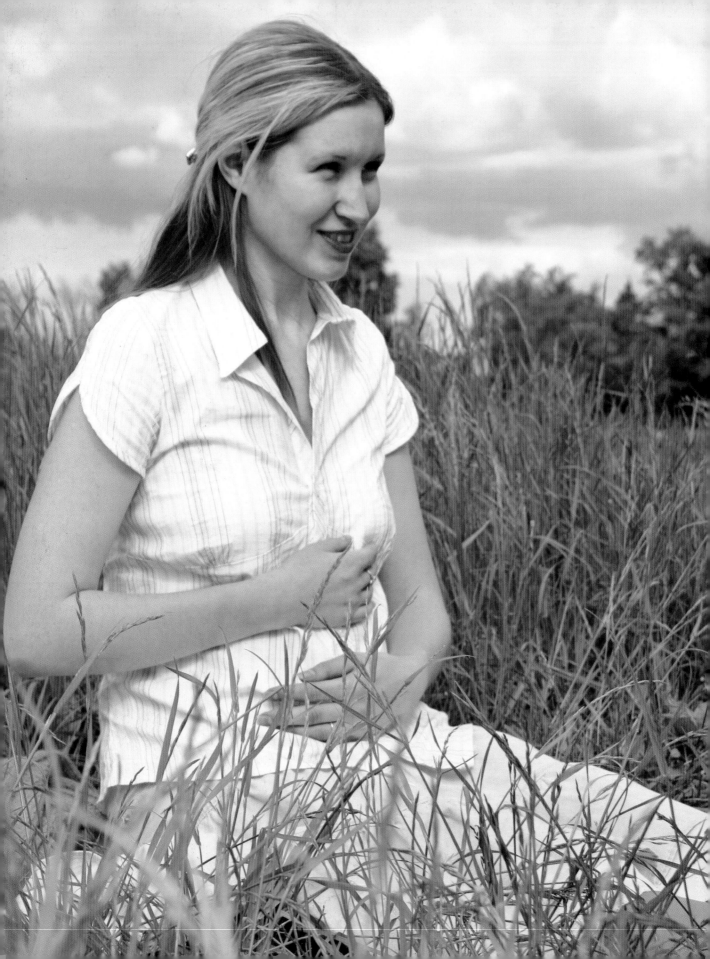

# Week 7

## ✎ CHECKLIST FOR WEEK 7

[ ] Watch what you eat for baby.
[ ] Find out what takes place during prenatal appointments.
[ ] Deal with insomnia.
[ ] Decide when to tell others about the pregnancy.
[ ] Cope with being pregnant after a previous loss.

## ⚲ WHAT TO WATCH FOR THIS WEEK

### Double Check

**One-sided pain:** One-sided pain in your abdomen that doesn't dissipate is a possible indicator of an ovarian cyst or ectopic pregnancy.

**Bleeding or spotting:** You should alert your practitioner to spotting because it raises the possibility of miscarriage, ectopic pregnancy, or blighted ovum (where a fertilized egg fails to grow). You needn't panic because spotting can be the normal result of having sex, a low-lying placenta, or loss of a twin, which is sometimes called vanishing twin syndrome.

**Back pain:** Pain in your back can be triggered by uterine cramping and stretching, or it might indicate a potential miscarriage or infection. Report severe pain and pain that does not abate to your midwife or doctor.

**Sudden disappearance of pregnancy symptoms:** If you've been experiencing pregnancy symptoms such as sore breasts, nausea and/or vomiting, and certain sensitivities that suddenly disappear, you should report this to your doctor or midwife. Symptoms such as these can come in waves, but when they vanish entirely, you need to find out if there is a hormonal issue present.

**Inability to keep food or liquid down:** Feeling nauseous and throwing up is typical during pregnancy, but getting dehydrated is a real and serious threat if you throw up too often and for too long. Report this condition to your practitioner right away.

*Report any strange or troublesome symptoms to your practitioner immediately.*

##  BODY BASICS

Your body isn't changing in the ways that you expect of pregnant women yet. Most women can feel something going on in their uterus, but they can't quite find words to describe it. Words such as heavy, tight, thick, and tickle get thrown around by women trying to pinpoint this feeling.

You may be dealing with the ongoing symptoms such as morning sickness, constipation, heartburn, exhaustion, and other not-so-fun parts of pregnancy. If you're having a rough time, you might be wondering why anyone would ever choose to be pregnant. The truth is, most women forget the intensity of the first trimester as their pregnancy progresses. They have a vague recollection of not feeling well, but pregnancy amnesia is responsible for making the population rate thrive.

## 🚼 BABY DATA

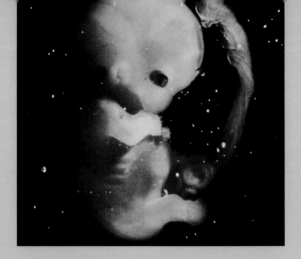

Your baby is growing rapidly and developing organs. This week your baby is working on its kidneys along with other organs. The crown-to-rump length is about ¼ inch (7 to 9 millimeters). Finger rays (the equivalent of pre-fingers) are also forming.

While your baby is a girl or a boy from the moment of conception, you can't physically distinguish the sex yet, even though the genital tubercle (what will become the penis or clitoris) is present.

Your baby's face is not very baby-like yet. This week the nasal pits are developing, and the eyes are very large and lidless. The intestines are forming inside the umbilical cord and will move into your baby's abdomen.

If you were to have an ultrasound at this point in your pregnancy and you were really in your 7th week, you should see a fetal pole with a heartbeat. If you don't, chances are you are not as far along as you thought and a repeat ultrasound in a week's time will tell a different story.

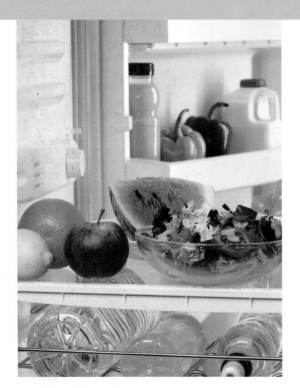

*Eating a variety of foods, choosing from many colors and families, will help you fulfill the nutrient requirements you and your baby have during pregnancy.*

PREGNANCY PARTICULARS

## Watch What You Eat for Baby

Pregnancy is often touted as the time that you get to eat for two. It's probably better to think of it as the time in your life when what you eat is twice as important, but you don't need to eat twice as much food. In fact, you probably only need an average of 300 extra calories a day when pregnant.

Three hundred calories is the equivalent of an extra snack. It's always better to make sure that you're eating something that is good for you than to waste those calories on a candy bar. This is where many moms go astray. They use the extra calories to fill their bodies with junk food rather than any number of healthy options. Good choices include fresh fruits and vegetables or protein such as peanut butter, nuts, or cheese.

# PREGNANCY AFFIRMATION FOR WEEK 7

Being pregnant is a big change for me. I am up to the challenge.

There are also lists of things that you should avoid during your pregnancy. Some are no brainers such as alcoholic beverages, but there are other categories of foods that aren't as commonly thought of as problematic including raw fruits and vegetables that haven't been washed and soft, unpasteurized cheese, such as Gorgonzola or Brie.

The general rules are that all of your foods should be washed thoroughly before you eat them. Your meats should always be cooked medium to well done to ensure that all of the bacteria have been destroyed. Avoid raw fish such as sushi and sashimi. Not heeding these precautions can needlessly expose you and your baby to food borne illnesses. Talk to your practitioner about any specific food allergies you have prior to pregnancy.

## Find Out What Takes Place during Prenatal Appointments

Prenatal visits are not only an opportunity for you to ask questions and to seek advice and support but also a chance for your practitioner to watch how your baby is growing and how your body responds to pregnancy. This is done by taking a series of measurements throughout the course of your pregnancy. Some measurements are external factors such as your weight or how large your uterus is growing, and others involve screening your urine for protein and checking your blood pressure.

What happens at prenatal visits throughout your pregnancy varies only slightly. Typically they include the following:

- Weight check
- Blood pressure check
- Urine screening
- Lab work, as needed
- Uterus measuring
- Listening to your baby's heart (after week 12)
- Discussing your questions and concerns
- Vaginal exams (rarely, because they can cause infection)

Your particular health profile and the health of your baby may indicate that other screenings are appropriate or necessary. Be sure to ask if you have questions about what to expect from your prenatal care.

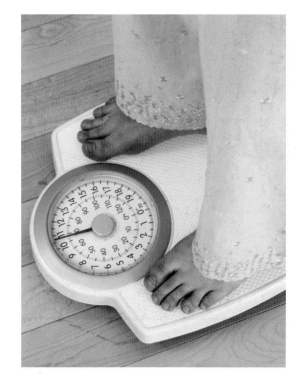

*Weight gain in the first trimester is fairly limited. You should aim to gain weight slowly and steadily, avoiding large gains made quickly when possible.*

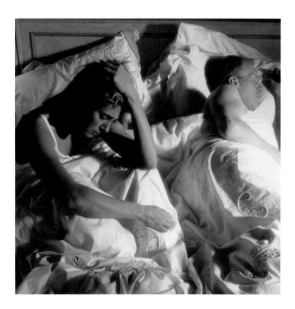

*Insomnia can be an early symptom of pregnancy. Various exercises and relaxation techniques can help, sometimes it's just a passing issue.*

## Deal with Insomnia

Most women will have difficulty sleeping at some point in their pregnancies. Insomnia generally takes two forms: not being able to fall asleep or waking up and not being able to get back to sleep. Either form can really disrupt your sleep schedule, and some women are unlucky enough to experience both forms.

While you're not yet experiencing the extreme pregnancy sensations that will keep you awake in the later months, such as a large abdomen and a kicking baby, what you may feel is extreme fatigue without the relief of sleep, a racing mind that keeps you awake, or simply an unexplained inability to sleep.

To help relieve your insomnia, try some or all of the following:

- Exercise during the day but not prior to bedtime.
- Avoid caffeinated beverages after mid-afternoon.
- Do not eat just before going to bed.
- Practice relaxation or meditation before bedtime to clear your mind.
- Drink warm milk before going to bed.
- Take a warm bath before going to bed.
- Read before you fall asleep.
- Keep to a set bedtime.
- Don't take too many or overlong naps.

If you find that you're not able to get back to sleep or if the above strategies don't help, you should avoid just lying in bed and stewing over the problem. Yes, you can't sleep, and it's not fair. But after about twenty minutes, you should get up and do something for a while. You might watch television, read, write a letter, or catch up on the mail. After twenty to thirty minutes, try to sleep again, and hopefully you will be more successful. Be sure to talk to your practitioner about sleeplessness if it becomes a common occurrence.

## Decide When to Tell Others about the Pregnancy

There is a huge difference between telling your husband that you're pregnant and telling, say, your family. And beyond family and close friends, there is the question of when to tell the rest of the world. For starters, let's think about your boss.

Most experts agree that telling your boss you are pregnant in the first trimester is probably not advisable unless your job needs to be adjusted because of your pregnancy, in which case it is imperative that you tell him or her immediately. In other cases, you should wait until your pregnancy is well established and you have mentally worked out some of the details of your maternity leave and how your work will be handled while you're pregnant and while you're gone.

Telling the rest of the world is a personal decision. You have to remember that telling anyone creates the possibility of a leak, so take that into consideration before confiding in others, particularly people who aren't that close to you.

This advice is especially recommended for kids who have trouble keeping secrets. Don't tell your older kids until you're ready for the announcement to be shared far and wide. In fact, this is a great way to spread the news if you aren't interested in spreading it yourself.

## Cope with Being Pregnant after a Previous Loss

If you have been pregnant before, and your baby died either through miscarriage, stillbirth, or infant death, pregnancy may be a particularly difficult time for you. You may not feel all of the happy emotions that you felt with your previous pregnancy, and your concerns may be great. It is important that you find a way to share these concerns with your spouse, with others in a support group, or with your practitioner so they don't build up inside, which can lead to depression. They do not make you a bad parent.

While it may not be easy to view this pregnancy as separate from the past, try to find differences when you can and celebrate milestones as they arrive. For example, if you had a miscarriage early in a prior pregnancy, celebrate when you pass that week. Try to rejoice in aspects of your new pregnancy, such as seeing your baby's heartbeat or feeling your baby kick.

Be sure to talk with your practitioner about getting support and help from him or her and from others as well. Your doctor or midwife should provide suggestions for what you can do to help ease your fears. But he or she can only help if you open up and talk honestly about your feelings.

While you may be leery of joining a support group, many couples find them very beneficial. They offer a place where it's okay not to be excited simply about being pregnant and a chance to talk to others who have been in the same place as you, even if they are further along in their journeys. If you can't find a local group to join, look for an online community on the Internet.

**HOT MAMA**

Brushing your teeth may trigger gagging in early pregnancy, but that doesn't mean you should skip oral hygiene. The following tips can make toothbrush time less traumatic:

- Buy a new toothbrush with soft bristles.
- Switch from a mint-flavored toothpaste to something that doesn't nauseate you.
- Go easy on the back of your tongue and use less pressure.
- Adjust the water temperature to make sure it's comfortable for your stomach.

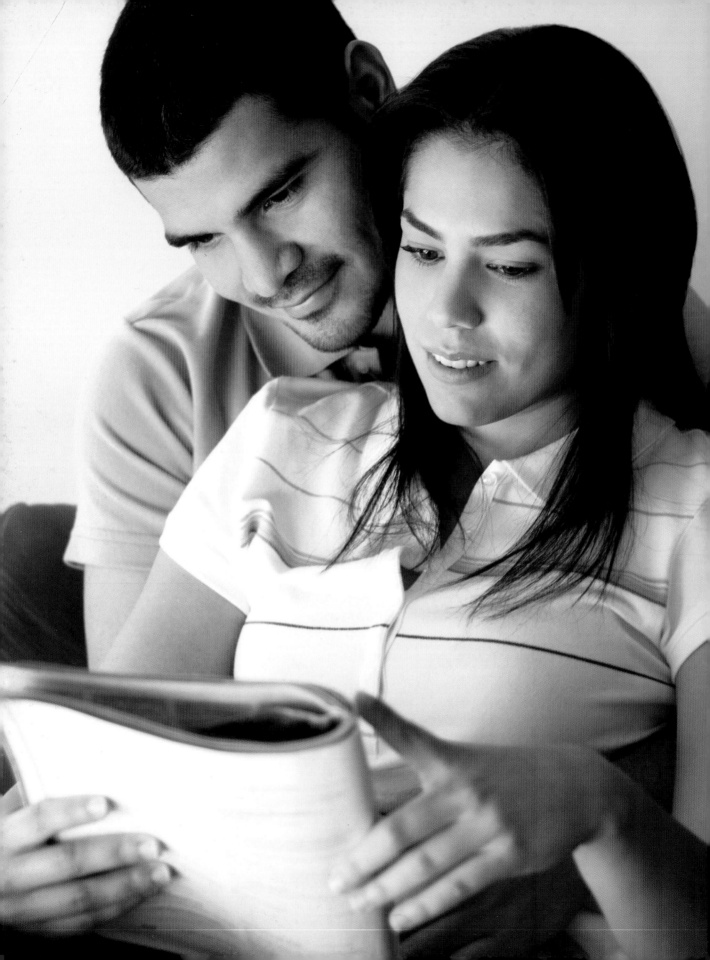

# WEEK 8

## CHECKLIST FOR WEEK 8

[ ] Monitor your first trimester weight gain.

[ ] Don't worry about being vegetarian.

[ ] Be familiar with the signs of miscarriage.

[ ] Prepare for wild and weird pregnancy dreams.

[ ] Learn about common lab work in the first trimester.

[ ] Watch out for hyperemesis gravidarium.

[ ] Consider where you'll give birth.

## WHAT TO WATCH FOR THIS WEEK

### Double Check

**One-sided pain:** One-sided pain in your abdomen that doesn't go away is a potential sign of an ovarian cyst or ectopic pregnancy.

**Bleeding or spotting:** You should alert your practitioner because the possibility of miscarriage, ectopic pregnancy, or blighted ovum (where a fertilized egg fails to grow) is present. The spotting could, however, be the result of having sex, a low-lying placenta, or loss of a twin (vanishing twin syndrome).

**Back pain:** Explanations for back pain range from uterine cramping to miscarriage, and it can also be a sign of infection or that your uterus is stretching. If you pain is severe or does not abate, contact your midwife or doctor.

**Sudden disappearance of pregnancy symptoms:** If you've been having a lot of pregnancy symptoms such as sore breasts, nausea and/or vomiting, and sensitivities to smell, and they suddenly disappear, you should see your doctor or midwife. Symptoms can fluctuate, but it's concerning when they vanish suddenly and completely.

**Inability to keep food or liquid down:** Throwing up during pregnancy isn't a problem unless it happens so frequently that you risk becoming dehydrated. If this applies to you, contact your practitioner immediately.

*Report any strange or troublesome symptoms to your practitioner immediately.*

##  BODY BASICS

You have now missed your second period. Your first prenatal visit is probably coming up soon. This visit will be one of your longest visits because of the added amount of history taking that is required. Sometimes the prenatal history is taken by a medical assistant or a nurse rather than the doctor or midwife. Be sure that you talk to the practitioner about anything you feel is significant, even if he or she doesn't directly ask you about it.

Your pregnancy symptoms continue this week. Hang in there! The first trimester ends in a couple of weeks, and you will no doubt start to feel better.

Your baby is nearly a centimeter long crown to rump, around ⅓ inch (eight to eleven millimeters). This is when the gonads become specifically testes or ovaries. Last week, fingers were big; this week, it's toes. In addition to toes, your baby's bones are beginning to harden in spots, known as ossification. Your baby is starting to develop elbows.

One of the most thrilling developments this week is that spontaneous movement begins. This means that your baby is beginning to use the joints and will try to wave, kick, and flip. An ultrasound now reveals quite the little acrobat—even when you can't feel all that is going on inside your body—a very odd sensation indeed.

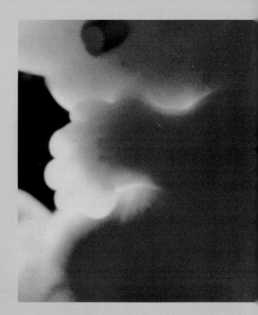

## Monitor Your First Trimester Weight Gain

Most women don't like to focus on weight gain during pregnancy. After all, when have you ever wanted to gain weight? But the fact of the matter is that weight gain in pregnancy is not only normal but also healthy and necessary. The good news is that the first trimester is not a time of substantial weight gain.

In fact, of the three trimesters, the first is typically the time you will gain the least amount of weight. Some mothers even lose a little weight because of dietary changes and changes in their appetites. (It is important to note that purposely losing weight is to be avoided in pregnancy because of the potential risks of reducing the appropriate amount of nutrients to your baby.)

The average first trimester weight gain is about four pounds—one pound more if you're underweight and one pound less if you're overweight. Remember that your baby and uterus haven't grown very big yet. If you've experienced a bigger weight gain than this, you might talk to a nutritionist to evaluate your diet if you can't pinpoint an obvious explanation such as a drastic change in exercise or food intake. Most health insurance will cover this as a benefit; if your does not, look for someone at a local hospital who offers this service as an out-reach program for pregnancy.

## Don't Worry about Being Vegetarian

In the past, pregnant women who didn't eat meat were told that their diets was harmful to a growing baby. Today we know that vegetarians and vegans can enjoy healthy pregnancies. Still, many vegetarian women are concerned that a lack of meat will affect their pregnancies in a negative way. This is simply not true. While lean meats, for some, can be a good source of protein, many foods that supply you with protein are not meat based.

If you have been a vegetarian for numerous years and have maintained a healthy lifestyle, you will probably not need to make any changes in

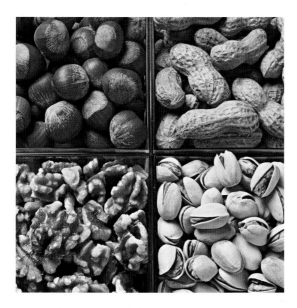

*Nuts can be a great snack during pregnancy. They are filled with protein and good fats. They also store nicely in your purse or backpack for quick snacking.*

# My baby
# feels my presence.

Eating a healthy diet without meat is not difficult. Maintaining a food log is highly recommended for all pregnant women to help them assess their diet, and for a new vegetarian, it is essential. Your practitioner or nutritionist can help you evaluate your diet for inadequacies and help make suggestions to guarantee that you and your baby are getting all the nutrition you need.

## Be Familiar with the Signs of Miscarriage

The loss of a pregnancy prior to 20 weeks is known as a miscarriage. It is nothing you want to worry about, but most pregnant women will worry about it at some point.

The following are signs to look for because they indicate the possibility of a miscarriage:

- Bleeding
- Cramping
- Backache
- Complete loss of pregnancy symptoms

If you experience any of these signs, you should immediately call your midwife or doctor. Many times there is nothing that can be done. It is estimated that about 1 in 5 pregnancies will be lost to miscarriage, including many before a positive pregnancy test.

your pregnancy diet. If you choose to become a vegetarian during pregnancy, that's fine, but you should seek guidance from your practitioner and possibly a nutritionist.

Some women find that during pregnancy the thought of meat makes them feel ill, and they wish to avoid it. Again, meat is not a necessary part of a healthy diet for pregnant women. Seeking the support of a nutritionist who has experience working with vegetarians is useful to many women.

Because protein is the building block of every cell, it is essential for a healthy pregnancy. Protein is available in many sources; in fact, almost everything has at least some protein in it. The main sources of protein for vegetarians include:

- Nuts and nut butters, such as peanut and almond
- Beans
- Tofu
- Meat replacement products, such as tofu and other soy products

However, it is possible to have the signs of miscarriage and not actually miscarry. For instance, vaginal exams and vaginal ultrasounds can cause bleeding, which is a sign of miscarriage but doesn't really pose a threat to the pregnancy. This is known as a threatened miscarriage. (Any bleeding from the vagina is called a threatened miscarriage because it may or may not cause a threat to the pregnancy. Other terms used to describe bleeding can be associated with other symptoms such as an open cervix, which is more ominous than simple spotting or bleeding that may be caused by other issues, including the sensitivity of the cervix to mere touch as with a vaginal exam, transvaginal ultrasound, or with sexual intercourse.)

## Prepare for Wild and Weird Pregnancy Dreams

Pregnant women will be quick to tell you that their dreams can be pretty wild. Wild can mean very vivid, realistic, weird, or thought-provoking. Dreams can provide insight into what you're thinking or worried about—such as dreams about leaving your baby at the store or forgetting to feed her. Some women dream about babies that look like small animals or about having more babies than they are gestating, such as ten or twelve.

Your dreams are a pleasant way to free your mind of things that are worrisome. This is true even if you are not consciously aware that you are worried about something. You might even enjoy these sneak peeks into something like the sex of your baby or even how many babies you have in your uterus. Mother's intuition is usually spot on, even when it takes the form of dreams. So don't be so quick to dismiss them as meaningless.

Occasionally these dreams will become incredibly worrisome or keep you up at night to avoid returning to the dreams. If that is the case, you should talk to your doctor or midwife to get a referral to a counselor who can help reduce your rate of dreams and help you sleep more peacefully.

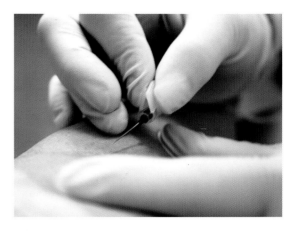

*Lab work needn't be worrisome. Be sure to know what blood work is being done, why, when, and how you can expect the results. This can prevent some concern later.*

## Learn about Common Lab Work in the First Trimester

Lab work or blood work is ordered at various stages of your pregnancy. At your first prenatal visit, you may feel like you've been ordered to donate blood based on the number of vials that get filled. The following basic tests are ordered for almost everyone:

- BLOOD TYPE AND RHESUS FACTOR: This is to see what your blood type and rhesus factor are, so that your practitioner can know about potential complications should your partner be a different rhesus factor, from you.

- RUBELLA TITER: This test is to see if you're immune from this childhood illness that can cause problems with the pregnancy if contracted. If you are not immune, you will need to avoid people who have rubella and be immunized after giving birth.

- VDRL STATUS, SUCH AS SYPHILIS AND GONORRHEA: These are tests for various sexually transmitted infections (STIs) that can cause problems during pregnancy or birth.

- IRON LEVELS: This is to check for anemia, which is when your iron levels are lower than normal. This affects how much oxygen you get, causing you to feel tired, sluggish, and even short of breath. It is fairly common in pregnancy, particularly at certain points because of the large expansion of blood volume you go through to help nurture your baby inside the uterus. Low iron can potentially cause problems during your birth and postpartum as well.

You may also have more specific lab work done if you have chronic issues or other problems, which includes the following:

- Liver function tests
- Thyroid levels
- HIV/AIDS status (This is mandatory in some states.)
- hCG levels

Be sure to discuss any blood test that's been ordered with your doctor or midwife. It may be that they need information to adjust your current medications, or it may be that they are looking for something specific. They should always be willing to take the time to explain what is going on with your lab work.

You should also remember to ask not only what they are testing and why, but how the results will be given and when the results will be made available. Some practices have a special line you can call for lab results, or they may ask you to wait until your next appointment to discuss the results. Sometimes, however, an immediate answer is needed to treat you promptly. For example, if your thyroid hormone levels are low, you should start treatment as soon as possible. Waiting a month between appointments would be detrimental.

## Watch out for Hyperemesis Gravidarium

Throwing up during pregnancy is awful, but it's also fairly common, and you're entitled to complain. An abnormal level of nausea and vomiting is called hyperemesis gravidarium. Technically this is defined as the loss of at least 5 percent of your body weight, and it affects only 1 out of 300 women.

If you have been diagnosed with hyperemesis, you will most likely be given a variety of treatments until one is found that works for you. While many cases of hyperemesis can be treated on an outpatient basis, some are severe enough to require treatment in the hospital.

Treatments include the following:

- Alternative therapies, such as vitamins, talk therapy, and acupuncture
- Various medications
- IV hydration
- Total parental nutrition (Using an IV to feed someone so she doesn't have to worry about food or digestion)
- Tube feedings

If you have reason to believe you might be suffering from hyperemesis, be sure to bring it up with your doctor or midwife.

## Consider Where You'll Give Birth

Where you give birth is a very important decision. There are a number of places available for you to give birth, including the following:

- Home
- Free-standing birth center
- Hospital birth center
- Hospitals (various levels)

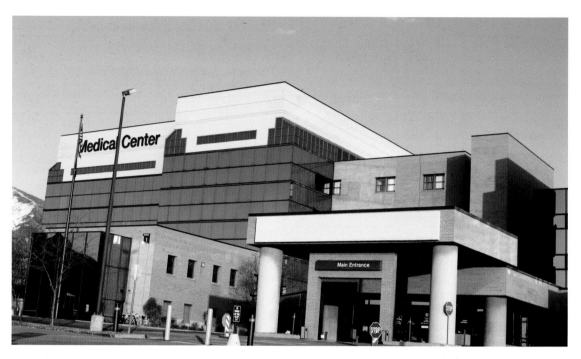

*Your choice of where to give birth is important. Be sure to take tours and discuss your options early. Don't hesitate to let them know you are shopping around.*

## MEMORABLE MOMENTS

"I wanted to tell everyone I met so badly. But my husband and I agreed that we should wait until we were out of the first trimester to make the announcement. Sometimes I would tell strangers, just to relieve the pressure building up inside me."

Unfortunately not all communities will have the resources to fund or support each type of place of birth. You may have only one or two options where you live, or you may have the full range of options from which to choose. You need to understand the perks of each before deciding which appeals most to you.

HOME BIRTH: Women who choose to give birth at home do so for a variety of reasons, including a desire to avoid unnecessary interventions during labor and birth and a wish to control their environments. Home birth may be an option for you if you have practitioners who practice at home, and you meet their requirements, which usually include being healthy with a low-risk pregnancy. During your pregnancy, you will be screened constantly for signs of not being low risk, at which point you would transfer to the care of a different birth place.

FREE-STANDING BIRTH CENTER: A free-standing birth center is not located within a hospital and is typically not on hospital grounds. A centralized location for care providers, it has very little medical equipment other than the basics for dealing with emergencies. It is a place for healthy women having low-risk pregnancies to safely have babies with practitioners who choose to practice there. Typically women giving birth here are choosing to minimize certain interventions in birth.

HOSPITAL BIRTH CENTER: A hospital birth center gives expectant mothers less autonomy than a free-standing birth center, and it may be housed on a separate floor of a hospital. Some hospitals may call their maternity wards "birth centers," but they lack the philosophy that birth is normal. "Normal" is a term used to describe a birth that proceeds physiologically the way the body is meant to, free from routine interventions such as epidurals and Cesarean sections. A belief in and support for normal births is what tends to set birth centers of all kinds apart. Ask if your hospital's birth center has separate staff trained to assist in helping you labor with minimal intervention.

HOSPITAL: The majority of women give birth in hospitals of all levels, from hospitals with only well newborn nurseries (for infants who are not ill) to hospitals with Level III Neonatal Intensive Care Units (NICU). Each hospital will have its own philosophy of birth and care for a variety of women. Some hospitals see more high-risk patients than others, so be sure to ask if that matters to you. Hospitals have all sorts of interventions and medications available and are accustomed to using them. If you choose to give birth in a hospital and want to minimize the use of medication, be sure to plan ahead for pointers from the hospital on navigating that path.

**HOT MAMA**

Resist the temptation to run out and buy maternity clothes. You will have plenty of time for that in later weeks, and it is considered a fashion faux pas to wear them too soon. Instead consider baby doll style tops and loose-fitting pants if you're feeling bloated due to constipation or other gastrointestinal distress.

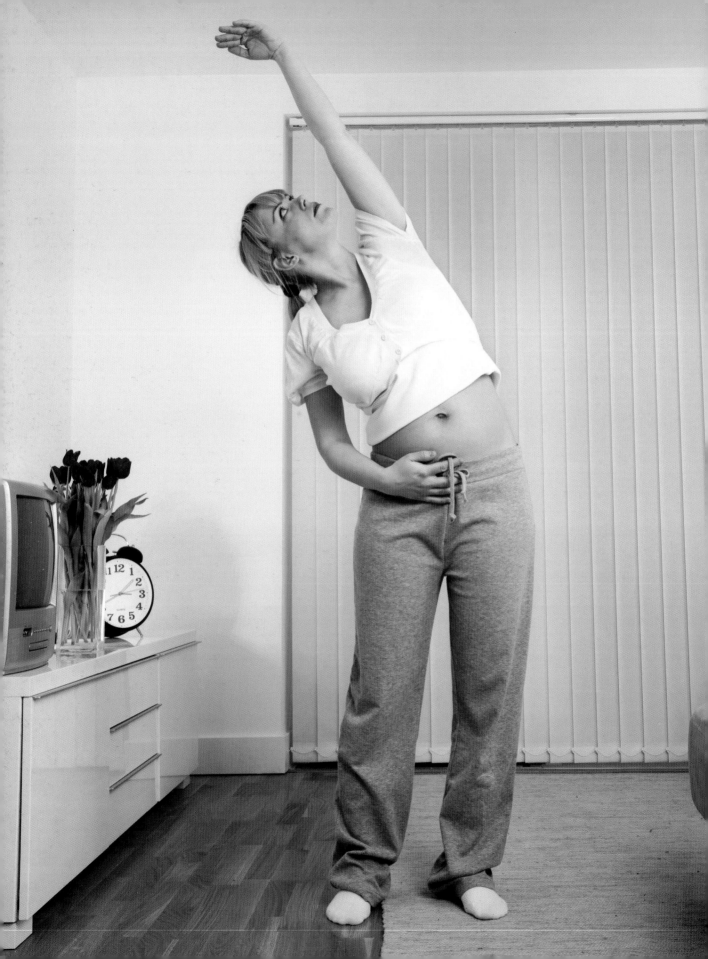

# WEEK 9

## ✎ CHECKLIST FOR WEEK 9

[ ] Exercise for two.
[ ] Look forward to showing.
[ ] Watch out for weird pregnancy symptoms.
[ ] Figure out if you're having twins.
[ ] Choose your practitioner.

## ⌕ WHAT TO WATCH FOR THIS WEEK
*Double Check*

**One-sided pain:** A constant pain on one side of your abdomen can suggest the presence of an ovarian cyst or ectopic pregnancy.

**Bleeding or spotting:** You should alert your practitioner to red or brown spotting because it can mean a miscarriage, an ectopic pregnancy, or a blighted ovum (where a fertilized egg fails to grow). Not all spotting is bad, though, because it can also be caused by sex, a low-lying placenta, or loss of a twin (vanishing twin syndrome).

**Back pain:** Pain in your back can be a sign of uterine cramping and potential miscarriage, and it can also be a sign of infection or that your uterus is stretching. Report severe pain and pain that does not abate to your midwife or doctor.

**Sudden disappearance of pregnancy symptoms:** If you have suffered from a host of pregnancy symptoms, including sore breasts, nausea and/ or vomiting, and sensitivities to smell, it's worth contacting your doctor or midwife if they suddenly disappear. Fluctuations are normal, but a complete loss may indicate a hormonal issue. Blood work can test your levels of various hormones to identify any problems.

**Inability to keep food or liquid down:** It's a fact that many pregnant women throw up—especially during their first trimesters. But in extreme cases, dehydration can result, which is a serious health threat and should be brought to the attention of your practitioner.

*Report any strange or troublesome symptoms to your practitioner immediately.*

##  BODY BASICS

Well, a few weeks into this and you're probably adapting to whatever symptoms of pregnancy you've been experiencing. Experience is the key here. That, and some good advice. Pregnancy is not as easy as it appears in the movies or from a distance, but the end of the first trimester is near, and hopefully the challenges of the first trimester will pass.

## 👶 BABY DATA

Your baby is continuing to grow and develop. After a growth spurt, your baby now measures just over half an inch (thirteen to seventeen millimeters) from crown to rump. The toe rays are beginning to have toes, and they are wiggling more.

If you were to look via ultrasound at your baby at this point, you would see the arms and legs and the baby moving. If you were to touch the outside of the uterus, your baby's home, your baby would move away from the touch.

The organ systems are still growing, and the bones are still hardening. This work will continue for weeks to come.

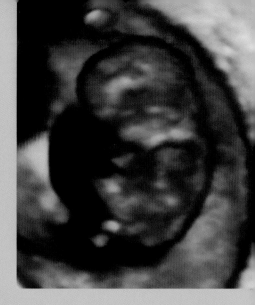

## Exercise for Two

Exercise is incredibly important in pregnancy. Not only does it contribute to an easier pregnancy by keeping weight gain and side effects such as back pain at a minimum, but it also can provide benefits in labor. Women who have exercised during pregnancy tend to have faster and easier labors, not to mention shorter recoveries. This means you will bounce back from having a baby faster.

The following are a few simple rules to exercising when pregnant:

- Stay well hydrated before, during, and after exercise.

- Don't do anything that hurts.

- Continue doing most of your pre-pregnancy regimen, but talk to your practitioner before starting new exercises.

- Avoid anything that could cause you to lose your balance or get kicked in the abdomen.

- Stop immediately and call your practitioner if you have bleeding, shortness of breath, or pain.

- Watch your heart rate. The general rule of thumb is to keep your heart rate from going higher than 140 beats per minute, but this may be different for women who are extremely active. Ask your practitioner for the appropriate range for your fitness level.

Pregnancy may spur you to exercise in a way you haven't before. Many women find that pregnancy is a good time to start thinking about the optimal lifestyle habits that they want to instill in their kids. While you shouldn't use pregnancy as a time to start something like running marathons, it can be a great time to explore low-impact forms of movement such as walking, prenatal yoga, and swimming.

With the help of your body's signals, your practitioner, and your fitness trainer or coach, you can find an exercise plan to help both you and baby grow toward fitness. The circumstances under which you would need to avoid exercise completely, even if only for a brief period, include the following:

- Bleeding

- Threatened preterm labor, or a history of it

- Some instances of multiple pregnancies

- Intrauterine growth restriction, which is when fetal development slows beyond what is normal due to a physical restriction in growth or lack of nutrients

It's important to find something that you really enjoy so you'll stick with it and reap all the benefits that exercising in pregnancy can offer you and your baby. This is also a wonderful time to get your husband and/or friends on board to do something you all can enjoy and feel good about together. If you start with group walks in the park now, once the baby arrives, you can bring your sling or stroller along as you continue a lifelong habit of health.

## Look forward to Showing

Few things are more thrilling than the protruding abdomen of a pregnant woman. It's even better when that belly belongs to you. So you're probably waiting to feel that expansion in your own body and clothes.

The problem is that it doesn't happen soon enough for most women, and usually not in the first trimester. This is because your uterus is still safely tucked into your pelvis. But don't assume you're crazy because your clothes seem to be fitting differently than before and you swear you're feeling something.

Some of your pregnancy symptoms, such as bloating, gas, and constipation, can make your intestines feel expanded, which can make your clothes feel tight or fit differently. Plus as your uterus grows, while it's still in the pelvis, your intestines have to move somewhere—so why not up and out? This may require some wardrobe alterations on your end, but it's probably not enough to require maternity clothes.

## Watch out for Weird Pregnancy Symptoms

When you're reviewing the list of common pregnancy symptoms, some tend to be familiar, such as morning sickness and heartburn. But there are others that may surprise you, such as nasal stuffiness, sensitivity to smells, emotional highs and lows, and food aversions.

PREGNANCY AFFIRMATION
FOR WEEK 9

## Pregnancy is a normal and natural state for my baby and me.

As the hormones begin their work of supporting your pregnancy and helping your baby grow, your body will change and react differently than you may have expected. The dance of the hormones is doing its job, and your body is taking part in the process.

The following are several lesser-known pregnancy symptoms and how you can best handle them:

NOSE TROUBLE: Nasal stuffiness and nose bleeds are fairly common in pregnancy. Keeping your nasal passages well moisturized and snorting saline solution (store bought or homemade) can help alleviate these side effects.

BURPING AND BELCHING: The gastrointestinal tract takes a huge hit during pregnancy. Not only is it dealing with the influx of hormones, but it is also taking a beating as the uterus rises and displaces your intestines. Don't be surprised if you frequently burping after a meal, often uncontrollably. If you are able to identify certain foods or drinks that seem to make matters worse, try avoiding them to see if the problem goes away.

INSOMNIA: The inability to fall asleep or stay asleep is a major annoyance in pregnancy. The real problem arises when you're exhausted and still can't get the sleep you need. Try relaxation before bed time, practice yoga, do your exercises earlier in the day, and avoid heavy meals before bed. If you find that you're still having trouble, ask your practitioner to help you pinpoint what the issue is—whether it's physical, mental, or emotional. Sometimes a racing mind or problems you're having during the day can keep your mind ccupied all night.

Any other symptoms that you are experiencing may or may not be a normal part of a healthy pregnancy. Don't forget to ask your midwife or doctor for advice for handling them. Your practitioner has lots of experience dealing with every possible pregnancy symptom and is likely to have some tried-and-true solutions for you.

## Figure Out If You're Having Twins

A frequent question of women during early pregnancy is: How many babies are in there? You may find yourself asking that question too. The following are the most common reasons that women believe that they may be having multiples:

- History of multiple pregnancy personally or in the family
- History of fertility treatments
- Rate of expansion of their abdomens
- A hunch or dreams

All of these are valid reasons to believe that you might be the mother of more than one baby. Your practitioner will likely take a detailed family and personal history as it relates to multiple pregnancies and decide what needs to be done. Sometimes an ultrasound is ordered early on to verify if you are indeed expecting twins (or more). Other times, you and your practitioner might decide to wait until other clinical symptoms of a multiple gestation arise. These might include:

- Uterus measuring large for dates
- Hearing more than one heartbeat during a routine exam
- Mother feeling lots of movement or that the "baby is all over the place"
- Abnormal numbers for certain blood work

Sometimes twins aren't found until later in pregnancy following additional testing, such as a screening ultrasound conducted at mid-pregnancy.

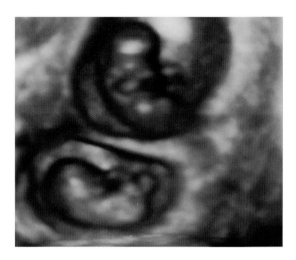

*Twins are most often diagnosed via early ultrasound. Talk to your practitioner about multiples if you are having symptoms.*

If you find you are having twins, it will probably come as quite the shock to you and your family. Try to let the information sink in before making any big decisions such as changing doctors or hospitals or making major purchases. Joining a local Mother of Twins Club or other multiple birth organization is a good place to start. You can also talk to your practitioner about his or her ability to cope with the special needs of a multiple pregnancy. It may mean that you should invite another practitioner to assist in your care depending on the practitioner you have already employed.

## Choose Your Practitioner

The practitioner that you choose should be able to care for you throughout your pregnancy and postpartum period. This will be someone with whom you will need to build a great deal of trust and someone with whom you develop a bond over the course of your prenatal care. Today's pregnant woman has many different types of practitioners from which to choose.

Obstetrician/gynecologist: These surgical specialists have dedicated their lives to taking care of women's issues, including pregnancy and birth. Many women choose to see an obstetrician for their pregnancy care. Most obstetricians work in hospitals, but a few do home births and work in birth centers. They usually work in groups of other obstetricians and may have a call schedule devised for doing births outside of office hours.

MATERNAL FETAL MEDICINE (MFM) SPECIALIST (PERINATOLOGIST): The MFM specialist is an obstetrician who has completed a fellowship beyond medical school and residency to care for extremely sick mothers and babies. They are often used as consultants for other practitioners to help guide the care of pregnant women who fall into this category. You may be in the care of a midwife and be asked to do a genetic screening with an MFM, or your regular doctor finds out you are carrying twins and would like a second opinion or extra screening. Many high-risk women wind up seeing an MFM for their entire pregnancies. MFMs most always practice in hospitals with NICU capabilities because of the nature of their patient population.

FAMILY PRACTITIONER: These doctors have the care of the entire family at heart and may specialize in births or may run general practices. This could be someone with whom you already have a close relationship and that makes it easy to continue receiving care from this person. Another benefit of using a family practitioner is that he or she can often continue on as your baby's doctor after birth. Family practitioners work in all types of birth settings.

CERTIFIED NURSE-MIDWIFE: A nurse-midwife is a nurse and a midwife, a combined profession in the United States. These women care for low-risk pregnant women and do well woman care. While they are also trained in well newborn care for the first year of life, the majority do not practice this skill, opting instead to defer to pediatricians. You will find nurse midwives practicing in all types of birth settings and can look for one at *www.mymidwife.org* or by contacting the American College of Nurse-Midwives. (See "Resources" on page 310.)

CERTIFIED PROFESSIONAL MIDWIFE: This type of midwife has been trained and passed rigorous board examinations by the North American Registry of Midwives to be awarded this credential. They care only for low-risk pregnant women, usually in home birth or birth center settings. They are also trained in screening women for problems to ensure that they receive the care that they need from the right source, even if that means transferring care when appropriate. Most certified professional midwives are affiliated with physicians or physicians groups or will work with a physician of your choosing. Contact Midwives Alliance of North America or *www.mana.org* to learn more and get referrals. (See "Resources" on page 312.)

DIRECT ENTRY MIDWIFE: A direct entry midwife may or may not have formal training, and many train as apprentices to other midwives. She may be studying to be a certified professional midwife. You will most often find this type of provider in a home birth or birth center setting, caring for low-risk pregnant women.

**HOT MAMA**

Did you know that pregnancy even changes your eyes? The progesterone and fluid retention triggered by pregnancy has the ability to alter how you see, both by changing the shape of your eye and increasing dryness.

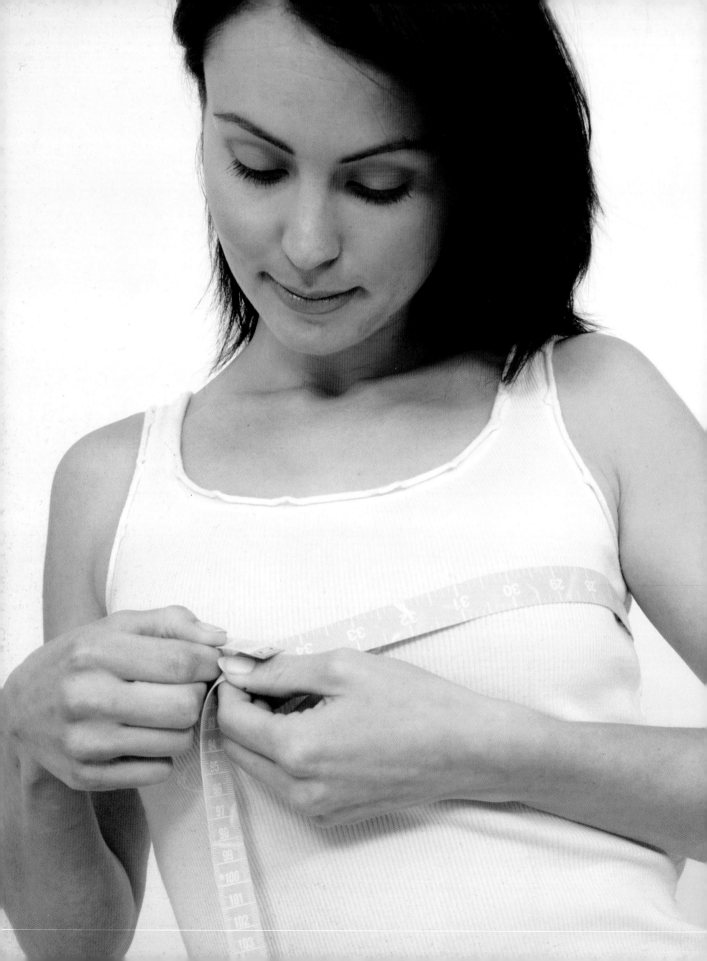

# WEEK 10

## ✎ CHECKLIST FOR WEEK 10

[ ] Buy a new bra and almost-ready-for-maternity clothes.

[ ] Eat for a healthy pregnancy.

[ ] Take an early pregnancy class.

[ ] Tour birth facilities.

[ ] Discuss family leave policies and protocols.

[ ] Try a new exercise or exercise class.

[ ] Take a picture and measure your abdomen.

## ⌕ WHAT TO WATCH FOR THIS WEEK

*Double Check*

**One-sided pain:** One-sided pain in your abdomen that doesn't go away is a potential sign of an ovarian cyst.

**Bleeding or spotting:** You should alert your practitioner because the possibility of miscarriage or blighted ovum (where a fertilized egg fails to grow) is present. There are perfectly normal explanations too: sexual intercourse, a low-lying placenta, or the loss of a twin.

**Back pain:** If you suffer from severe and persistent back pain, contact your midwife or doctor. It might be a sign of uterine cramping or stretching, or it might suggest a potential miscarriage or the presence of an infection.

**Sudden disappearance of pregnancy symptoms:** If your symptoms—sore breasts, nausea/vomiting, heightened sensitivities—suddenly disappear, you should report this to your doctor or midwife. While these things do come in waves, a complete loss may indicate an issue with progesterone and other hormone levels.

**Inability to keep food or liquid down:** While you may have expected to throw up occasionally while pregnant, the risk of dehydration can be real for many pregnant women. You need to report this to your practitioner.

*Report any strange symptoms to your practitioner immediately.*

##  BODY BASICS

While you are almost out of the first trimester, some of the nastiest physical symptoms may be persisting. Feeling extremely tired, as in "I can hardly lift my head off the pillow" and "I dream of taking a nap at 10 A.M.," is a perfectly normal way to feel at this point in your pregnancy. But don't fear; relief is in sight!

If you've not yet found the solution to counteract morning sickness, be sure to keep trying different strategies. (See Week 6) Even if you never find the cure, searching for one could provide you with enough distraction to make it through.

If you find that your abdomen is starting to poke out a little, you're probably feeling either excited or worried. The bad news about your swelling abdomen is that it is not actually the baby, but rather your bowels, which are being displaced by the growing uterus and feeling a bit more sluggish, like you do, thanks to pregnancy hormones.

Your baby and your body work in conjunction to grow and thrive. Your job is to continue to nourish your body with healthy food, movement, information, and a positive attitude.

## 🍼 BABY DATA

Your baby's head is still a large portion of his total body, but your baby is more recognizably human this week. Measuring about 1.38 inches (3.5 centimeters) from the top of the head to the rump (CRL), your baby is growing quickly. Imagine if you will that your baby's arms are about as big as the "I" on this page. The tiny toes that you long to count are now formed. Your baby's ears are formed, even on the outside. The baby's eyes are still open, but the eyelids are beginning to fuse. Once fused, they will stay fused until about 25 to 27 weeks into your pregnancy. While your baby doesn't weigh much, just four grams or about the weight of four paper clips, it is a good start.

As your baby enters the fetal period this week, you quietly pass an important milestone. All of the major organs are nearly completely

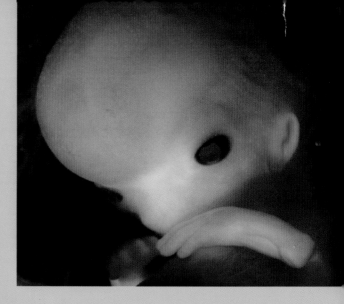

formed. The risk of major malformations is over, although your continued care and attention is still needed for the subtle yet crucial processes such as brain functioning, cognitive development, reflex growth, and breathing development.

PREGNANCY PARTICULARS

## Buy a New Bra and Almost-Ready-for-Maternity Clothes

Have you noticed the veins that may have started to appear on your breasts and belly? This is how your body maps out ways to bring more nourishment to these areas. You probably aren't thinking ahead to breastfeeding yet, but those veins are there to help your breasts work extra hard to lay down the foundations of successful nursing. This work is why your breasts may be tender in the early weeks of pregnancy and why your breasts have started growing.

Now is the time to think about purchasing a new bra. Take yourself bra shopping, keeping in mind that your breasts may change sizes several times throughout your pregnancy and during breastfeeding. Look for a bra that provides comfort and good support. If you can limit the amount of bouncing and shaking, you can also limit some of the soreness that goes along with early pregnancy breast development.

In addition to needing a new bra, you may find that your clothes are getting a little uncomfortable. It might be that you're beginning to have trouble snapping the top button on your pants, or maybe your jeans are a bit too snug. While you're not quite ready for maternity clothes, there are solutions!

You can raid your husband's closet for larger shirts or even wear your own shirts untucked. You can also try to layer clothing, such as a solid color shirt underneath and a button down, left unbuttoned, worn as a jacket over the top layer. There are also a whole range of clothes sold for that almost ready for maternity clothes set. These belly covering garments look simple and work beautifully. Made of elastic fabrics, they do a miraculous job of helping to hold up your pants if you're not quite ready to ditch the pre-pregnancy jeans, but you can't quite button them anymore. These fashion items last the entire pregnancy and well into the postpartum period as well, making them a terrific value when it comes to clothes shopping for pregnancy and postpartum. You can find them at some maternity clothes stores and at select retailers online.

## Eat for a Healthy Pregnancy

You might be concerned about weight gain in pregnancy and the fact that the recommendations for what is and isn't appropriate seem to change on a daily basis. The good news is that with a few simple guidelines, you can navigate your way through the maze of nutritional data while helping ensure a healthy pregnancy weight gain. (See Week 3 for specific nutrient guidelines.)

Throw out the old adage that you are eating for two. By this point in your pregnancy, the baby weighs just a few grams, and you've probably put on very little weight, if any. Add about 300 extra calories a day—the equivalent of one snack. A snack could be a healthy snack bar and a piece of fruit, a handful of almonds, or a small sandwich full of lean protein, such as turkey or cheese. Make every bite count—you could snack on a candy bar but would you feed it to your baby? By preplanning snacks and having them ready at hand, you gain more control over what you eat.

Avoid diseases such as listeria, E. coli, and toxoplasmosis. Handle food safely by washing it and cooking it thoroughly when appropriate, in other words don't eat raw fish or undercooked meats.

Select your cheering squad carefully—family, friends, coworkers, and practitioner. Invite people into your corner who offer you healthy snacks, give you sound advice, and set proper examples to keep you motivated and on track. Don't be afraid to call in reinforcements like a dietician if you have special needs or a lot of questions.

Consider taking a cooking class. This gives you new things to try, and you can include your partner in the fun.

## Take an Early Pregnancy Class

Early pregnancy classes teach you how to have a safe and healthy pregnancy. Topics that are covered are usually only glimpsed in your prenatal visit. Some of these topics include nutrition, pregnancy fitness, prenatal testing, and safety in pregnancy. This will also help you formulate questions to take with you to a prenatal visit with your practitioner. For example, if you've had an early pregnancy class and the instructor teaches the basics of watching your heart rate in pregnancy and mentions that women who are already working out have a higher tolerance for raising their heart rates during pregnancy, you will need to ask your doctor or midwife if your fitness level is one that would qualify for this exemption.

Early pregnancy classes are taught in a variety of locations. At many hospitals and birth centers early pregnancy classes are taught by nurses or childbirth educators. They may even include a hospital or birth center tour. These classes are beneficial, but they may also be a marketing tool for the facility. Before signing up for the class, be sure to talk to other parents who have already done so. Their candid feedback will give you a sense of how useful and practical the information is for your needs.

Other places to find early pregnancy classes include pregnancy fitness facilities, private childbirth educators and even some nutritional/health centers. Your practitioner may also have a recommendation. If you have special needs—such as a chronic illness or multiple pregnancy—you may even consider finding someone to teach you a private class. (Check "Resources" on page 310 for certifying agencies.)

## Tour Birth Facilities

The truth about birth tours is that they are marketing tools. Hospitals know that if you choose their facility to give birth, you are likely to return for other medical needs in your life. This makes the maternity tour a huge marketing opportunity. Many hospitals sink a fair bit of time and effort into their tours.

Tours can be lead by a labor and birth nurse, a local educator, or other staff member. They will typically show you a labor and birth suite, where you will spend your postpartum time, the waiting room or family room, and other amenities. Your job is to ask hard questions about their policies that matter most to you, such as the following:

- What are the visiting policies for husbands and other family members, both during labor and postpartum?

- Will you have to go to a triage area when you are in labor or will you be shown directly to a private room?

- How many private rooms do they offer postpartum and how are they assigned?

(See page 307 for complete list of questions.)

Even if there is only one hospital or birth center where you live, or if the practitioner that you have chosen only uses one facility, touring this facility gives you an idea of what to expect when you arrive to give birth and helps you feel more familiar and comfortable with the surroundings as you imagine your birth during your pregnancy.

Your tour will provide you with some basic details on how to get around and what is offered during your pregnancy in terms of classes and services. This also gives you a chance to ask questions that are specific to you and find out what the exceptions are to their standard policies and how to go about arranging them to make your stay what you'd like it to be.

## Discuss Family Leave Policies and Protocols

Now that you're approaching the end of the first trimester, it's time to start planning ahead for your postpartum leave from work, if necessary. Many women erroneously believe that they should start planning their postpartum leave in the third trimester. This is too late in the process, and you may not have time to plan for it adequately and thoughtfully.

For example, if your place of business requires that you take unpaid leave or that you use your vacation concurrently, you will need to plan for this financially. You might choose to revise your family budget or apply some or all of your personal vacation during the pregnancy (including possibly skipping a previously planned vacation). You may also be eligible to apply for "free" days from the employee vacation pool, but that takes time to arrange. (This is where employees donate vacation time they cannot use to a general pool for other employees who have a medical or family need demanding extra time off.)

Don't be concerned if you are uncomfortable about announcing that you are pregnant. You do not have to be pregnant to access this information from your company. In fact, many women and men do this before pregnancy, so it's not a suspicious request at all. If you're still worried, simply ask for a manual of company policies in general or refer to your employee handbook for a generic guide. Remember that women are afforded certain protections under the Pregnancy Discrimination Act (part of the Title VII of the Civil Rights Act of 1964). While the protections vary state to state, you can learn more about the Pregnancy Discrimination Act at the Equal Employment Opportunity Commission website *www.eeoc.gov/facts/fs-preg.html*.

## HOT MAMA

As you reach the end of your first trimester, you may actually be looking forward to having a baby bump. Go to your local maternity store and have fun trying on a few outfits. The secret is that you can use the belly extender pillow found in most dressing rooms. Check out your profile for what is to come, even if you don't wind up buying any clothes that day. Take several pictures on your cell phone and send them to your husband!

## GIRLS, BOYS, AND GENETIC TESTS

If you're interested in finding out if your baby is a girl or boy before giving birth, the external genitalia are just now starting to look different, though it's still too early to tell without prenatal genetic testing. Early amniocentesis and chorionic villus sampling (CVS) are the genetic tests offered at this point in pregnancy.

Both of these tests look at genetic material from your baby and are more invasive than ultrasound and maternal serum (blood) screening tests. These tests are usually reserved for couples that are at a greater risk of genetic abnormalities either because of a previous personal or family medical history. Recent scientific studies have shown that early amniocentesis and CVS carry similar risks to your baby. CVS can still be performed earlier in pregnancy than an amniocentesis, but the small difference in timing may not be as important as it once was for these tests. A discussion with your partner, genetic counselor, and your practitioner can help you sort through the options.

Nuchal Translucency Screening (Nuchal Fold Screening) for Down Syndrome is also possible from week 11 through week 14. Be sure to talk to your doctor or midwife about this simple screening tool if you are interested. This screening is performed by doing an ultrasound and measuring the fold of skin at the back of your baby's neck. A thicker nuchal fold means a higher risk of Down Syndrome. This is one of the earliest, noninvasive measures to screen for Down Syndrome. Because it is done early it can also leave time for more in depth testing like the CVS or early amniocentesis.

## HEARING YOUR BABY'S HEARTBEAT

At your next prenatal appointment, when you are nearing the end of the first trimester, your doctor or midwife may try to hear the baby's heartbeat with a small handheld device called a Doppler. Sound waves are bounced through the uterus and reflect that sound back. An ultrasound and the Doppler, which is another high intensity form of ultrasound, are the only two ways to see or hear the heartbeat this early in pregnancy.

Be sure to bring someone with you to this appointment to share in the excitement. While the sound of the galloping of your baby's heartbeat is really neat, it can sometimes be hard to record. If you want to try, bring something with a small microphone rather than trying to capture the sound on your cell phone.

At later prenatal appointments, your midwife or doctor may also use something called a fetoscope, which is a specialized stethoscope for listening to babies in utero. You can use a fetoscope or stethoscope at home during the later weeks of pregnancy as well. These are not regulated medical devices and can be purchased in many local stores and online.

Be leery of places that rent Dopplers to consumers. The Food and Drug Administration discourages selling this medical device over the counter because of the risks of misuse and overexposure to ultrasound for your baby. Your practitioner is the only person who should be prescribing its use for you in your home.

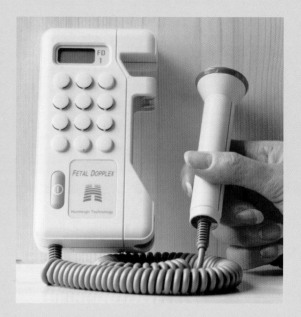

*How you hear your baby's heartbeat will depend on your practitioner and how far along you are in pregnancy. Ask what they commonly use, like this Doppler.*

If you are looking for reassurance of your baby's health, look no further than your own doctor or midwife. Most practitioners will allow you to come in as often as you need to feel assured. Their feedback is the most valuable because that they know you, your medical history, and your baby's history. This type of care is more reassuring than trying to use a Doppler at home, alone, and not always knowing exactly what's going on.

# WEEK 11

## ✏ CHECKLIST FOR WEEK 11

[ ]  Get Dad involved with the pregnancy.
[ ]  Avoid certain foods.
[ ]  Join online groups of pregnant women.
[ ]  Decide how to tell people your good news.
[ ]  Avoid extra stress.

## 🔎 WHAT TO WATCH FOR THIS WEEK

*Double Check*

**One-sided pain:** One-sided pain in your abdomen that doesn't go away may suggest the presence of an ovarian cyst.

**Bleeding or spotting:** You should alert your practitioner to spotting that occurs at this stage because the possibility of miscarriage or blighted ovum (where a fertilized egg fails to grow) is present. You may discover that it is the result of having sex, a low-lying placenta, or the loss of a twin (vanishing twin syndrome).

**Back pain:** While pain in your back can be a sign of uterine cramping and potential miscarriage, it may also be a sign of infection or of your uterus stretching. Report severe pain and pain that does not abate to your midwife or doctor.

**Sudden disappearance of pregnancy symptoms:** If you've been having a lot of pregnancy symptoms such as nausea, vomiting, sore breasts, and sensitivities, and they vanish suddenly, report it to your doctor or midwife. Symptoms tend to come and go, but a complete loss may indicate a problem with your hormone levels.

**Inability to keep food or liquid down:** Throwing up during pregnancy is to be expected, but severe cases result in a woman becoming dehydrated. If you've been unable to keep food or liquids down for some time, contact your practitioner.

*Report any strange or troublesome symptoms to your practitioner immediately.*

##  BODY BASICS

As you round out the first trimester, you should notice outwardly visible changes—most notably your abdomen. Your uterus is just about ready to grow out of the pelvis and into the abdominal cavity. This is when changes in your appearance are hard to miss.

You may still be experiencing your pregnancy symptoms full force. If this is the case, hang on! The first trimester's end brings a big measure of relief for most mothers.

## 🍼 BABY DATA

At this stage of development, your baby's head is approximately half the size of his or her body. This is very normal. At the time of birth, your newborn's head will still be a good portion of the body because of the brain growth going on.

Your baby is continuing to grow this week, now weighing in at about seven grams, which is equivalent to seven paper clips. It's hard to imagine something so tiny having all of the parts your baby has. This week, we add fingernails to the list. Your baby will also spend some time this week developing the iris, the colored portion of the eye that controls light intake. Your baby's eye color is genetically determined, although it can be hard to tell what that color is at birth; it takes time for it to develop.

If you were to have a prenatal appointment this week, you would most likely be able to hear your baby's heartbeat with a Doppler.

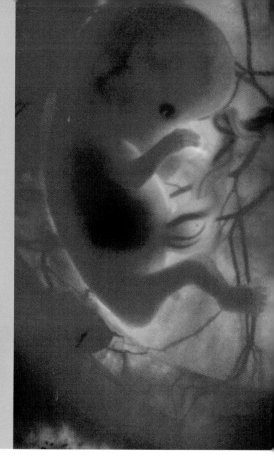

**PREGNANCY PARTICULARS**

# Get Dad Involved with the Pregnancy

It can be difficult to involve your husband with the pregnancy during the first trimester. He may want to help, but there isn't much he can do at this point. It can be confusing and even upsetting when you've both put a lot of time and effort into planning the pregnancy and discussing the many details, and now that your dream has come true, you find yourself feeling a bit abandoned and on your own.

Do not despair! This is a fairly common feeling for women in their first trimesters. While the pregnancy feels very real to you both internally and externally, to those around you, not much has changed. This makes it more difficult for people to jump into the game and focus on what's going on in the way you can. The following are some ideas to include your spouse, and others, in your pregnancy:

- Have him accompany you to your prenatal appointments.
- Read books together.
- Take an early pregnancy class together.
- Take a tour of your birth place together.
- Write a journal together.
- Enlist him to photograph your changing body.

It is also important to do something as a couple that isn't baby related. This can be challenging when your mind and body tell you to focus completely on the baby.

It is also possible that your husband has legitimate reasons for seeming like he isn't involved or as involved as you would like, such as the following:

- He doesn't know what to do to be involved.
- You've accidentally excluded him or made him think you have everything under control.
- He's nervous and doesn't know what to think or do.

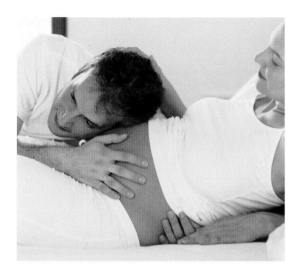

*Your partner may be really into pregnancy or not so much so. Don't fret, just be sure to keep the lines of communication open.*

These are common ways for dads to feel. By being sensitive to his feelings and offering practical suggestions for getting him involved, you can help him to overcome his reluctance and apprehension. When the second trimester arrives and you begin to show, it becomes easier for many dads to take part in pregnancy-related activities as the pregnancy and baby become more real to them.

## Avoid Certain Foods

You have probably been avoiding certain foods that made your stomach churn for the past few weeks. One theory is that food aversions are a protective mechanism for women in pregnancy to avoid substances that may harm their babies. Whether or not your body is signaling you to avoid certain foods, you should eliminate the following categories of food for the duration of your pregnancy:

- Raw and undercooked meats and fish
- Unwashed vegetables
- Excessive amounts of fish (more than twelve ounces per week to avoid overexposure to mercury and other toxins)

## PREGNANCY AFFIRMATION FOR WEEK 11

## I feel healthy and confident about my pregnancy.

- Soft, unpasteurized cheeses, such as blue cheese or Brie
- Alcohol
- Foods to which you are allergic or that irritate your system

These restrictions require women to make adjustments to what they eat and drink, but most find quite manageable. If you are accustomed to eating meat rare, you simply need to start ordering and preparing it medium well. Restaurants should be happy to work within your specifications and may carry warnings on their menu as reminders.

The reason that you want to avoid these foods is because of the potential of contracting a food borne illness such as listeriosis or salmonella. Ensuring that your food has been properly washed and cooked will protect you from many of the potentially nasty consequences of consuming food that has been insufficiently cleaned or cooked.

## Join Online Groups of Pregnant Women

One of the fun parts of being pregnant is enjoying the camaraderie of other women who are also expecting. A great place to start is with an online group.

The advantage of joining an online group is that you can usually find a large group of women all due at the same time as you. That gives you a pool of people to talk to about what you're going through emotionally, mentally, and physically. (Check out the online communities at *pregnancy.about.com* and *www.mothering.com* to get started.)

An online community of women can also share ideas and ask questions of one another throughout the pregnancy, forming a close bond, despite the geographical distance that may separate them. It is also really neat to compare regional and geographical differences in pregnancy attitudes, birth, and baby care. This can be a tremendous source of new ideas—and new friendships—in your life.

Some of the groups are run via electronic discussion boards, where messages are left in threads and you respond when you log on. Other groups are run via email, meaning that you receive email as members conduct discussions and answer one another's queries.

While these groups won't take the place of real life friends, they are a great way to spend time commiserating with and learning from other women in your same boat—especially when you're up at 2:00 in the morning with no one to talk to!

You can start with an online group, but there are many other places where you can connect with women who have due dates near yours, including the following:

- Childbirth classes
- Prenatal exercise classes
- Your practitioner's office
- Specialty groups, such as twins clubs

## Decide How to Tell People Your Good News

The time is finally approaching that some have chosen to wait for—to begin sharing news of your pregnancy. If you haven't told anyone, you have a lot of work to do. If you have told a few people, you may have a bit less pressure to get ready.

Deciding how to share your big announcement is entirely personal. Perhaps you'd prefer not to make a big scene and just let the news leak out slowly. One couple began the leak by sharing the news with their preschool daughter. It didn't take long before this excited little girl had told almost everyone who would listen, "I'm going to be a big

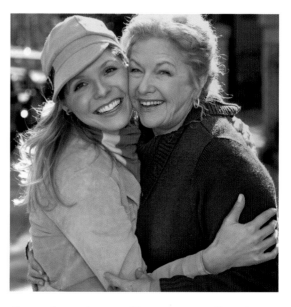

*Sharing the good news and having it received happily is a great moment. Be sure to celebrate.*

sister!" Theirs was a low-key strategy that took the hard work out of their hands—while giving their daughter a special role in the pregnancy.

Some couples prefer to take the "Ask me and I'll tell you" route. If the topic comes up naturally in conversation, they're happy to share the news. That approach may play out differently for everyone. For some, it looks like this:

"Would you like a glass of wine?"

"No thanks, I'm pregnant."

Or perhaps:

"You still have a few holiday pounds you're carrying . . ."

"Yes, but the baby likes them."

Sincere or snarky, you're the ones to decide, but as you start to show, the news will become harder to hide. You should decide who needs to be told before the secret gets out. This usually includes people who may be offended if you don't share the news with them personally. This list may include the following:

- Family members
- Close friends

- Clergy
- Boss and/or coworkers

## Avoid Extra Stress

Stress is a normal part of pregnancy, particularly with all of the changes that you are going through. The goal is not to panic about stress. It is normal to feel it from time to time, even in the most well planned and perfectly executed pregnancy.

Remember that you have more control over the stress in your life than you think. Small steps can be taken to reduce stressors and to help you alleviate unnecessary or excessive stress. Doing so will help you have a more pleasant and positive pregnancy.

Another reason to acknowledge whatever stress you're under and deal with it head on is that it can exacerbate pregnancy symptoms, feelings of fear, preterm labor, and small-for-gestation-age babies.

In attempting to reduce your stress level, look at the various activities you engage in. Figure out how to cut back or cut out those that are no longer bringing you pleasure and possibly making you feel stressed.

You can also learn about relaxation and how to incorporate it into your daily routine. Relaxation can have a huge impact on how you perceive and deal with stress, which is a helpful tool when changing or eliminating activities isn't an option.

The simplest relaxation method is counting to ten. Don't knock it before you give it a good-faith effort. When you feel your stress level rising, or before you go into a situation where you anticipate becoming stressed, take a moment to stop.

Here's another technique: Draw a deep breath in through your nose and slowly exhale through your mouth. Do this ten times. Some women find that closing their eyes enhances their sense of relaxation, while others like to visualize a peaceful scene or recall a calming, happy memory.

By practicing these methods and experimenting with other forms of relaxation, you will be doing a great deal to manage your stress. If you are anxious to learn more stress-relieving techniques, you can also take classes in relaxation and meditation. In addition, certain yoga classes and childbirth education courses should teach these types of activities.

**HOT MAMA**

Pointed-toe shoes may be stylish, but when you are pregnant, style must sometimes yield to good sense. You avoid shoes with pointed toes—and high heels—because of the loss of balance issue, particularly after the fourth month when your center of gravity changes. The right shoe choice will protect your legs from aches and pains.

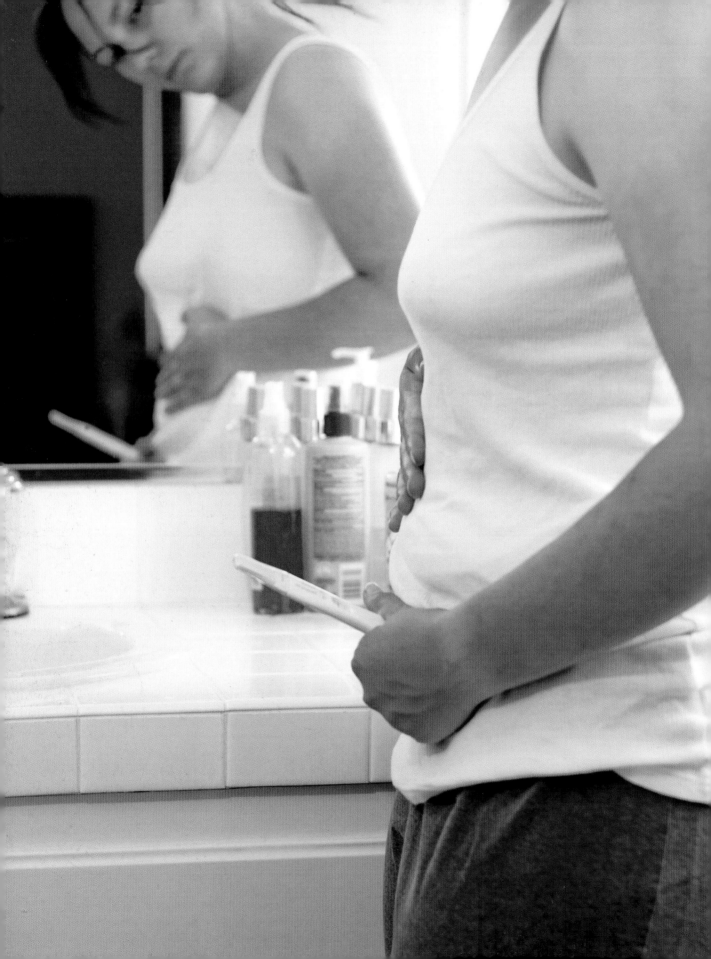

# WEEK 12

## ✎ CHECKLIST FOR WEEK 12

[ ]  Learn about disappearing pregnancy symptoms.

[ ]  Sleep in a comfortable, safe position.

[ ]  Get a pregnancy massage.

[ ]  Find out when you'll start to show.

## ♀ WHAT TO WATCH FOR THIS WEEK

### Double Check

**One-sided pain:** When you have one-sided pain in your abdomen that doesn't go away, it's important to rule out the possibility of an ovarian cyst.

**Bleeding or spotting:** Alert your practitioner if you see bleeding or spotting because it may indicate the possibility of miscarriage or blighted ovum (where a fertilized egg fails to grow). Or, you may find that it was caused by sex, a low-lying placenta, or the loss of a twin (vanishing twin syndrome).

**Back pain:** Report severe pain or pain that does not abate to your midwife or doctor. It may be a symptom of your uterus stretching or cramping, or it might suggest a possible infection or miscarriage.

**Sudden disappearance of pregnancy symptoms:** Fluctuating symptoms are not cause for alarm, but symptoms associated with pregnancy symp-toms such as sore breasts, nausea and/or vomiting, and sensitivities to smell that suddenly disappear should be reported to your doctor or midwife.

**Inability to keep food or liquid down:** A certain amount of nausea and throwing up accompanies many pregnancies. However, when a woman throws up so much that she risks dehydration, the practitioner should be alerted to the problem.

*Report any strange or troublesome symptoms to your practitioner immediately.*

##  BODY BASICS

Good news abounds this week! For starters, many women begin to feel relief from the nausea, vomiting, and extreme exhaustion that plagued their early pregnancies. This isn't to say that you'll wake up one morning and the queasiness is gone, but most women notice a gradual return to normalcy. It may occur to you, one day, that while you still feel nauseous, it's been days since you've actually vomited.

Some of this change is the result of the placenta, which has been busy growing all along, beginning to take over the production of hormones for your pregnancy. This is good news if you've been dealing with the pain of a corpus luteal cyst, which is a cyst at the site on the ovary where you ovulated that sustains the pregnancy until the placenta takes over. These cysts are not harmful and should begin to subside this week as the placenta takes over, meaning less pain for you.

If this is not your first pregnancy, you might begin to show this week, but just a bit, meaning your clothes might feel snug at the waist. This is because the uterus stretches more easily after your first pregnancy.

The best news of all is that once you've made it to 12 weeks, the risk of miscarriage is drastically reduced. Talk to your midwife or doctor more about specific risk factors for you.

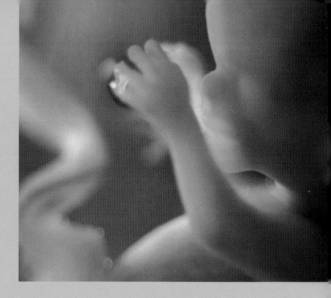

## 🍼 BABY DATA

Weighing in at fourteen grams this week, your baby is growing by leaps and bounds. The total length from head to toe is about three and a half inches (8.9 centimeters). While growing, your baby is also moving around and practicing moves that are both spontaneous and that involve reflexes.

The structure of your baby's brain is now in place. What will happen between week 11 and birth is a period of rapid growth. After birth, babies undergo a dramatic spurt of brain growth until it begins to slow in their toddler years.

## Learn about Disappearing Pregnancy Symptoms.

As you end the first trimester, pregnancy symptoms such as morning sickness and exhaustion that may have been troubling you for the past couple of months will begin to lessen. Sometimes they even disappear completely. This can mean a whole new lease on life. You no longer have to plan everything around your nap schedule, nor do you need to watch where you are and what you eat for fear it might come back up.

Earlier in pregnancy, disappearing pregnancy symptoms can indicate a potential problem. Sometimes it means that your hormone levels are falling too quickly because the pregnancy is failing, which is known as miscarriage. Toward the end of the first trimester, however, most pregnancy symptoms will naturally start to lessen and even disappear.

## Sleep in a Comfortable, Safe Position

The position that you sleep in is probably not something that you have given much thought. But as your pregnancy progresses, you will most likely need to reconsider not only how you sleep but also the pillows you sleep on. After about the fourth month of pregnancy, it is usually recommended that you do not sleep on your back. This is because the weight of the uterus can slow the blood flow in the vena cava, which is a major supplier of blood to your body, thereby restricting the amount of blood circulating throughout your body.

Most women are unable to rest comfortably on their backs during pregnancy anyway, but with stomach sleeping out of the question in later months, it might be time to consider your sleeping arrangements. The following are some things to consider:

- Get comfortable. Use all the pillows you need to cushion and prop up various parts of your body.

- Don't stress. You may occasionally wake up and find that you've been sleeping on your back

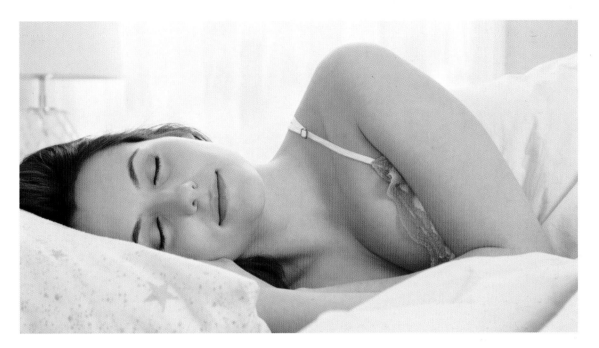

*Occasionally, you may find you wake up on your back. Don't let this bother you, because chances are nothing has happened.*

- Do not fear; your body woke you up so that you could move, just as it should.

- Start training now. If you're a stomach sleeper, make a concerted effort to begin sleeping on your side, even if it is only for part of the night. This will make the adjustment easier when you need to shift to side sleeping later in the pregnancy.

- Angling is fine. You can lie mostly on your back propped with pillows that tilt you to one side. This is a good arrangement for preventing a problem with blood flow.

Sleep is an important part of pregnancy and beyond. Each trimester presents its own issues and challenges as you move toward giving birth. Then there will be new sleep challenges when you bring home your newborn!

## PREGNANCY AFFIRMATION FOR WEEK 12

# My body and mind are open to the experience of pregnancy.

## Get a Pregnancy Massage

Massage is a great way to promote comfort and relaxation in pregnancy. A good massage can reinvigorate your body and increase blood flow while relieving some of the common aches and pains associated with pregnancy. Pregnancy massage is something that virtually all mothers-to-be can appreciate.

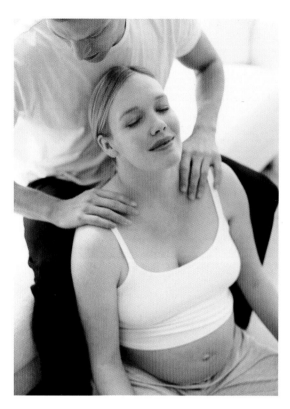

*A good massage is a great way to reconnect and help you relax. Also, try to use this time to talk about nonbaby related things.*

Be sure that when you sign up for a massage that you'll be treated by a therapist who has experience working on pregnant women and who also has received special training. This will help ensure both your comfort and your safety during the massage.

Many massage therapists will not perform pregnancy massages in the first trimester. So this treat is a perfect way to celebrate the end of your first trimester. Most massages require appointments, so you will need to plan ahead.

During a pregnancy massage, you will lie on a special table designed for massage. You will undress to your comfort level, and the massage therapist, after taking a brief history of your medical needs and massage preferences, will begin the treatment by rubbing you with various oils and lotions. There may be music or ambient noise to heighten the relaxation benefits of your massage. Always be sure to speak up and tell your therapist if you're hot, cold, or uncomfortable, if the stroke is too strong or not strong enough, or if you're not feeling well for any reason.

You will not be asked to lie on your stomach, unless the table has a specially supportive cutout for pregnant bellies. Some women do not find these design features comfortable. You can also request that special pillows be used as you are turned from side to side to work on your back.

When your massage is done, you should drink lots of water to help flush toxins from your body after the massage and give yourself some time to sit quietly. If the experience is pleasurable, you should treat yourself to massages throughout your pregnancy and consider using it as a wonderful pain-relieving tool during labor.

**MEMORABLE MOMENTS**

"Twelve weeks! I couldn't believe it. I had buckled down for what seemed like the long haul to this stage in pregnancy. This is when I would feel 'safe,' and we could share the good news. I felt a huge sense of relief to have reached this date, even if it was all trumped up in my head."

## Find Out When You'll Start to Show

Most women are anxious for their swelling bellies to show as a signal to the outside world that they are indeed pregnant. Fortunately or unfortunately, most women do not show in the first trimester, prompting some to wear T-shirts that read: "I'm not fat, I'm pregnant!" There is an exception for very slender women, women having their second or third (or more!) child, and women who are expecting multiple babies.

Because the uterus is tucked inside the pelvis until after the 12th week of pregnancy, there simply isn't much to show. However, as you begin the second trimester, your baby and your body begin to grow outwardly more rapidly. By around the 16th week, you will definitely be aware of changes in your body, and most people will notice something going on. By week 20, maternity clothes or other major clothes revisions are in order. From that point on, your abdomen grows exponentially.

At your prenatal visits, your practitioner will measure your uterus through your abdomen. This is known as a fundal height measurement. This measures from the top of your pubic bone to the top of your uterus, the fundus. This measurement should be within a centimeter or two of how many weeks pregnant you are at the time. So for example, if you are 20 weeks pregnant, your uterus should measure about twenty centimeters, give or take a few. You can see how this would cause your belly to show in the latter trimesters of pregnancy.

It is important to note that all bellies do not look alike. The reason is that not every woman is shaped the same, and differences in the length of your torso and the space inside your body will determine how your belly is shaped. Another factor is how your baby is positioned—head up, head down, or sideways—which at this point is subject to change on a moment's notice.

**HOT MAMA**

If you're feeling that your pregnancy shape puts you somewhere in between your normal clothes and maternity clothes, it might be time to buy a special outfit to make you feel better about your body and your wardrobe. Some women like to buy a clever maternity T-shirt that announces your joy to the world, while others are merely looking for something more comfortable to wear to accommodate their expanding waistlines.

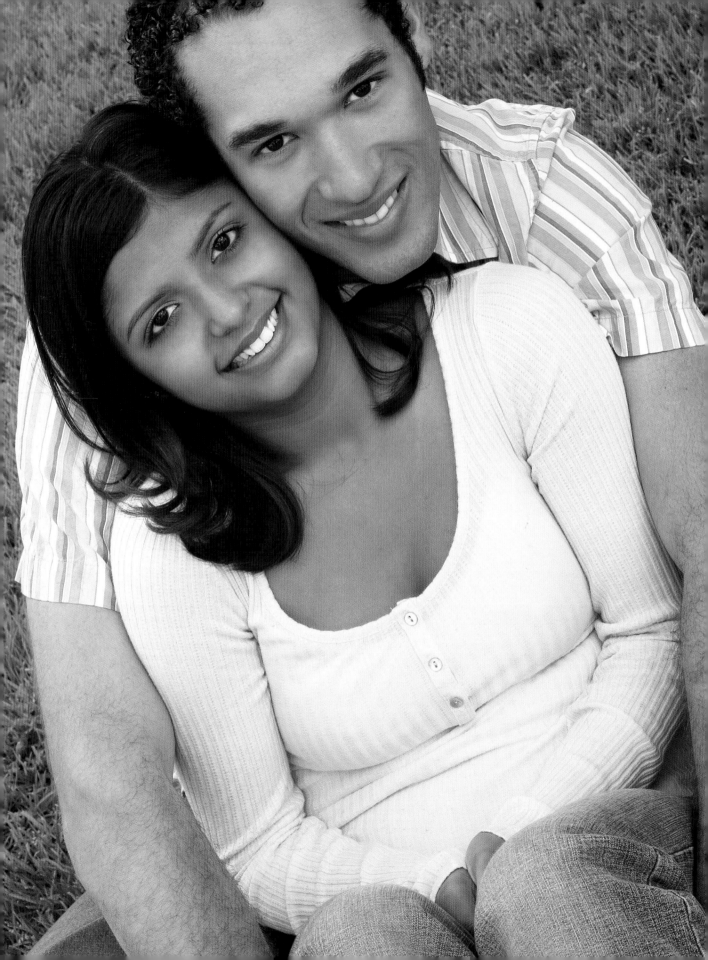

# WEEK 13

## ✏ CHECKLIST FOR WEEK 13

[ ] Interview childbirth educators.
[ ] Learn how your practitioner measures your uterus.
[ ] Know how sex changes in the second trimester.

## ⚲ WHAT TO WATCH FOR THIS WEEK

**Back or abdominal pain:** Pain in your back or abdomen can be brought on by contractions or premature dilation of the cervix, a sign of potential preterm labor.

**More than six contractions per hour:** This can be a sign of preterm labor. It can be normal to have contractions, just not at this frequency.

**Gush of fluid from the vagina:** This can be a sign that your water has broken prematurely. Your practitioner can determine if fluid leaking from your vagina is amniotic fluid or normal vaginal discharge.

### Double Check

**Bleeding or spotting:** Reddish or brown spotting at this point in pregnancy can happen after sexual intercourse, a vaginal exam, or vaginal ultrasound. You may be warned in advance of this possibility should you have this type of exam or activity. Bleeding or spotting that occurs unrelated to these activities should be reported immediately to your practitioner, because it may be a sign of infection, premature dilation of the cervix, or issues related to your placenta.

*Report any strange or troublesome symptoms to your practitioner immediately.*

##  BODY BASICS

The good news this week is that hopefully you are experiencing fewer of the less-than-pleasant symptoms associated with the first trimester. Some women gradually start to feel better around week 11 or 12 and then it dawns on them that it's been days since they've become ill. For other women, the transition is more sudden. They seem to wake up one day and discover that the pregnancy symptoms that were driving them nuts have vanished. Either way spells relief. If you continue to suffer with morning sickness or other symptoms, it is regrettable, but still normal at this point.

## 🍼 BABY DATA

Your baby is blissfully unaware that you both have moved on to the second trimester. He or she is just happily paddling around inside your uterus. Even though their babies weigh in at about an ounce now, most mothers still cannot feel their movements.

Other internal happenings include the intestines moving into the abdomen from the umbilical cord. The intestines are also working on their internal structure as the villi form inside. The villi help the baby with digestion by encouraging food to move inside the intestines for the rest of the baby's life. In other intestinal news, the pancreas has started secreting insulin. Your baby also has all twenty teeth formed under the gums.

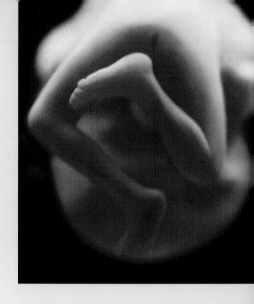

## Interview Childbirth Educators

The goal of childbirth classes is for expectant parents to leave class with an understanding of their options in terms of prenatal care and the birth process and the skills to put their choices into effect. Classes are also an avenue for developing a great support network, starting with your childbirth educator and your classmates.

This is why your choice of a childbirth educator is so very important. The instructor that you choose should be open, honest, and knowledgeable. Your instructor should have experience with the information, either by assisting other couples as a doula or through personal experience. Why are you looking for a doula rather than a nurse? It's because a nurse has so many other responsibilities while a woman is in labor that she cannot focus solely on the woman and her family.

*A baby care class is a great idea, even if you think you know what you're doing. It's an easy way to catch up on the latest in parenting news.*

**MEMORABLE MOMENTS**

"Week 13 was a blur. I'd spent so much time in the first trimester thinking about pregnancy, mostly because I was either feeling ill or terribly excited. But as I began to feel better, I found that I thought less about the pregnancy. Someone asked if that bothered me, but oddly it felt comforting, as in I was adjusting nicely to the idea rather than fretting."

How do you find the right childbirth educator for you? Ask the following questions:

- When are the classes offered?
- How many couples are in each class? Is there a maximum? Minimum?
- How much does the class cost?
- What does the fee include?
- What certifications does the instructor hold in this area?
- What subjects are covered in the classes?
- What is the instructor's birth philosophy?
- Is it possible to speak to former students and other references?
- What happens if I miss a class?

## PREGNANCY AFFIRMATION FOR WEEK 13

### Pregnancy is a growing experience for me in more ways than one.

Many instructors claim to teach childbirth education classes. They may be mothers, they may be nurses, they may even be educators, but the true mark of a childbirth educator is affiliation with and rigorous testing by a certifying organization. This ensures that she has a basic knowledge as defined by her organization and that she knows how to teach about giving birth and parenting. The problem with using someone who doesn't hold an international or national certification is that you may not get what you need out of the class.

### Learn How Your Practitioner Measures Your Uterus

Your uterus will grow at a predictable rate. This rate is measured using a tape measure that your practitioner uses at each prenatal visit. Typically this will start between weeks 13 and 20, depending on your practitioner's preference.

They are measuring the distance between the top of your pubic bone and the top of your uterus, the fundus. At about 20 weeks, your fundus should be about twenty centimeters from your pubic bone. The "give" here is two centimeters in either direction. This test is not painful and it can be repeated multiple times without risk to you or your baby.

This measurement will be taken at every prenatal visit, and you will see a steady increase as your baby grows. Each week should be close or equal to the number of centimeters (i.e., your uterus should be 16 centimeters at 16 weeks).

## Know How Sex Changes in the Second Trimester

The second trimester brings many changes, including your sexual relationship. One of the biggest and best changes is that you are starting to feel a bit more human. For most pregnant women, the round-the-clock nausea, exhaustion, and moodiness that punctuated the first trimester is gone or fading. All of this leaves you feeling more romantic.

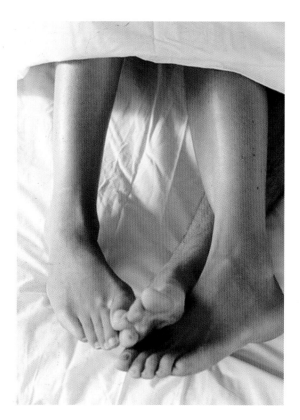

*Sex is a great way to reconnect, but sometimes you don't feel like it. Be sure to talk about your feelings so that your partner doesn't feel left out.*

You also should not be worrying about the possibility of a miscarriage any longer, which is a worry that can certainly have a negative effect on your sex life. So as you grow more confident in your pregnancy, your sex life is likely to experience a boost as well. The same can be said for your partner, who is also likely feeling more confident and less worried.

At this point, you need not make any physical changes to your sex life. (You do not have to use different positions to accommodate your expanding abdomen.) Whatever side effects you may have from being pregnant can actually enhance sex. For instance, most women experience an increase in lubrication, and many find that achieving orgasm—even multiple orgasms—becomes easier, due to the increased blood flow to the region.

The major exception is toward the very end of pregnancy when you may measure smaller because the baby has dropped into your pelvis.

Many things can influence the measurement, including the baby's position, the fluid levels, and an accurate due date. If you stray more than the two centimeters from the target, however, your midwife or doctor may order an ultrasound to check on these factors.

You may still be enjoying the relief from not having to count cycle days and trying to get pregnant. This freedom can be a great benefit for many couples, while the opposite is also a benefit: not having to worry about getting pregnant and the freedom from birth control. Your focus can be on each other and the pleasure you bring to your relationship.

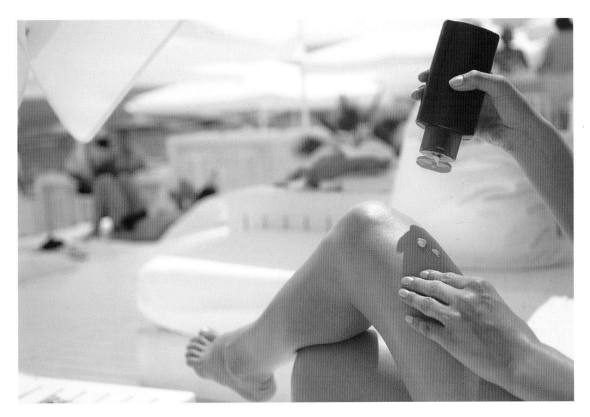

**HOT MAMA**

*Sun protection is very important in pregnancy. As your body changes so does your skin, meaning you might be at greater risk for a sunburn.*

During pregnancy, your skin can become extremely sensitive. Consequently, you should use sunscreen to protect your skin from exposure to harmful rays. You don't have to apply the strongest sunscreen. Even choosing a lotion or makeup that contains a mild sunscreen can really make the difference in keeping your skin tone even. It can also prevent more serious skin problems in pregnancy such as chloasma (hyperpigmentation of the facial skin).

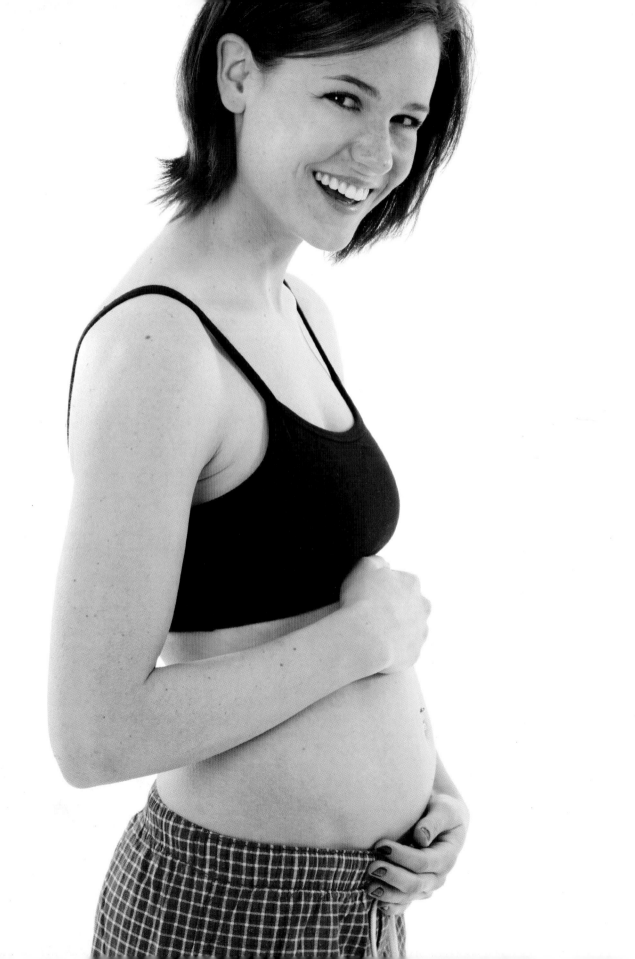

# Week 14

### ✎ CHECKLIST FOR WEEK 14

[ ] Start planning the nursery.
[ ] Decide if you want to know the sex
of your baby.
[ ] Research amniocentesis.
[ ] Watch out for depression.

### ⚲ WHAT TO WATCH FOR THIS WEEK

*Double Check*

**Bleeding or spotting:** Reddish or brown spotting
at this point in pregnancy can happen after
sexual intercourse, a vaginal exam, or vaginal
ultrasound. You may be warned in advance of
this possibility should you have this type of
exam or activity. Bleeding or spotting that occurs
unrelated to these activities should be reported
immediately to your practitioner, because it may
be a sign of infection, premature dilation of the
cervix, or issues related to your placenta.

**Back or abdominal pain:** Pain in your back or
abdomen can be brought on by contractions or
premature dilation of the cervix, a sign of
potential preterm labor.

**More than six contractions per hour:** This can
be a sign of preterm labor. It can be normal to
have contractions, just not at this frequency.

**Gush of fluid from the vagina:** This can be a
sign that your water has broken prematurely.
Your practitioner can determine if fluid leaking
from your vagina is amniotic fluid or normal
vaginal discharge.

*Report any strange or troublesome symptoms to
your practitioner immediately.*

###  BODY BASICS

Your pregnancy symptoms should be slowly
disappearing if they haven't already done
so. With less energy devoted to these pesky
symptoms, you'll have more energy to focus
on your to-do list. You may, however, encounter
what's come to be called "fuzzy brain" or
"pregnancy brain." It's simply a feeling that you're
not really paying attention or that you've become
forgetful. You might forget—midsentence—what
you're saying, misplace your keys, or blank on
an important date or commitment. Using a
portable calendar helps. Otherwise, be ready to
smile and apologize when fuzzy brain strikes.

When you're feeling energized (and not
suffering from pregnancy brain), you may want
to write things down for those times when you
may not be quite so clear-headed. Using a large
binder with tabbed indexes for what needs to be
done is a good idea. Mark tabs for categories
like including the following:

- Baby's stuff
- Medical info
- Childbirth classes
- Doulas
- Pediatrician search
- Child care

These are just some basics to get your started
as you begin to organize your thoughts about
pregnancy and giving birth.

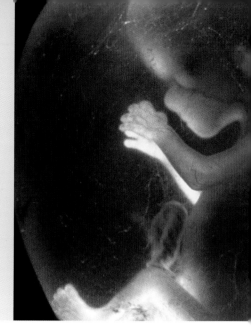

## ☺ BABY DATA

Your baby is just about five inches (13 cm) long! You baby's kidneys are producing urine, which is being excreted into the amniotic fluid that surrounds the baby inside the uterus. Amniotic fluid completely surrounds your baby, and it allows your baby to move about the uterus, practicing flips and turns. Your baby also "breathes" the liquid in and out to practice for extrauterine life. Amniotic fluid is the ultimate renewable resource, replacing itself every few hours.

**PREGNANCY PARTICULARS**

## Start Planning the Nursery

Your nursery planning may be something that you've given a lot of thought to prior to pregnancy, or it may be something that you suddenly realize requires some attention. Either way it is not one decision but a serious of decisions that need to be addressed.

Begin by deciding if the baby will have his own room. If this is your first baby, you may have a guest bedroom or spare room that can be converted to a nursery. Or you may only have one bedroom with which to work. If this is not your first baby, you may have to think about moving children into the same room together.

Some families find that after evaluating their living arrangements, a move is in order. Moving while pregnant can be very difficult, but it can be much easier than moving with a newborn. For optimal timing, moving in the second trimester is best. Your move may involve buying a house or moving from one rental property to another. Moves are stressful under any circumstances, so plan carefully to minimize as much stress as possible on your pregnancy.

Once you know where you will be living and have defined your baby's space in your mind, you can begin to plan for the nursery. You'll need to choose paint colors or wall paper, furniture, themes, and decorations. The following are some things to keep in mind when planning a nursery:

- Infant safety (babyproofing)
- Maternal safety (such as climbing on ladders and inhaling paint fumes)
- Your theme (How long will your theme last? For example, if you choose Winnie the Pooh, when would you have to remove it because it's too young for an older child?)
- The type of furniture you prefer
- Activities in the room (such as feeding and changing)

Envisioning the type of activity that will take place in the room will influence what you need to plan for. In other words, do you see yourself feeding the baby in the room or elsewhere? Will the room include a diaper-changing area? Where will baby clothes be stored?

In these early months of planning, it is best to consider every option. Look at many different types of furniture. Talk to parents about what they bought that turned out to be essential, sort of useful, or a waste of money. Between their input and your own wish list, you can plan your budget accordingly.

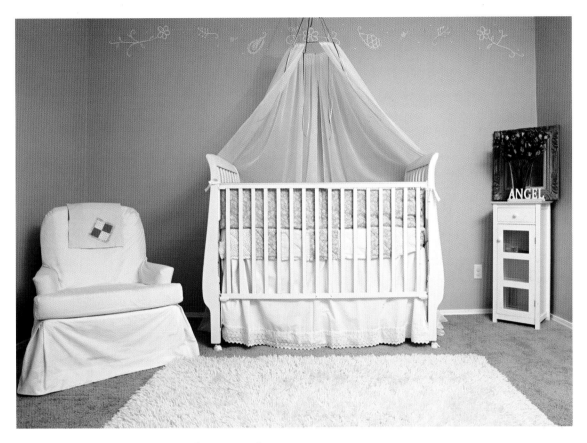

*Your baby's room can be a lot of fun to plan.  Start early to avoid last minute delays.*

A nursery can expensive. But it doesn't have to be, nor does every item have to be purchased all at once. But the process of planning ahead for the baby's living and play space is part of the bonding experience for many parents. Have fun imagining your ideal nursery, where you, your husband and your baby will share lovely times together.

## Decide If You Want to Know the Sex of Your Baby

The decision to find out if your baby is a girl or a boy is a very personal one. Unfortunately it is also one that generates lots of vocal opinions. It's hard to walk around with a pregnant belly without someone asking if you know what you're having. And if you don't, the opinions fly in both directions.

PREGNANCY AFFIRMATION
FOR WEEK 14

# I am feeling good and looking good in pregnancy.

The truth of the matter is that you and your partner get to decide what is right for your family. Keep the following things in mind when trying to figure out what works best for you:

WHY DO YOU WANT TO KNOW? There is no right answer to this question. It is posed merely to get you to think about the answer. Sometimes when moms consider this question, they realize that they are merely going along with the flow and that they really do not care either way. Other times, you will have clear reasons that will cement your choice.

The following are some typical answers:

- Preparing for a girl or boy baby

- Picking a name ahead of time or only having to worry about one set of names

- Having to make fewer decisions (for example, you needn't worry about circumcision if it's a girl)

- Avoiding surprises

- Having a strong preference and needing time to adjust if it's not your first choice

HOW ARE YOU GOING TO FIND OUT? This question goes beyond whether or not you are planning to use genetic testing such as amniocentesis or chorionic villus (CVS) sampling versus ultrasound. CVS and amnio carry risks to the baby/pregnancy that ultrasound typically does not. But you get additional and more accurate info with that greater risk. If you're doing it for sex knowledge only, it's most likely not worth the risk unless you're trying to look for a sex specific genetic issues, at which point you'd most likely be looking at genetics too.

DO YOU AND YOUR SPOUSE PLAN TO FIND OUT TOGETHER? If you can't be together for an ultrasound or to receive the results from genetic testing, can you find a way to learn the information together? Some couples ask to have the information written down and sealed in an envelope. Then they open it together at an arranged time.

WHOM WILL YOU TELL? Along with how you will find out, you should also address the question of whom you plan to tell. More and more couples are choosing not to share the information with others, even in their own families. They cite various reasons for withholding the information—from enjoying keeping the secret between themselves to an intrusion of privacy and letting the baby be an unknown and a fun surprise for others.

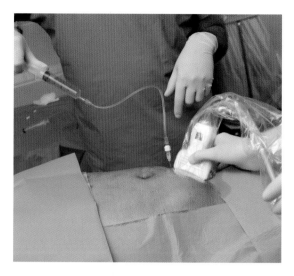

*Amniocentesis can be used to help look at your baby's genetic make up, including the sex of your baby.*

HOW WILL KNOWING AFFECT YOUR PLANNING FOR BABY? Some couples believe that knowing will help them plan better for their baby. This may or may not ring true for you. Do you really want to invest in an entire pink or blue wardrobe before you even know your baby's complexion or hair color? Is painting a room really that important? Again, there aren't right answers, except those that matter to and work for you.

WHAT WOULD HAPPEN IF THE INFORMATION TURNED OUT TO BE INCORRECT? This is something that most people don't like to entertain. And yet, it's not uncommon at births for people to be surprised by an unexpected announcement. You might laugh the idea off, but for families who have placed considerable thought, time, and emotional energy in getting to know a "certain" baby, it can be a devastating blow. It has nothing to do with whether or not you love your new baby, but simply that you have bonded with a baby that isn't coming. Some parents wind up genuinely heartbroken when this happens, and it can even require therapy.

WHAT HAPPENS IF ONE PARENT WANTS TO KNOW AND THE OTHER DOES NOT? This is a tricky situation to be in. It seems impossible to make both people happy. If the parent who wants to know can manage to keep it a secret from the other, go for it! The trick here is that the person who knows can't tell anyone else, and he or she has to convincingly debate all the name possibilities, not just boy or girl names. Should you slip up by showing less or no interest in one category of names, the secret's out. In this situation, some families decide to go with whatever the mom wants to do, and naturally, some dads don't approve of this approach.

WHAT WOULD BE DIFFERENT AT THE BIRTH IF YOU DID OR DID NOT KNOW? Some people are very tied to finding out what they're having at the moment of birth. They imagine being swept up in the moment and relying on the anticipation to get them through the last few rough patches of labor. You might even be able to picture the moment that your husband, your practitioner, or a nurse says, "It's a …!"

There can be a lot of anticipation built into that moment. How will knowing the sex in advance change it for you and your family?

ARE THERE VARIATIONS THAT WORK FOR YOUR FAMILY? Some families decide against finding out because they do not want to have to give up all the exciting details. These families may feel that by finding out the baby's sex before birth, they will be required to share the name they've chosen and other information with close relatives and friends. This is not necessarily true. Many families learn if the baby is a girl or a boy and then keep silent on details such as the name.

In the end, this is a decision that only you can make. The problem is that once you decide, you can rarely go back. So you might want to delay finding out as long as possible. For example, have your practitioner seal the information in an envelope at his or her office. Then it will be available should you want it, but it's not sitting around for anyone else, such as your mother-in-law, to open.

Keep in mind that what worked for you in one pregnancy may not be what you want in this pregnancy. Perhaps you found out the sex of baby number one, but this time you may prefer to be surprised (or vice versa).

## Research Amniocentesis

Amniocentesis has been the long-standing choice for most genetic testing issues that require a decisive test rather than a screening test. This means that you will know definitively whether or not your baby has a medical condition, rather than knowing the odds of it happening, which is what a screening test such as a triple screen will tell you. An amniocentesis is performed with ultrasound supervision. The ultrasound guides the needle away from the baby as well as the placenta. The procedure involves inserting a large needle through the uterus and into the amniotic sac. A small sample of fluid is removed from around the baby.

Because the fluid around the baby contains skin cells that slough off the baby, these cells can be analyzed for genetic material. Using the genetic material, scientists can make a genetic map of your baby to check for some genetic problems such as Down syndrome, sickle cell anemia, Tay-Sachs disease, and other genetic diseases.

Normally when you have an amniocentesis, a specific issue is being checked for, so your screening will not test for all of the hundreds of potential problems. Because an amniocentesis can tell you if your baby is a boy or a girl, it can also tell you about sex-linked disorders, such as Turner's syndrome.

An amnio test is about 99 percent accurate, barring lab error. However, there is a small risk that the test will sample the mother's cells and not the baby's. Other risks include infection, premature rupture of the membranes, and miscarriage, even if the baby was genetically healthy. Though these risks are small, about 1 in 200, they are real and should factor into your decision whether or not to proceed with testing.

## Watch out for Depression

It is estimated that about one in ten pregnant women suffers from depression. Feeling depressed is so different from what they expected that pregnant women will often fail to seek treatment. But depression in pregnancy is real, and it can have serious negative side effects on both mother and baby, including low weight gain, self mutilation, self medication, and even suicide.

The signs of depression are many, and they can include the following:

- Problems with sleep (too much or too little)
- Changes in appetite
- Lack of concentration
- Loss of energy
- Inability to make decisions
- Restlessness or agitation
- Suicidal thoughts or actions

As you can see, many of these conditions could easily be written off as normal pregnancy symptoms. Doing so can lead to potentially serious consequences for all involved. If you think your pregnancy symptoms go beyond what is considered normal, speak up. Hopefully your practitioner is watching for signs of depression in pregnancy, and if your husband or close family members suggest there might be a problem, take it seriously.

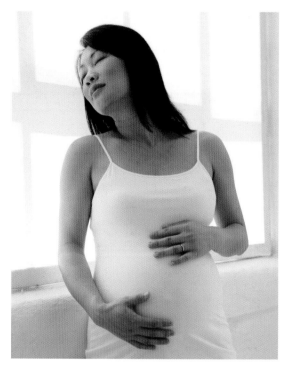

*Pregnancy depression is nothing new, though it's not often talked about. Be sure to discuss with your practitioner any issues you are having with depression.*

There are many ways to treat depression in pregnancy that are both effective and safe. You, your practitioner, and the baby's practitioner can decide together what the best course of action is. This may include counseling, light therapy, medication, or a combination. You should discuss the benefits of each treatment with your team, including the ramifications it may have on your pregnancy, your birth, and your postpartum period.

## HOT MAMA

While you might not be showing all that much, many women begin to notice that by the end of the day, their abdomens are really sticking out. Some of this is intestinal, and some of this is bloating. Either way it can be tricky to dress for two different sizes from morning till end of day. Wearing clothes that are elasticized in the waistband is one solution. Or you could wear a long sweater or large shirt that covers your pants so you can unbutton your pants as the day progresses and your belly expands outward.

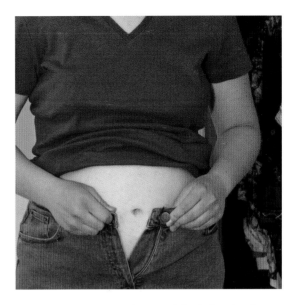

*One morning you may wake up and the clothes that fit just yesterday don't fit any longer. Welcome to maternity clothes!*

The good news is that this is only a temporary issue, demanding a temporary solution. Soon the size of your stomach will stabilize, and you'll be fully covered with maternity clothes.

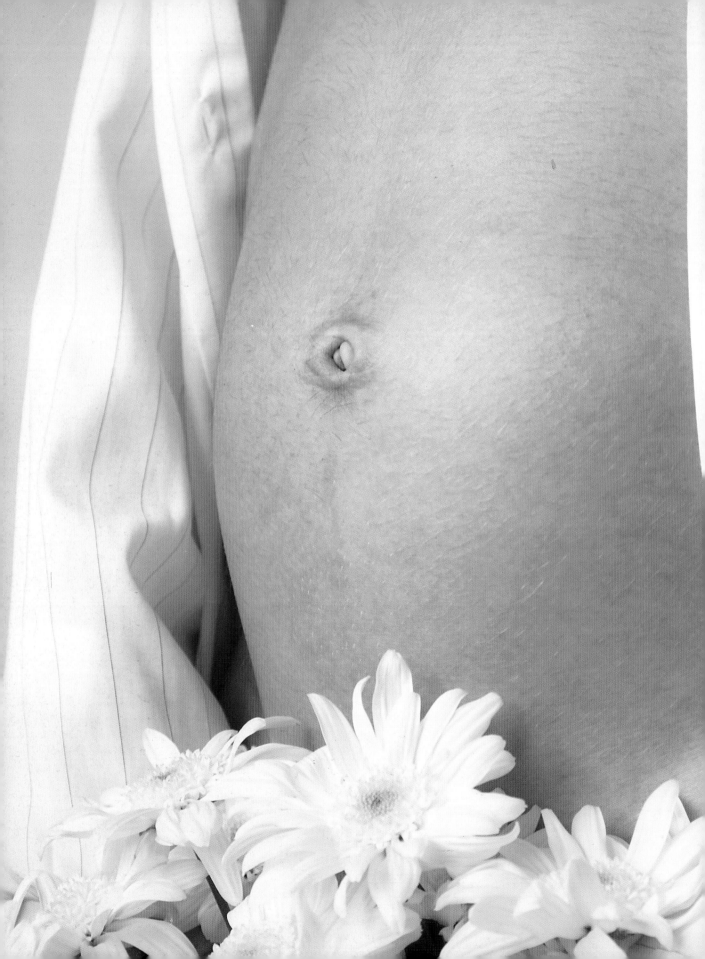

# WEEK 15

## CHECKLIST FOR WEEK 15

[ ]  Reevaluate your hair care.

[ ]  Check for a birth network in your area.

[ ]  Learn about maternal blood screening for certain defects.

[ ]  Be prepared in case you get sick while pregnant.

## WHAT TO WATCH FOR THIS WEEK

*Double Check*

**Bleeding or spotting:** Bleeding or spotting is the normal result of having sexual intercourse, a vaginal exam, or vaginal ultrasound. You should be told in advance of this possibility prior to this type of exam or activity. Bleeding or spotting unconnected to sex or vaginal exams should be reported immediately to your practitioner, because it may be a sign of infection, premature dilation of the cervix, or issues related to your placenta.

**Back or abdominal pain:** Pain in your back or abdomen can be a sign of contractions or premature dilation of the cervix, a sign of potential preterm labor.

**More than six contractions per hour:** It can be normal to have contractions at this point in your pregnancy, but at this frequency, the possibility of preterm labor is present.

**Gush of fluid from the vagina:** This can be a sign that your water has broken prematurely. Your practitioner can determine if fluid leaking from your vagina is amniotic fluid or normal vaginal discharge.

*Report any strange or troublesome symptoms to your practitioner immediately.*

## BODY BASICS

Just as your baby's heart is working hard, so is yours. Did you realize that your heart will increase in size and output during pregnancy? By the end of pregnancy, your heart will have a 30 to 50 percent increase in output to keep up with the energy and oxygen needs of your growing baby. This can sometimes make you feel extra tired or funny—as if something is off in your body that you can't quite put a finger on. If you have heart issues—such as skipping a beat, beating irregularly, or racing too quickly—be sure to talk to your practitioner about it.

Perhaps this week is when you feel crammed into your regular clothes. If so, skip your normal clothes and dive in to some maternity clothes or some in-between clothes. Few things can interfere with your concentration—or your mood—like fretting over too tight pants!

## 🍼 BABY DATA

If you were to catch a glimpse of your baby today, it would look very different from a newborn. You would see a very thin-skinned baby the size of a Barbie doll. The skin is so thin that you can see the blood vessels peeking through. This is also one of the last weeks that you can see most of the baby in one image of an ultrasound. Past this point, your baby is simply too big.

The scalp hair pattern has developed, cowlicks and all. Your baby still only weighs about seventy grams, or the weight of seventy paper clips, which is light for such a long body. But remember that body fat is one of the last things to develop on your baby. The good news is that your baby's heart is pumping blood, nearly twenty-five quarts a day! That may sound like a lot, but by the time his or her birth day arrives that number will be about 300 quarts.

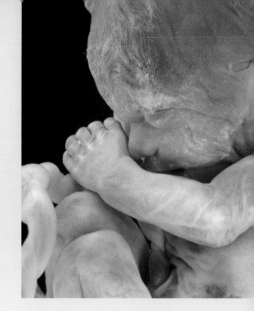

# Reevaluate Your Hair Care

Pregnancy is supposedly a time when your hair looks its best. It looks full and lustrous—without any change in how you are treating it. Some attribute this to prenatal vitamins; others claim that it is due to the fact that their hair follicles aren't releasing the hairs that would normally fall out because the body is too busy growing a baby.

Either way, your hair can be a source of pride during pregnancy—or a source of stress. If, before getting pregnant, you received regular perms or colored your hair on a regular basis, pregnancy may throw you for a loop.

Stress no more! The good news, particularly if coloring your hair is the issue, is that most people, including the American College of Obstetricians and Gynecologists, agree that coloring your hair in pregnancy is not harmful to you or your baby. This means that you can color to your heart's delight.

The not-so-good news is that some women report that the color doesn't take as well or look the same. This is thanks to pregnancy hormones. You may still be concerned about hair coloring even with all the professional reassurances. If so, consider taking one of the following alternative routes:

- Skip coloring in pregnancy.
- Color only after the first trimester.
- Use a natural source of color, such as henna.

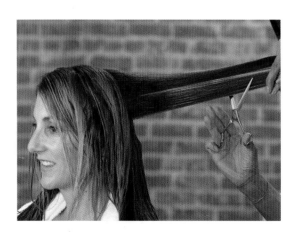

*Your hair may behave differently in pregnancy. Try a trusted hair professional for a consultation and cut before you go too wild.*

Perms can be a bit trickier in pregnancy. First, the strong-smelling perms should be done in a well ventilated area. If you're perming yourself, you should wear gloves to minimize your contact with the chemicals. Even with these precautions, however, you may be less than thrilled with the results. Pregnancy may be when you want to take the test curl very seriously. Most every home perm product recommends that you test a section before doing your whole head. Lots of people ignore the suggestion, but in this case, it could save you from a hair disaster. If you have concerns, consider seeking a hair stylist who has experience working with pregnant women.

No matter what you decide to do with coloring and perming, take the time to treat your hair well. You can even consider a new hair style, but avoid doing anything drastic. That's because you have limited options for fixing a problem and the hormone factor may lead you to freak out more than if you weren't pregnant. The goal here is maintenance with a little pampering thrown in—not a wild new style.

## Check for a Birth Network in Your Area

A birth network is a collection of birth professionals who gather to provide educational support and meetings for local pregnant women and families. Often, they offer classes taught by local practitioners on specific subjects related to pregnancy, birth, and newborn care.

This is a great opportunity to meet local birth professionals and other like-minded individuals. Many birth networks offer opportunities to meet local practitioners, such as a meet-the-pediatrician night or a meet-the-doula night. Other topics might include local resources for breastfeeding or child care. This local flavor can really be helpful as you talk to other mothers and fathers about what has been helpful in your area. This is something no generic pregnancy website or book can do.

PREGNANCY AFFIRMATION
FOR WEEK 15

✚

## Being pregnant is enlightening and fun.

You won't find a listing in the phone book for birth networks. Sometimes you might find a birth network on the Internet or from word of mouth. Your childbirth educator, doctor, or midwife may also connect you to a birth network. Or you can find birth networks online at *www.birthnetwork*.org and *www.lamaze.org*.

## Learn about Maternal Blood Screening for Certain Defects

Most practitioners will offer you a maternal blood screening between weeks 15 and 17 of your pregnancy for neural tube defects (such as spina bifida and anencephaly), Down syndrome, and Trisomy 18.

The blood screening has different names, based on how many of the hormones that you are screened for. For example, it is called a "triple screen" if you are tested for three of the five hormones, a "quad screen" if you are tested for four of the five hormones, and a "penta screen" if you are tested for all five. The generic term is a "multiple marker test," the multiple markers being the substances being tested for in your blood.

Depending on your practitioner and the lab that they use, you can be tested for up to five different substances in your blood, including the following:

- Alpha-fetoprotein (AFP)
- Human chorionic gonadotropin (hCG)
- Uncojugated estriol (uE3)
- Dimeric inhibin A (DIA)
- Invasive trophoblast antigen (ITA)

It is important to remember that this is a screening—not a definitive diagnosis. Based on your age, the gestational age of your pregnancy, and a series of blood work, you will be given a risk calculation that defines your baby's risk for a particular disorder. A positive test, or a high risk ranking, may make you want to seek additional testing. The additional testing is typically more invasive, such as an amniocentesis, which yields more specific results.

One of the problems with this series of tests in the past has been the high false positive rate to this screening. The more items screened for, the better able you are to get a realistic answer to your questions. If your practitioner or lab only tests for three substances, you may want to ask where you can go to get the full penta screen. If you have the screenings done more than once, it is recommended that you have them done at the same lab because labs can vary slightly.

This test is offered, not required. Just thinking about the screening can give some mothers mental stress and strain. Some choose to skip it entirely. Others go directly to genetic testing, which provides more definitive answers.

If you have any questions, don't hesitate to talk to your midwife or doctor. You may ask about your risk factors based on your age and history or even discuss the possibility of genetic testing. There are also alternative screenings offered, including ultrasound screening at various points in your pregnancy.

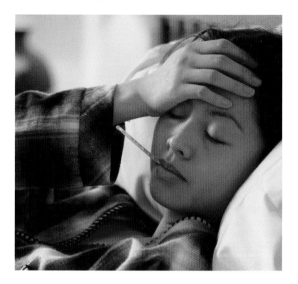

*Nine months is a long time for most people to go without being ill, expect to experience some illness. Check with your midwife or doctors before treating even common illnesses.*

## Be Prepared in Case You Get Sick While Pregnant

No matter how healthy you try to be, you will most likely find yourself feeling sick at some point in your pregnancy. There are a few considerations when you are pregnant and dealing with an illness such as a cold, sinus infection, or flu.

FEVER: When pregnant, you want to avoid raising your body temperature over 101 degrees Fahrenheit, and that includes having a fever. You can't avoid getting a fever, so you need to know how to treat it. In general, a "normal" fever will not harm your pregnancy. In other words, if you have the flu and you run a fever, you have not endangered your baby's life or brain capacity. Only a prolonged rise in body temperature or hitting extremes can cause problems. Talk to your doctor or midwife about which medications they recommend for fever reduction.

MEDICATIONS: Before heading off to the medicine cabinet to deal with whatever symptoms you have, you should talk to your practitioner for advice. Many common over-the-counter medications aren't appropriate for pregnancy. When taking an approved medication, use the least amount and choose the simplest formulation. (Of course, you will have already talked with your practitioner about how to take medications such as asthma medications and inhalers that are critical for your survival.)

RECOVERY TIME: Sometimes when you get ill during your pregnancy, it takes awhile to recover. It can be that your body is already weakened in the pregnant state or that you are simply dealing with so much at once. Some mothers think it's because they aren't able to take their normal medications. The truth is, most viral illnesses (such as colds) run their course, and the medicine we throw at them don't work on anything but our minds. If a pregnant woman develops a bacterial infection (such as bronchitis), however, antibiotics will be employed regardless of gestational status.

VACCINATIONS: Not many vaccinations are safe for pregnant women, but the major exception is the flu vaccine. This vaccine is recommended for all pregnant women, regardless of your trimester. (In other words, get a flu vaccine when it's recommended, which is usually in the fall, no matter where you are in your pregnancy.) However, you should avoid the flu vaccine if you have other reasons not to take it, such as allergies to flu vaccine components.

Take it for granted that it's unlikely that you will make it through all nine to ten months without becoming sick, even if it's only a cold. The best thing you can do is to be prepared for illness. Get a list of approved medications for the most common ailments before illness strikes. This will give you peace of mind and will prevent middle-of-the-night phone calls for minor problems.

You should also stock your medicine cabinet with nonmedicinal tricks. For instance, before reaching for a decongestant to treat a stuffy nose, try saline drops or a steamy shower. It can also be helpful to use a cool mist humidifier and apply warm compresses to the affected areas of the face and sinuses.

These tricks will be helpful later in learning to care for your baby, because very few medications are approved for use with infants.

**HOT MAMA**

If it's time to start shifting over to maternity clothes, be sure to do it before you have a wardrobe malfunction. Trying to use rubber bands and other types of emergency measures for clothes that don't fit anymore is risky. They could backfire and potentially be quite painful (not to mention embarrassing).

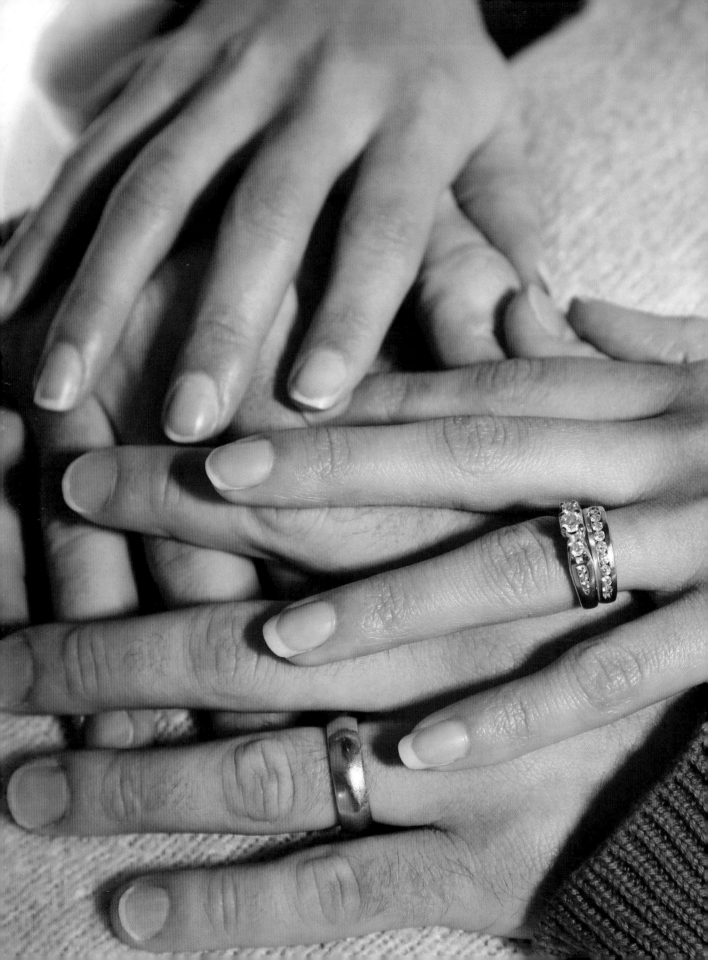

# Week 16

## CHECKLIST FOR WEEK 16

[ ] Feel your baby move.
[ ] Get ready for food cravings
[ ] Plan for a vaginal birth after Cesarean.
[ ] Do Kegel exercises.
[ ] Know the warning signs for pregnancy-induced hypertension.

## WHAT TO WATCH FOR THIS WEEK

*Double Check*

**Bleeding or spotting:** After sexual intercourse, a vaginal exam, or vaginal ultrasound, it is normal to experience some bleeding or spotting. However, if you spot without having had sex or been given an exam, it may be a sign of infection, premature dilation of the cervix, or issues related to your placenta. Contact your practitioner right away.

**Back or abdominal pain:** This type of pain or discomfort may be the result of contractions or premature dilation of the cervix, which is a sign of potential preterm labor.

**More than six contractions per hour:** This can be a sign of preterm labor. It can be normal to have contractions, just not at this frequency.

**Gush of fluid from the vagina:** To determine if this means your water has broken prematurely, make an appointment to see your practitioner. The fluid may be normal vaginal discharge.

*Report any strange or troublesome symptoms to your practitioner immediately.*

## BODY BASICS

Hopefully you are enjoying some of the glow of pregnancy. Remember, not every expectant mom feels happy all the time. Even if you don't feel physically sick, it is normal to have a few days or weeks where you feel blah or cranky. Some women want to know what all the fuss is about in pregnancy. Everyone says you should enjoy it, but what if you don't all the time?

Don't feel guilty if you don't feel 100 percent connected to your pregnancy at every moment. Some women need time to let the idea settle in their minds—even if they went to great lengths to get pregnant. Hang in there, feelings of uncertainty or ambivalence will surely pass.

## 🛒 BABY DATA

You are not the only one going to the bathroom every hour. Your baby's bladder fills and empties about once an hour from this point on. This is good practice for your baby's kidneys. Zometimes, via ultrasound, if you catch your baby at the right time, you can even witness this. Around now, sometimes ultrasound can begin to hazard a guess as to whether your baby is a girl or a boy. However, there are more mistakes earlier, so take a guess now with a grain of salt.

Your baby still only weighs about three ounces (85 grams) and is just over six inches (15 centimeters) long. His or her features are becoming more babyish. One good example is that the eyes and ears are assuming a more normal placement. Your baby also has complete fingernails at this point!

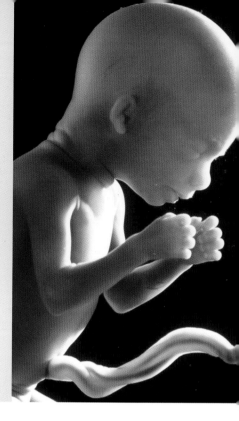

## Feel Your Baby Move

Most moms will tell you that feeling the baby move is one of the best things in pregnancy. However, it is also one of the things that will lead to a host of questions in your pregnancy. Here are some common questions and answers about fetal movement.

WHEN SHOULD I FEEL MY BABY MOVE? The first movements of your baby happened weeks ago. But as your baby has grown bigger, you may begin to feel your first movements, called quickening. Quickening usually happens between 18 and 22 weeks for first-time moms. It can happen sooner if you know what you're feeling for or if you are thin.

This range is the average. Obviously some mothers will feel their babies sooner, and other mothers will feel them later. If you are concerned or if you reach 24 weeks and still haven't felt your baby move, you should talk to your doctor or midwife. The most common explanation for a lack of fetal movement is that the baby's position or the position of the placenta is blocking your sensations of the movement.

WHAT DOES A BABY MOVING FEEL LIKE? If you haven't had a baby before, you may not know what you're looking for when they baby moves inside your uterus. Some women describe fetal movements as feeling like butterflies or bubbles are trapped inside them. Others report that they felt rhythmic bouncing or tapping.

Some women report that they are able to feel their babies better when they are lying still and focusing on what they are feeling. You might hear people tell tales of pressing on their bellies while laying down or drinking carbonated beverages to try to stimulate their babies to move. The best advice is to stop and pay attention if you think you feel small movements.

HOW DO I KNOW IT IS THE BABY AND NOT GAS? Because the first movements you feel are likely to be light, you may wonder if you're feeling bubbles of gas in your intestines. Gas typically doesn't feel rhythmic and is often associated with pain and/or flatulence. If neither is present you only feel the movement for a brief time, chances are that it is your baby and not your dinner.

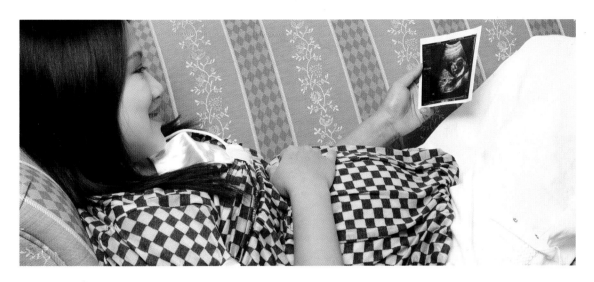

*Some women fall in love with the babies at the sight of an ultrasound, while others are left wondering how to determine which part is heads and which is tails. Both are normal.*

CAN THE BABY MOVE TOO LITTLE? Once you feel your baby move, you will begin to worry about the quality and quantity of movement. You have to remember that after the first movements, you may not feel your baby moving regularly for awhile. This is completely normal.

If you are worried that your baby isn't moving as much as you think is normal, you can talk to your practitioner about it. Most of the time, however, it is simply that your baby is still small and shielded by the uterus or the placenta. Your baby can still turn somersaults at this point in pregnancy, so small changes in his or her position will affect how you feel movements.

CAN THE BABY MOVE TOO MUCH? Along with the fear of your baby moving too little, you might wonder why you feel your baby move so much. Some mothers question frequent movement as the sign of something wrong from strokes in utero to fetal signs of attention deficit hyperactivity disorder. The good news is that lots of movement is simply the result of your baby's temperament and activity level, the position of the placenta, the position of the baby, and your body type.

## PREGNANCY AFFIRMATION FOR WEEK 16

### My baby and I are growing.

WHEN WILL MY HUSBAND FEEL AND SEE THE BABY MOVE? Even though you will feel the baby much earlier, movements strong enough for others to feel and see usually come much later. Typically between 26 and 28 weeks is when others will be able to enjoy the movements you've been feeling for weeks.

The scenario goes like this:

YOU: "Oh feel the baby move!" (You grab his hand and put it on the spot where baby has been moving wildly.)

HIM: "Ohhh..." (expectantly)

BABY: stays still

This will play itself out time and time again before someone else can feel the baby move. This is because the movements have to be much larger to be felt all the way through your body. This can be frustrating for you and the others in your life who are anxious to feel the baby. On the flip side, don't be concerned if others don't want to feel the baby move or don't seem to share your excitement. Feeling a baby move inside the uterus is not everyone's cup of tea.

WHAT IF I'M HAVING MORE THAN ONE BABY? If you are having more than one baby, you may expect to feel more movement. Some expectant mothers of multiples do note that they feel a lot of movement and movement that feels "all over" rather than in one spot. This is because you can feel punches, kicks, and turns from multiple babies. It is often difficult—and sometimes disconcerting—when you cannot identify which baby is making which movement. Later, as the babies become more fixed in their positions, doing fewer flips, you can sense which baby is moving.

Some twins and other multiples move in tandem; think of small fist fights inside your uterus. Other multiples move one at a time, or one right after the other. You may also notice that one baby moves differently than the other. This is quite normal. Discuss the differences with your practitioner. Some multiples do not move as much as others because of a variety of reasons, such as personality, muscle tone, and position.

In short, when it comes to fetal movement, it is up to you to pay attention and feel the baby. Later in pregnancy, fetal movement becomes the best indicator of fetal well-being, and you will be asked to do fetal kick counts. Rather than view this as a medical event, think of it as a way to bond with your baby.

## Get Ready for Food Cravings

Food cravings during pregnancy are not just an old wives' tale. The wild food combinations that you've no doubt heard about—such as the classic pickles and ice cream—may sound like a joke. But the truth is, many women say that they genuinely crave certain foods during pregnancy.

Scientists have long tried to pin down exactly why pregnant women crave certain foods or food combinations, but because of the wide variances in the particular foods and the women experiencing the cravings, it's been a difficult and not terribly conclusive process. The findings suggest that some women crave things that their bodies need, such as protein or certain vitamins. Other women have more emotionally based cravings. They want a milkshake and use the pregnancy to justify it, or they feel depressed and reach for a piece of chocolate.

Food cravings can be a constant in your pregnancy. The big question is whether or not to give in to them. The answer depends on what you are craving, how often you crave it, and how it affects the overall stability of your diet. For example, craving ice cream every night is probably not something to give in to. However, craving oranges or salads is probably fine as long as you are eating a variety of other foods.

Some cravings, however, are a serious problem. The condition is called pica, and it involves a craving for nonfood substances. It typically indicates a vitamin deficiency and makes women crave anything from ice to dirt and rocks. Some women crave laundry soap or even burnt matches.

*Cravings can be normal, but may not be for what you expect. Some women crave fresh fruit, meat, or even cereal. Don't stress about the occasional shake.*

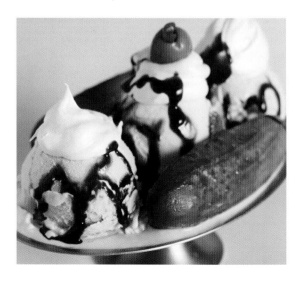

Report this type of nonnutrient craving to your practitioner immediately so that you can receive nutrient therapy.

The opposite of a craving—food aversion—is one of the body's protective mechanisms. It is the reason you may not want to eat or drink alcohol, caffeine, or foods that aren't good for you. Sometimes even smelling or thinking of a particular food makes you nauseated or lose your appetite. Typically this doesn't interfere with your ability get the nutrients that you need, but it may cause you to avoid some foods that you previously loved, even if they don't seem so harmful. Some examples of common food aversions include spaghetti sauce, cheese, and eggs.

## Plan for a Vaginal Birth after Cesarean

If your first baby was born via Cesarean, you fall into a special category for giving birth known as vaginal birth after Cesarean or VBAC (pronounced vee-back). Because some practitioners and places of birth may not allow you to have a VBAC at their facility, you should look into this up front in case you want to make other plans.

A VBAC is considered very safe for the vast majority of moms and babies. In fact, compared with a Cesarean birth, it carries far fewer risks for both parties. In fact, a VBAC offers many benefits, including easier recovery, reduced postpartum stay, fewer neonatal intensive care admissions, less postpartum infection, and lower cost.

Risks from a prior Cesarean include the following:

- Increased risk of placenta previa in subsequent pregnancies
- Slight increased risk of uterine tearing in pregnancy and labor (Inducing labor greatly increases this risk.)
- Increased interventions for fear of problems

You and your practitioner will decide the safest way for your baby to be born. This will involve a discussion of your preferences, your hospital or other birth place, your capabilities, and potential emotional and physical issues in labor and birth. Your practitioner should be completely supportive of your decision to have a VBAC. Hemming and hawing means that he or she does not totally support your decision to labor and give birth vaginally and may lead to unnecessary surgery. Be sure that your practitioner is completely on board with a VBAC and committed to helping you have the safest birth possible.

To prepare for a VBAC, educate yourself about labor and birth in general and after a Cesarean in particular. Consider taking special VBAC classes or hiring a doula who specializes in VBAC. There are many VBAC-related consumer support groups, including the International Cesarean Awareness Network (ICAN) *www.ican-online.org*. This group has an online email group and runs local meetings in cities all over the world. More than 85 percent of women who go forward with VBAC plans are successful.

Ask your practitioner the following questions about VBAC:

- How many VBACs do you do in your practice?
- What is the success rate?
- Are there added interventions done in a VBAC birth?
- Do you have special rules or preferences for VBAC moms?
- What will you do to support me in a VBAC?
- Can I speak to other moms who have had VBACs in your practice?
- Do you have classes, books, doulas, or educators to recommend?
- Can you share some of the current research on VBAC with me?

Ask your place of birth the following questions about VBAC:

- What VBAC policies do you have in place?
- Do you require continuous fetal monitoring or anesthesia for VBACs? If yes, how do I get an exception?
- How many VBACs do you do each year?
- What is the success rate for VBACs at your facility?
- Do you have a special VBAC class?
- Do you have a VBAC waiver that I must sign? When will I see this? If it is in labor, can I have a copy now?
- What community resources do you recommend for VBAC?

## Do Kegel Exercises

The Kegel is a special exercise for your pelvic floor. You have a muscle known as the pubococcygeal muscle (sometimes shortened to "pc muscle") that resembles a hammock between your pubic bone and tail bone. This muscle holds up your internal organs, including your uterus and bladder. (Men also have Kegel muscles.) You can feel this muscle work by stopping the flow of urine while using the bathroom.

Once you have identified this muscle, it is time to learn to exercise it. You can do this by simply squeezing and releasing the muscle. This is easy to do while driving or sitting at a desk or table. Practice this exercise and increase the number of times you're able to do it. After mastering that basic exercise about 50 to 100 times per day, you are ready to move on. Now, try squeezing and holding for 3 to 5 seconds, and then release. After you've got that down, the next level is like an elevator, where you tighten slightly, hold, tighten more, hold until you get to the highest level of tightening, and then slowly go back down.

Why are Kegels important? First, keeping your pc muscle strong will give you lifelong support for your internal organs. It will also help you to avoid

### WHERE IS YOUR PLACENTA?

You might have given a lot of thought to where your placenta is located. But as you start to wonder when you will feel the first flutterings of your baby's movements, your placenta may play an integral part as to when that happens. This is because the location of your placenta may block how much you feel your baby moving.

You can't locate your placenta on your own, but your doctor or midwife can listen for the placenta with a stethoscope or Doppler. You can see also where your placenta is located during an ultrasound.

Your placenta can be on top of the uterus (fundal). It can also be on the front of the uterus, known as an anterior placenta. If it's in the back, it is called a posterior placenta. A placenta near the bottom of the uterus or over the cervix is called a placenta previa.

If you have an anterior placenta, you may feel fewer movements, particularly early on. This is because the placenta does not have nerve endings and cannot feel the movements. The thickness of the placenta also acts as a barrier to your baby's movements. Remember, your baby weighs only a few ounces, and even a body slam can be hidden by the thick, healthy placenta.

problems with urinary incontinence. Also, doing Kegels helps you identify this area and strengthen it for giving birth. By being able to have some control over the area, many women are able to push their babies more effectively. Doing these exercises postpartum will help restore the health and blood flow to the area. It is one of the first exercises you're allowed to do postpartum, beginning almost immediately after birth.

## Know the Warning Signs for Pregnancy-Induced Hypertension

Pregnancy-induced hypertension (PIH) affects about 5 to 8 percent of first-time mothers and a smaller percentage of second- or more-time moms. Hypertension simply means high blood pressure, and some women have chronic hypertension before they become pregnant. PIH, however, relates to women who did not have chronic high blood pressure prior to pregnancy but develop some form of it during pregnancy.

Your practitioner will be monitoring you throughout pregnancy for this disorder during your prenatal visits. This is one reason that they test your urine—protein in your urine is a sign of it. They also look for signs of swelling (which is a symptom of PIH), and they check your blood pressure and weight at every visit to look for changes that might indicate a problem.

Signs of PIH include the following:

- Sudden swelling, particularly in the face and hands
- Swelling in your legs that doesn't go away after twelve hours of rest
- Increase in blood pressure
- Protein in your urine
- Weight gain of about five pounds (2¼ kilograms) in one week with no explanation
- Visual disturbances, such as spots or floaters
- Severe and/or sudden headaches

These are the major symptoms and signs of problems, but there can be other less common symptoms. If your practitioner suspects that you are having an issue with PIH, you will go through additional testing, which may include more frequent visits, a twenty-four-hour urine collection, and a special test for your baby.

PIH can cause major complications in pregnancy, including strokes and convulsions, so it should be taken very seriously. Sometimes it is safer for a woman with severe PIH to give birth to

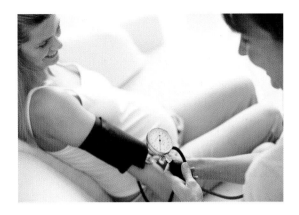

*Measuring your blood pressure is a normal prenatal care routine. Be sure to ask how your blood pressure is doing and what it means, so that you can be active in your care.*

her baby early than to wait for labor to begin. You and your practitioner will decide what is the best course of treatment for your pregnancy.

### HOT MAMA

If you are trying to draw attention away from your pregnant belly because it is at that awkward in-between stage, accessorize with larger jewelry such as earrings or necklaces. A striking pair of hoop earrings or a colorful chunky necklace will draw the eye upward and away from your abdomen.

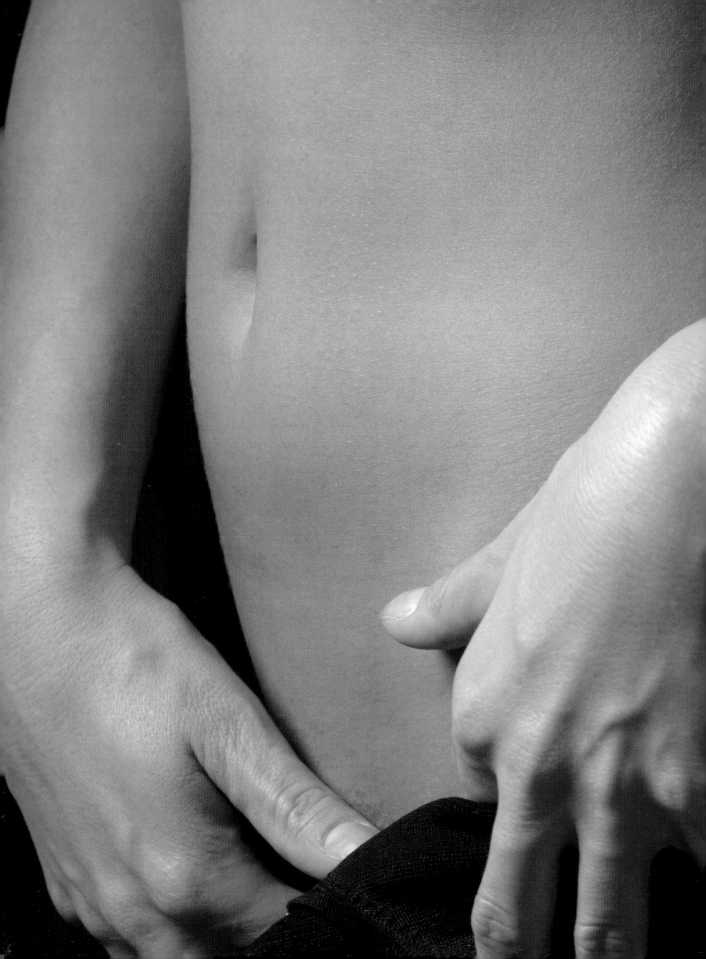

# WEEK 17

 **CHECKLIST FOR WEEK 17**

[ ] Buy a birth ball.
[ ] Start planning for your maternity leave.
[ ] Find out about chloasma.
[ ] Try a new pregnancy exercise.
[ ] Check on your life insurance.

## WHAT TO WATCH FOR THIS WEEK

*Double Check*

**Bleeding or spotting:** Bleeding or spotting at this point in pregnancy can follow sexual intercourse, a vaginal exam, or vaginal ultrasound. Hopefully you were told this might happen prior to being given this type of exam or activity. Should you experience bleeding or spotting unconnected to these activities, report it immediately to your practitioner, because it may be a sign of infection, premature dilation of the cervix, or issues related to your placenta.

**Back or abdominal pain:** If you have pain in your back or abdomen, it may be the result of contractions or premature dilation of the cervix, a sign of potential preterm labor.

**More than six contractions per hour:** Contractions that occur at this rate at this point in your pregnancy may be a sign of preterm labor.

**Gush of fluid from the vagina:** This can be a sign that your water has broken prematurely. Your practitioner can determine if fluid leaking from your vagina is amniotic fluid or normal vaginal discharge.

*Report any strange or troublesome symptoms to your practitioner immediately.*

## BODY BASICS

As your uterus inches up toward your belly button, you will start to notice a bulge in your lower abdomen, if you hadn't already. This is your baby's home! You may or may not need maternity clothes yet, depending on your regular wardrobe and body type.

This week you may notice you have fluid leaking from your breasts ever so slightly. Or you may notice an orange-colored film over your nipples. This is colostrum, your baby's first milk, and it will likely continue through birth. You may or may not notice it every day. If it becomes worrisome, mention it to your practitioner. If you are more worried about it leaking through to your clothes, you can wear disposable or washable nursing pads inside your bra.

## 🍼 BABY DATA

It has been fifteen weeks since conception. Your baby weighs about five ounces (142 grams) and is roughly the same size as the placenta at this point. From here on out, your baby will surpass the placenta in size, although the placenta continues to grow.

Brown fat is the substance that helps keep your baby warm after birth. It is built up under the skin. This week your baby started laying down some brown fat, which will continue to develop until birth.

Your baby is developing reflexes in the uterus. One of the big milestones this week is that your baby can hear loud noises outside of the uterus. You may actually feel your baby startle when you hear a loud or sudden noise.

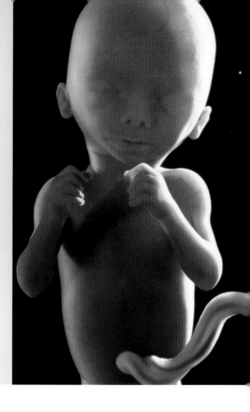

*A birth ball can be a great place for you to sit while watching television, doing your work, or even practicing relaxation. It's also a great labor tool!*

**PREGNANCY PARTICULARS**

## Buy a Birth Ball

A birth ball is the same thing as an exercise or physiotherapy ball. A birth ball is very useful for the duration of pregnancy and not simply the labor and birth portion. You can use a birth ball to replace your desk chair or to help you exercise.

The benefits of using a birth ball in place of your regular chair are many, including helping you with your posture. Because posture is a key factor in reducing back strain and pain in pregnancy, you will want to pay attention to this even in your everyday life, such as when you're sitting at a desk. When you sit on a birth ball, you are forced to sit up straight, which helps align your back and pelvis. Sitting on a birth ball at your desk, dining room table, and wherever you sit will improve your posture, which means less backache.

In addition to using a birth ball as a chair, you can do exercises on it. You can rent or buy videos devoted to birth ball exercises, including ones that are just for pregnancy. They focus on stretching, aerobics, and improving your overall health.

Many women choose to use birth balls while giving birth. Many hospitals and birth centers supply their own balls to patients in labor. If your hospital or birth center does not, you will need to provide your own.

Birth balls come in three sizes. The one that's right for you is based on your height, according to the following guide:

- 4'8" to 5'5" takes a 55-centimeter ball
- 5'6" to 6'0" takes a 65-centimeter ball
- 6'0"+ uses a 75-centimeter ball

You should make sure that you select a birth ball that is meant for sitting on and will bear your weight. Some people have been tempted to purchase less expensive balls that are meant as children's toys. This can be dangerous for you to sit and exercise upon.

## Start Planning for Your Maternity Leave

Maternity leave sounds like a vacation, but truthfully it can be a nightmare if you don't plan appropriately. Much of what needs to happen while you are on maternity leave, whether it is for six weeks or six months, should be planned for before you leave. This will drastically cut down on frantic calls and emails when you do not have a lot of time or energy to take care of work issues. Advance preparation will also earn you Brownie points for taking care of work issues and not leaving your coworkers in the lurch.

Planning ahead should start with your daily tasks. Ask yourself, what is it that you do every single day? If it's hard for you to break it down because you are on auto-pilot once you walk into the office, try taking notes for a few days and then convert your notes into a simplified schedule. Be sure to include tasks such as checking email and

*Early planning for your time off can help ease your financial and employment woes, not to mention giving you time to enjoy your new baby!*

PREGNANCY AFFIRMATION
FOR WEEK 17

✚

# I am feeling strong and confident about my pregnancy.

phone messages. It's helpful hints such as, "The management really likes you to change your voice mail daily" that make everyone really happy.

Once you have some of the basics down, start to think about ongoing projects that will not be tidied up before you leave. List everyone involved with the project and gather the information that someone else will need to step up to the plate and move forward.

Gather all of your notes into a binder, which should include your daily schedule, projects database, and other relevant papers. Consider adding a quick directory of people you work with,

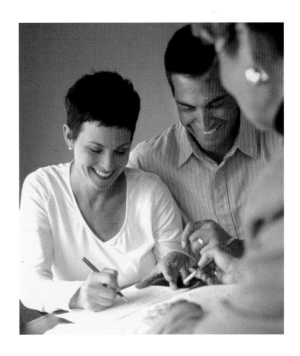

their job descriptions, and what they can help with on the project list. You may also choose to include a list of helpful resources, which could include books, databases, and computer programs. Be sure to include any necessary passwords or login information, particularly for your voice mail. You might also include your personal contact information and when you think would be a good time to contact you.

Begin to collect this information around your fourth or fifth month of pregnancy, sooner if you are expecting multiples. This will ensure that you have enough time to complete it. That way if you need to leave before the ninth month, you have the process started, even if it is not completely finished.

## Find Out about Chloasma

Some pregnant women will notice a darkening of the skin on their faces, particularly in the area over the nose, on the cheeks, and the forehead. This is known as the mask of pregnancy, or chloasma, and it typically shows up around the fourth or fifth month.

Chloasma occurs because of an increase in the secretion of melanotropin in pregnancy. There is nothing that can be done, except to cover it up with makeup. Avoiding the sun and wearing sunscreen will prevent the problem from getting exacerbated. About 45 to 70 percent of pregnant women experience chloasma.

The good news is that the dark pigmentation will fade after birth. How long it takes to fade varies, but it's usually not more than a few months. Some dermatologists may recommend treatment if you are still having issues after several months. Be sure to talk to your doctor or midwife for a referral.

## Try a New Pregnancy Exercise

If you have been faithfully exercising throughout your pregnancy, you might need to shake up your routine. This might be a great time to try something new. Don't make a drastic change, but how about buying a video in the category you already like or trying a new yoga class to work on relaxation?

Trying something new can also help you jumpstart a flagging desire to exercise. Just breaking out of a routine and giving yourself options can be a boost. No matter what you try, remember to watch for discomfort or signs of problems. In other words, make sure to listen to your body.

If you have the option, swimming is a wonderful exercise during pregnancy. The benefits of swimming are many, and it feels amazing to be able to move fluidly in the water without carrying the weight of your growing body.

If you aren't sure what exercise to try, consider talking to other pregnant women or women who recently had children. Your practitioner might also have a good idea about what would be helpful and fun for you.

## Check on Your Life Insurance

Many families do not think about life insurance until they are expecting a baby. This is because having a child changes how you think about the rest of your life. Some women say pregnancy puts them in touch with their mortality, making them focus on what will happen as they age.

If your husband is looking for something to take care of during your pregnancy or you think this task would be up his alley, it is a great way to involve him in the process.

You will want to factor many things into your decision about life insurance, including the following:

- How much money would it take one spouse to comfortably raise your child?
- What happens if you both die at the same time?
- What are your current debts?
- What is your annual salary?
- What are your spending habits?
- Are you factoring in college?

Now is a wise time to talk to a financial advisor or insurance agent about your choices for life insurance. Your life insurance options include whole, variable, and universal. While a rule of thumb is that your policy should be five to ten times your annual salary, the necessary calculation is not that simple for most people.

## HOT MAMA

As you start shopping for maternity clothes, do not be tempted to buy bigger sizes than you'd normally wear. Maternity shirts, pants, dresses, and even bathing suits are designed to match the size you were wearing pre-pregnancy. So if you were a size 8 or 10 before getting pregnant, you should shop for maternity clothes in that size. This will ensure that your wardrobe fits and flatters you throughout your pregnancy.

## CHOOSING A PAINT COLOR FOR THE NURSERY

Picking a paint color for your baby's room is very important. You don't have to be an interior designer to know that color can radically alter the look and feel of a space. Therefore, you should think long and hard before committing to a particular color.

When picking a color, consider the following:

- The size of the room
- The shape of the room
- How long you want the paint to last
- Color of the furniture
- Color and tone of the decorations

The color will set the mood in the room. Some say that certain colors are associated with certain moods. Keep this in mind as you select colors. Ask yourself, how do various colors make you feel? For example, does yellow make you happy or hungry? If you're leaning toward mint green, does it make you think of your grade school walls? Remember that you are likely to spend many, many hours surrounded by the color you choose. Your baby will also spend time in the room, and the color needs to be suitable and soothing for your infant.

You should also give some thought to the quality of the paint. Some paints are washable, which is always handy when your baby becomes a toddler. Gloss or semi-gloss paints give off a slight shine, but they are more washable than matte finishes. Check with your local paint store to see what will work best with the room, the paint that's already on your walls, and your cleaning needs.

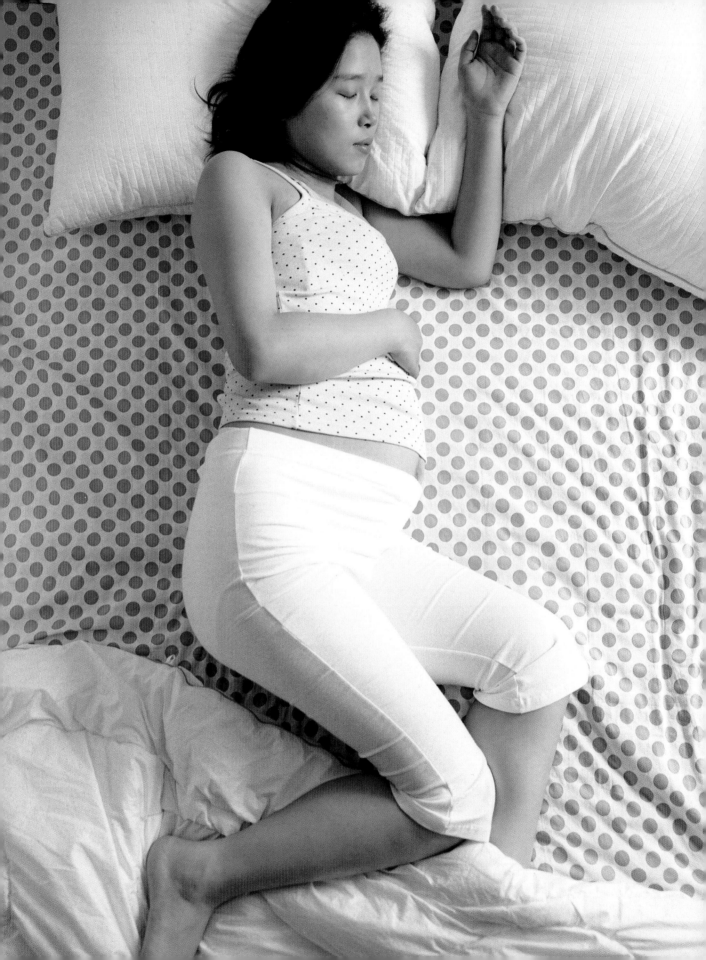

# WEEK 18

## CHECKLIST FOR WEEK 18

[ ] Start childbirth classes.
[ ] Try belly dancing.
[ ] Learn about round ligament pain.
[ ] Do a nutrition checkup.
[ ] Learn about linea negra.

## WHAT TO WATCH FOR THIS WEEK

*Double Check*

**Bleeding or spotting:** Bleeding or spotting (red or brown) at this point in pregnancy can happen after sexual intercourse, a vaginal exam, or vaginal ultrasound. You may be warned in advance of this possibility should you have this type of exam or activity. Other bleeding or spotting should be reported immediately to your practitioner, because it may be a sign of infection, premature dilation of the cervix, or issues related to your placenta.

**Back or abdominal pain:** Pain in your back or abdomen can be a sign of contractions or premature dilation of the cervix, a sign of potential preterm labor.

**More than six contractions per hour:** This can be a sign of preterm labor. It can be normal to have contractions, just not at this frequency.

**Gush of fluid from the vagina:** Contact your midwife or doctor, who will know if the leaking fluid means that your water has broken prematurely or is normal vaginal discharge. *Report any strange or troublesome symptoms to your practitioner immediately.*

##  BODY BASICS

Your body is starting to experience pregnancy changes on the outside. You may have noticed over the past few weeks that your center of gravity has started to shift. You may find that you feel a bit off kilter and may be a bit more clumsy than usual. Typically it takes a week or two to adjust and to gain some of your balance back, only to experience another shift.

These developments may also have you sleeping less well. Because you are supposed to avoid back sleeping, you should use a range of pillows to feel more comfortable as you sleep. Some women use a number of regular bed pillows while others prefer a single large body pillow. The critical places to support are between your knees, under your belly, and under your back if you tend to roll in that direction. Getting creative with pillows will hopefully earn you more restful sleep.

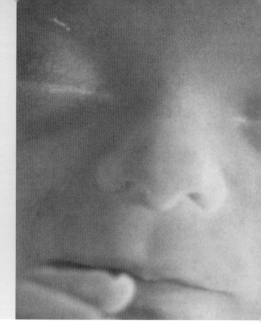

## 🍼 BABY DATA

Gotcha! Your baby is busy growing fingerprints. The finger and toe pads are growing, and the swirls and whorls that are characterized as hers and hers alone have started to grow. (Even identical twins have different fingerprints.)

Your baby is continuing the process of ossification, or hardening of the bones. This does not mean that your baby is becoming a heavyweight quite yet. But at seven ounces (200 grams), your baby is gaining weight at a much more rapid pace than before.

## Start Childbirth Classes

You might be thinking it's a bit early to start childbirth classes, but that is not the case. What you learn in a childbirth class will help inform the decisions that you make throughout the rest of your pregnancy. You will need this vital information as you move forward with your labor and birth plans.

Some classes are eight to twelve weeks long, meaning you want to ensure that you have enough time to complete the course. You also need time to process the information that you receive in class and to practice the relaxation and other comfort techniques, which can be difficult if you wait till

the end of your pregnancy to sign up. By giving yourself enough time to adequately take in and use the information, you will make the most of your childbirth classes and the friendships that develop.

If you schedule your classes toward the end of your pregnancy, you could even wind up missing classes should you give birth early, leading to gaps in your knowledge. To avoid the pressure or just the fear of missing classes, it is wise to schedule them earlier in your pregnancy.

Talk to your childbirth educator to see when classes start and which session works best with your due date. Many childbirth educators will let you continue to come to class after your first series runs its course if you are still pregnant. Some instructors offer a refresher weekend every month or so to help you stay on track with practicing. Be sure to ask if this is an option and you wish to continue coming to class. Scheduling your classes early also prevents you from missing a childbirth class all together because the classes are full.

## Try Belly Dancing

Belly dancing when pregnant can be a lot of fun! It is also a great form of exercise. Belly dancing is

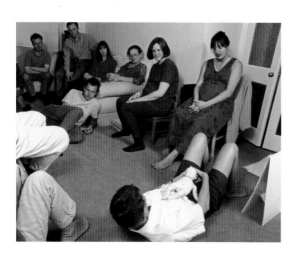

*Childbirth class is a great place to ask questions, learn the things books can't show you, and make new friends. Choose your class wisely.*

+

## My body is changing for the better of my baby.

gaining popularity and legitimacy as a way to keep fit. Anyone can try it, but there is something extra lovely about pregnant women showing off their bodies and moving their bellies.

The physical benefits of belly dancing are a great aerobic workout, plus stretching. In addition, many women report that they felt more confident and beautiful after learning how to belly dance. It is an amazing way to get to know your body. By having to move and twist, you can really see what your body is capable of, even in labor.

The only caution is to avoid vigorous moves such as rapid hip movements and hip snaps late in pregnancy (after the eighth month). If any moves feel wrong to you, don't do them.

A hormone called relaxin is released in pregnancy, making it easier to injure yourself if you aren't careful. Relaxin loosens the ligaments in your body, which makes birth easier because it helps your pelvis become more flexible. The problem is this added flexibility during pregnancy can lead to injury if you hyperextend or don't pay attention to how you move your body.

## Learn about Round Ligament Pain

The round ligament is one of the thick ligaments that anchors the uterus. As the uterus grows in pregnancy, this ligament stretches, thins, and becomes tense, much like a rubber band. The round ligament can be the source of pain in pregnancy. In fact, it is the leading cause of abdominal pain in pregnant women.

Sometimes with sudden movements, you will feel a sharp, stabbing pain as the result of this ligament being pulled on. This happens most often when pregnant women try to bend or twist at what was once their waist. You may notice this more on the right side than the left, because of the natural tendency of the uterus to lean toward the right.

Usually the pain from the round ligament is sharp and brief. If you have a dull ache that lasts for awhile, it may still be your round ligament, but it may be something that you should have checked out by your doctor or midwife.

A warm bath or shower can help ease the pain of a stressed ligament, as can warm compresses such as a rice sock. (See below.)

### HOW TO MAKE A RICE SOCK

A rice sock is a simple way to make a comfortable heating pad. Fill a thick, new, long sock with one to two pounds (1/2 to 1 kilogram) of regular white rice. Tie the end of the sock to prevent the rice from leaking out. Some people get fancy and add dried aromatic herbs, such as lavender.

Once the sock is securely fastened, microwave it for about two minutes. You now have a warm sock with radiant heat. The rice absorbs moisture and slowly releases it. The sock is great because it conforms to your body, unlike a stiff heating pad. And you don't have to worry about leaking, as with a hot water bottle.

These are safe to sleep with because they do not get warmer over time, and they don't stay hot indefinitely. It's a great way to ease the aches and pains of pregnancy or just warm your bed before you climb in.

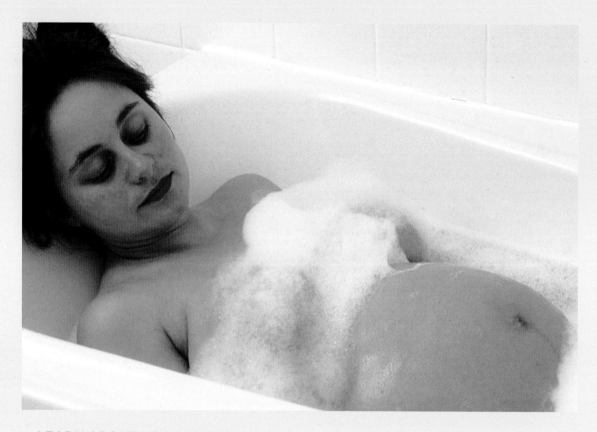

## LEARN ABOUT LINEA NEGRA

Linea negra literally translates to "black line." During the fourth or fifth month of pregnancy, you will notice the beginning of a single dark line (usually not black) running from your pubic bone upward on your abdomen. The line has always been there, called the linea alba, but you probably didn't notice it until the color made it more pronounced.

During pregnancy, the hyperpigmentation from the increase in estrogen and proges- terone cause the line to darken. It will usually begin to fade after birth as these hormones levels drop. For some women, the line remains faintly colored permanently.

Because the line does not darken for every woman in every pregnancy, the old wives started to speculate that the dark line is related to the baby's sex. Some say that if you have the line, the baby is a boy. Others refine that theory to say that if the line extends past your belly button, the baby is a boy. And if the line reaches to your belly button but no farther, then your baby is a girl. While amusing to consider, none of these theories has proven reliable in predicting the gender of unborn babies.

## Do a Nutrition Checkup

When you first get pregnant, you spend a lot of time worrying about everything, particularly what you eat. As you start to deal with the many issues associated with pregnancy, from morning sickness to sheer exhaustion, your focus shifts. You may find that you're eating very healthy foods but your diet lacks variety. Or perhaps you have worked so hard to keep from throwing up that you've fallen into the habit of shoving anything in your mouth that doesn't make you sick.

Now that you are well into your second trimester, it's a good time to look at your diet. Keeping a food log for a few days can be a good way to reevaluate what you are eating. You may find that writing things down makes you more conscious of what you're eating, which is why it is helpful to build a record over several days.

You may want to include the following in your food log:

- Number of fruits and vegetables per day
- Sources of protein
- Variety of foods
- Types of food (home cooked versus fast food and fresh versus frozen)
- Serving sizes

When you've gathered enough information, see what it tells you and where you need to make changes. You may find that you have certain trends or that you need to focus on certain aspects of your diet. If you're not up to doing the analysis yourself, share the results with a nutritionist and ask for feedback and advice. You should be able to ask your practitioner or insurance company for names of nutritionists.

Creating a new plan and incorporating changes is not always easy. The first step is awareness. Keep a written copy of your plan somewhere visible and ask for support from your husband, relatives, and friends. Slow and steady wins the pregnancy nutritional race.

**HOT MAMA**

Many pregnant women try to avoid bright-colored clothing. They fall for the "whole black is slimming" deal. While black may be slimming, you can only take it so far when you're talking about a pregnant belly. Instead, why not be bold and show off your true colors by dressing in shades you wouldn't normally wear? You may find several new colors that flatter you and make you feel happy. And that will have you smiling more, which is always a nice accessory.

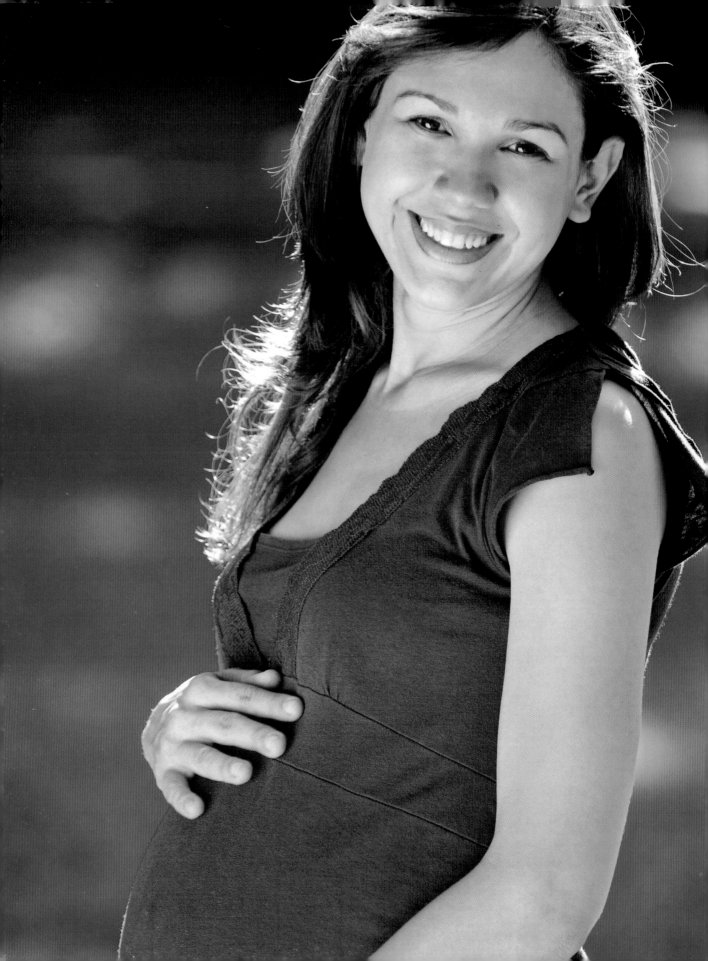

# WEEK 19

## ✏ CHECKLIST FOR WEEK 19

[ ] Buy a maternity outfit for special occasions.
[ ] Discuss circumcision.
[ ] Get a dental checkup.
[ ] Avoid baby-related reality television.

## 🔎 WHAT TO WATCH FOR THIS WEEK

*Double Check*

**Bleeding or spotting:** Bleeding or spotting that is not connected to having sex or being given a vaginal exam or vaginal ultrasound should be reported immediately to your practitioner. It may be a sign of infection, premature dilation of the cervix, or issues related to your placenta.

**Back or abdominal pain:** If you are suffering from persistent pain either in your back or abdomen, talk to your midwife or doctor to determine if you are having contractions or your cervix is dilating prematurely.

**More than six contractions per hour:** Contractions during the second trimester are not cause for alarm, but at this frequency, you may be having preterm labor.

**Gush of fluid from the vagina:** This can be a sign that your amniotic sac has broken prematurely. Your practitioner can determine if fluid leaking from your vagina is amniotic fluid or normal vaginal discharge.

*Report any strange or troublesome symptoms to your practitioner immediately.*

##  BODY BASICS

While you are probably feeling really great at this point in your pregnancy, there may be some small things that you find annoying. You might be experiencing heartburn, dizziness, or other issues. If any of these become worrisome, ask your practitioner for advice on treating the symptoms.

You may also find that you're beginning to think differently about how you live your life. These thoughts can cause you to look differently at your relationships. And this can be a time when you begin to think about how you want to parent. All of this thinking can make you feel anxious or confused. Not to worry; working through these weighty issues takes time, and pregnancy very conveniently provides you with nine months!

## 🍼 BABY DATA

During pregnancy, your baby, boy or girl, has been growing sex organs. Mature sperm won't appear in the male testes until after puberty, but if you are having a girl, she is developing primitive egg cells already. At birth, she will already carry every egg she will ever have in her lifetime.

Your baby weighs about eight ounces (225 grams) and is covered in fur. The good news is that most of this fine hair, called lanugo, will disappear before birth. You will occasionally see small patches of hair on the lower back and as long sideburns. Don't worry, you aren't giving birth to a baby Elvis! Your baby is also working on baby teeth this week.

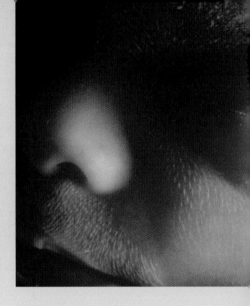

*We all need a special outfit, but in pregnancy it's never been more important. The right outfit can make you feel really great.*

## Buy a Maternity Outfit for Special Occasions

When you think of maternity clothing, you probably picture everyday outfits: the items that you would wear to work, for play, or just to lounge around the house. Every now and then you may decide that you want to dress up in pregnancy, or you may already have a special occasion on your calendar such as a formal party or a wedding.

Do not let the prospect of dressing up give you a panic attack. It is entirely possible to be pregnant and glamorous. And now that a number of celebrities have made pregnancy fashionable, there are many more flattering designs available for expectant women.

Consider the following when choosing a dressy outfit:

- Where do you intend to wear it?
- Is it a one-time function such as a wedding?
- Can you reuse the outfit for other functions?
- Is the outfit something you need to preorder? If so, how far in advance?
- Will the outfit look okay with flats or low heels?

- Can your outfit be altered? How long will that take?
- Does the outfit work for all seasons?
- How much does the outfit cost?

Many pregnant women choose fancy outfits that accentuate features that pregnancy has afforded them—or at least enhanced. This can include your newly found cleavage.

Your hair and makeup will also be something to consider when dressing up. Will you wear your hair up or down? This may alter which style of dress you choose. This will also influence the accessories that you choose.

Remember that getting gussied up, even when pregnant, should be lots of fun. Show off your blooming body and have a ball!

## Discuss Circumcision

The decision whether or not to circumcise a male child tends to elicit very strong feelings, both pro and con. It is therefore an important discussion to have early and often until you and your husband are both comfortable with the decision.

Circumcision is the medical procedure that surgically removes the foreskin from the glans, or the head, of the penis. Because many consider this a cosmetic procedure, it may not be covered by your medical policy. It is an outpatient procedure typically done in the hospital or at your practitioner's office within a month after birth.

The American Academy of Pediatrics (AAP) believes that circumcision is a personal decision and not a necessary surgery. The AAP supports religious circumcisions, such as the Jewish Brit Milah, or ritual circumcision, done on the eighth day of life.

If you decide not to have your son circumcised, you need to learn about genital care. You can find information on properly caring for an uncircumcised penis on the AAP's website *www.aap.org*.

If you decide to have your son circumcised, consider the following:

### PREGNANCY AFFIRMATION FOR WEEK 19

✚

## My baby hears my voice and is soothed.

WHEN WILL YOU DO THE CIRCUMCISION? Some say that it is easier for the baby if you wait until he is well established with breastfeeding and until natural clotting factors begin working on their own, which happens around the eighth day of life.

WHO WILL PERFORM THE SURGERY? Depending on where you live, you can find obstetricians, midwives, and pediatricians who do circumcisions. If you are having a religious circumcision, you will use a mohel or other religious figure who has been trained to do the procedure.

WILL YOU STAY WITH YOUR SON TO COMFORT HIM? Staying with your son to hold and comfort him during the procedure is possible and acceptable by many practitioners. It is a personal decision.

WILL YOU ALLOW REGIONAL ANESTHESIA FOR THE SURGERY? Some types of anesthesia can be used, such as the ring block or dorsal penile nerve block. Talk to your practitioner about which he or she uses. The AAP recommends that some pain control be used. Even during religious circumcisions, it isn't necessary to forego anesthesia.

WILL YOU PROVIDE YOUR BABY WITH ORAL ANALGESICS? Studies have shown that giving your baby acetaminophen (Tylenol) twenty to thirty minutes prior to the surgery can reduce the discomfort and crying.

WILL YOU BE NEARBY TO NURSE HIM IMMEDIATELY AFTERWARD FOR PAIN CONTROL? Nursing is a great source of comfort for babies. Nursing after painful procedures has been shown to reduce crying and promote relaxation.

If you have your son circumcised, be sure you understand the follow-up care that is needed for the penis. For example, ask his pediatrician the following questions:

- What amount of blood and pain is normal?
- How should you treat the pain?
- What can you to do promote healing?
- Under what circumstances should you call your practitioner?

You can find lots of information on circumcisions. The problem is finding neutral information. Read what you can and talk to as many people as possible as you form your opinions and ultimately make your decision.

## Get a Dental Checkup

It can be so easy to forget your biannual visit to the dentist. However, pregnancy is a time when your oral health is very important. For example, periodontal or gum disease has been linked to preterm labor. A timely visit to the dentist, therefore, is a must for all pregnant women.

The first trimester is not the ideal time to schedule a dentist's appointment. You may be suffering from ptyalism, which is an excess of saliva, or you might be feeling ill, and you may also worry about the safety of typical office procedures. Procedures such as dental x-rays and numbing agents for fillings or root canals are better left to the second trimester, and even then only when absolutely needed. Elective procedures can wait until after your baby is born. In fact, many dentists will require you to have a letter from your doctor or midwife stating it's okay to be treated if you require something beyond a regular cleaning.

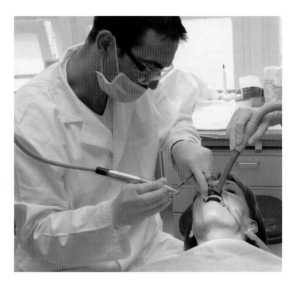

*Pregnancy is no excuse to avoid the dentist's chair. Be sure you get your regularly scheduled cleanings.*

You should report any medications you have been taking and any problems that you have been having to your dentist. This includes the following:

- Bleeding gums
- Sensitive teeth
- Swelling in your gums

Your dentist will let you know what is out of the ordinary and how to address it. You will also be told when to make your next visit, which usually will be a postpartum visit, unless you have a dental emergency.

## Avoid Baby-Related Reality Television

As tempting as it might be to watch baby-related reality or drama television while you're pregnant, it is best avoided. Life, and specifically birth, can rarely be summed up in thirty-minute minute segments. The real stuff gets thrown out on the editing room floor, leaving the viewer to believe that women go from smiling and nine months pregnant, to writhing in labor, to smiling again with sweet newborns—all in thirty minutes.

## HEAD OFF HEADACHES IN PREGNANCY

Headaches can be a huge problem in pregnancy. Sometimes when you experience headaches it is due to hormones. But other times it is your changing health habits. For example, eliminating caffeine from your diet makes you susceptible to headaches.

Because you can't reach for drugs at the first sign of a headache, you should work to prevent some of these headaches. Avoid any triggering foods, such as foods containing MSG. You should also avoid things that trigger headaches such as bright sunlight and loud noises.

If you have a headache, try some of the following mild headache pain relievers:

- Sleep
- Relaxation
- Dark room
- Quiet
- Caffeine

If you suffered from migraines before pregnancy, you should have a plan in place in case one crops up. Talk to your practitioner about how to handle migraines and ask him or her for a medication plan.

Some programs to avoid are medical dramas, which show only the scariest and most medically managed births because that's what sells. Do not believe for an instant that what you see on these shows happens to everyone, or even most people.

Many mothers-to-be think that watching this type of television show eliminates the need for reading childbirth books, talking with childbirth education and doulas, or any other type of support. These women are convinced that they have been shown everything they need and can therefore manage without additional help. Once again, thanks to heavy editing and other factors, these dramas are rarely realistic.

All that said, it is important for you to listen to birth stories, but get them from the women themselves. Listen to what worked for them, how they prepared, and how their realities differed from their expectations. This will give you more insight and power than anything you might see on TV. It will also probably be more locally relevant. After all, you can watch a water birth in some hospital on television, but that doesn't mean your local hospital will have a birth tub available for you.

### HOT MAMA

If you are a plus-sized mom, don't stress over maternity clothes. Stores offer plus-sized maternity lines, and you should start with brands that you already own and are loyal to. If you can't find what you need in retail stores where you normally shop, search online or call the company. You will be comfortably relieved that you sought out true maternity clothes rather than simply making due.

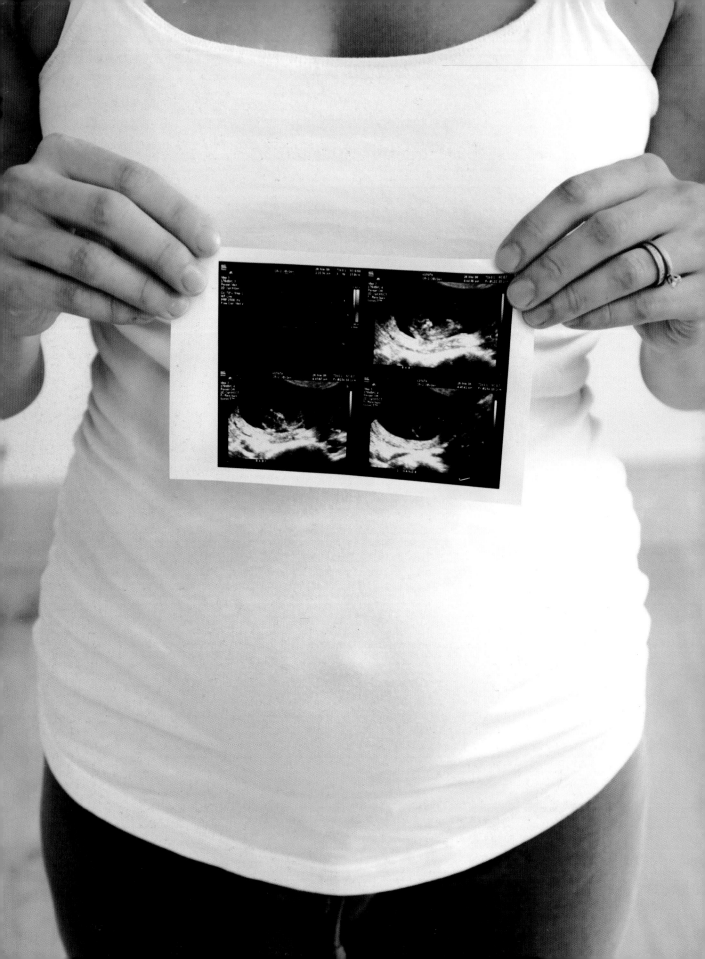

# WEEK 20

## ✎ CHECKLIST FOR WEEK 20

[ ] Talk to your practitioner about ultrasound screening.

[ ] Find out the sex of your baby, if you want to.

[ ] Learn to deflect unwanted advice.

[ ] Think about fetal movement.

[ ] Ask about the position of your placenta.

## ⌕ WHAT TO WATCH FOR THIS WEEK

**Headache:** Severe headaches should be evaluated by your practitioner. Headaches can be the normal result of pregnancy hormones, or they may be linked to other symptoms that together can be called pregnancy-induced hypertension (PIH) or even preeclampsia, which is a severe illness in pregnancy related to blood pressure, protein in your urine, and other complications.

**Blurred vision:** Report blurred vision immediately to your practitioner, with or without the presence of headaches, because it can also be a sign of PIH or preeclampsia.

### Double Check

**Bleeding or spotting:** You might notice some bleeding or spotting after sexual intercourse, a vaginal exam, or vaginal ultrasound. Report bleeding or spotting that results without having had any of these activities immediately to your practitioner, because it may be a sign of infection, premature dilation of the cervix, or issues related to your placenta.

**Back or abdominal pain:** Pain in your back or abdomen can point to contractions or premature dilation of the cervix, a sign of potential preterm labor.

**More than six contractions per hour:** Contractions of this frequency can be a sign of preterm labor, so you should contact your midwife or doctor to discuss.

**Gush of fluid from the vagina:** Your practitioner can determine if fluid leaking from your vagina is amniotic fluid, meaning your water has broken, or normal vaginal discharge.

*Report any strange or troublesome symptoms to your practitioner immediately.*

##  BODY BASICS

You are halfway through your pregnancy! This means that your uterus is about halfway to its highest point, which is usually around the point of your umbilicus or belly button. This means that the average measurement from your pubic bone to the top of your uterus is 8 inches (twenty centimeters). If you aren't already wearing maternity clothes for comfort, you will be soon.

The best part of the second trimester is that you are feeling much better than you did during the first trimester, yet you don't have many of the aches and pains that are common in the third trimester. You are looking unmistakably pregnant now as opposed to the well-fed look many moms worry about.

## 🍼 BABY DATA

Your baby weighs in this week at about ten ounces (285 grams), lighter than your average bottled drink! While your baby is still not very big weight-wise, he or she is about ten inches (twenty-five centimeters) long, roughly the size of a Barbie doll.

In addition to the fine hair called lanugo, your baby is covered in a thick creamlike material called vernix, which is made from skin cells. The vernix will cling to the lanugo and stick in the folds of your baby's skin. If your baby is born prematurely, you will see quite a bit of the vernix. If your baby is born at term or after, you see very little. You can sometimes find vernix in a baby's ears or in the creases at the arms and legs.

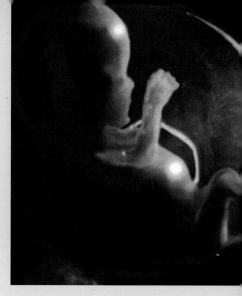

## Talk to Your Practitioner about Ultrasound Screening

Many mothers-to-be will be offered ultrasound screenings around the middle of their pregnancies. This screening is called the fetal anomaly screening, meaning that they are looking for major problems with your baby's anatomy.

This abdominal ultrasound may require that you have your bladder full at least for part of the ultrasound. Some practices ask that you drink thirty-six ounces (1 liter) of fluid prior to your appointment. For many pregnant women, this can be painful; other women do not experience any significant discomfort from a full bladder. If you are someone who finds it painful, rest assured this is a brief exam. The fluid in the bladder serves as an effective back drop for the ultrasound technician to see your baby. When the fluid is no longer needed, they allow you to empty your bladder, even if the test is not yet over.

During your ultrasound, you will lie on a table, and the ultrasonographer will wave the transducer over your abdomen. Images of your baby are shown on a screen from the sound waves bouncing back from the uterus.

If you don't want to find out the sex of your baby, you should mention that up front so that the ultrasonographer doesn't blurt it out or pan in so closely that you can see for yourself!

Your ultrasonographer will check for the following:

- Major organ systems
- Head circumference
- Abdominal circumference
- Femur length
- Placenta information
- Heart rate
- Gross abnormalities
- Position of the baby
- The sex of your baby

Mid-pregnancy is selected for the ultrasound because this is the point when many of the organs can be seen during the regular ultrasound exam. The uterus has also not become crowded yet, making it easier to detect problems. Your doctor or midwife can recommend a facility for the screening. Before you go, you will want to be sure that the facility you choose is covered by your insurance.

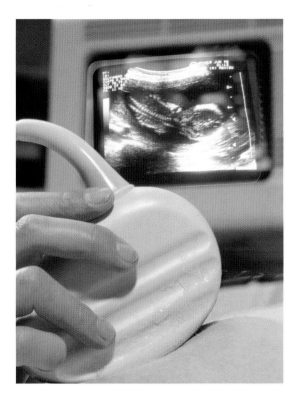

*During an ultrasound if you aren't sure what you're seeing, be sure to ask the technician for a running commentary.*

## PREGNANCY AFFIRMATION FOR WEEK 20

# I am enjoying my growing pregnant body.

when couples were told there were problems, and a follow-up exam showed everything was fine.

Even if you had an ultrasound prior to this screening, it might be a very exciting view of your baby. Do not be surprised if you need to have the ultrasonographer explain exactly what you are seeing on the screen. This what they do, and they will be happy to show you what they are looking for and what's displayed on the screen.

Make sure to bring your husband or partner with you to the screening. It can be thrilling to see your baby, even if the baby doesn't look like you imagined at this point. The images of older, black and white, 2D ultrasounds are familiar looking. But the newer 3D forms can be quite shocking if you ask many moms because babies look like clay forms. Be sure to ask for a couple of pictures and ask if they provide a DVD or CD of the experience. You may be required to bring your own blank DVD or CD, so ask before your appointment.

### Find out the Sex of Your Baby, if You Want To

One of the reasons that many moms give for wanting a mid-pregnancy ultrasound is to find out the sex of their babies. Reasons parents give for wanting to know include the following:

- Don't like surprises
- Want to plan the nursery
- Eager to choose a name
- Why not?

Not all women are offered this screening exam, for a variety of reasons, including the fact that not everyone believes it is helpful. Because this is a screening test and there is not universal belief that it should be done routinely, you may want to confirm with your insurance company that the ultrasound exam is covered.

If your insurance company does not pay for the exam, you could of course pay for it yourself. If you decide to pay for this exam out of pocket, be sure to use a facility that is set up for medical ultrasounds. Some couples may be tempted to get an ultrasound that is less expensive (and of inferior quality) done by technicians who are not medically trained but trained only for recreational purposes. Couples figure that they will be told if the exam reveals anything troublesome, but this is not always the case. There have also been cases

The point is that there are as many reasons for finding out as there are for people who choose not to find out. There are also regional variances in who finds out and who chooses not to. There are even larger variances by country, and some countries, including China and India, actually forbid prenatal sex discoveries. In some countries, it comes from the threat of infanticide.

Even in some places in the United States, you are not allowed to find out the sex of your baby before birth. It may be the hospital or facility rule or a rule established by the practice or your insurance. This comes from the threat of legal action should the "guesses" be inaccurate.

The majority of ultrasonographers are accurate in their findings. However, the following are some reasons why you might not be able to find out the sex of your baby:

- Baby's positioning precludes detection
- Type of ultrasound equipment
- Age of ultrasound equipment
- Gestational age of your baby
- Skill of the technician

It's also important to note that while ultrasound is the most common way to learn if your baby is a girl or a boy, it is not the most accurate. Genetic testing such as amniocentesis and chorionic villus sampling (CVS) are more accurate, but they also present greater risks. This is why they are not used simply to find out the sex of a baby.

There is no lack of old wives' tales for determining if you are having a girl or a boy. If you swing your wedding ring over your abdomen, supposedly if the ring goes side to side, you're having a girl, but if the ring travels in a circle, you're having a boy. Most of these make fun shower games, but some of them can be dangerous. In one test, the expectant mother mixes her urine with chemicals, which reportedly turn different colors depending on whether the baby is a boy or girl. You should also avoid scams advertised on the Internet and in the back of parenting magazine that offer to tell

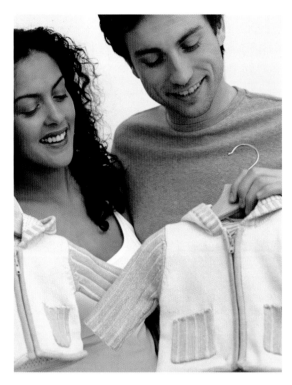

*It is important to acknowledge your personal desires regarding the sex of your baby. This can help you both as you decide whether to find out now or have a delivery surprise.*

you the sex of your baby. For lots of money, they promise you they can tell the sex of your baby with a small blood sample, dates on a calendar, or a urine specimen—all done through the mail. These are nothing more than ploys to get your money.

In general, whether couples find out or don't find out, the pendulum tends to swing both ways. One day it seems like everyone wants to know, and other days it seems like no one wants to know. With today's couples following celebrity trends of waiting until the baby's birth to find out the sex, more couples are choosing not to find out the sex of their babies beforehand.

## Learn to Deflect Unwanted Advice

For some people, there is nothing as exciting as a pregnant woman. Not only will complete strangers start touching your belly without permission, but they will also ask you all sorts of personal—and sometimes inappropriate—questions.

You may not be able to avoid this type of intrusion, but having a game plan can reduce the number of times it occurs and the duration of the conversations. The following are some tips for how to respond:

When offered some piece of advice on pregnancy: "Thanks, I'll talk to my midwife about that idea."

On having someone touch your belly: Touch his or her belly back and ask, "Did you have a big lunch today?"

On getting asked personal questions: "Have you had your most recently scheduled colon screening?"

The telling of a birth horror story, if you listen to it: "Thanks for sharing; I'll be sure to take that into consideration."

The telling of a birth horror story, if you don't listen to it: "I've been advised to avoid negativity for the baby's sake."

The idea is to remember that you are entitled to set boundaries and to protect your personal space and personal information. If you want to discuss what your nipples look like with your best friends, that's fine. But you don't have to answer when the woman from the next cubical asks the same question. Having prepared answers at the ready can help you stay calm and in control.

## Think about Fetal Movement

At the halfway point, you may be feeling your baby move. The baby has been moving for many weeks, even though you've been unable to feel it up until this point. There are many ways to describe what it feels like to have your baby move. Some women say it's bubbles or butterflies, but other women feel more like quick jabs in the gut. No matter what you feel, you may wonder at first if it's your baby. You might think it's something else completely, including an upset stomach, gas, or your imagination.

If this is not your first baby, you might feel your baby really early, but if it is your first baby, it might take a couple more weeks before you feel anything. Your practitioner won't be concerned about the lack of fetal movement until after about week 26. If you are concerned, talk to your doctor or midwife.

There are many reasons that you may not be feeling your baby move. It might simply be how your baby is turned inside the uterus or even the placement of your placenta. Your weight can sometimes be an insulating factor as well.

Taking matters into your own hands to try to increase the likelihood that you'll feel your baby is quite simple. Consider drinking something bubbly to make more noise in your stomach. Lay on your side and place your hands over your abdomen and wait for the show to begin. You may have to try this for several days in a row before you are lucky enough to catch your baby in the act.

## Ask about the Position of Your Placenta

At your prenatal visit this month, be sure to ask about the position of your placenta. This can be determined easily via ultrasound or by listening with a Doppler or fetoscope. If your placenta is in the front, it is said to be an anterior placenta. This can make it more difficult to hear your baby with a Doppler or fetoscope because you have to listen through the placenta. It can also insulate you from feeling some of baby's movements while your baby is still small.

You may also have a posterior placenta. This means that the placenta is located on the back wall. You will typically not notice anything different about fetal movements or hearing your baby if your placenta is posterior.

You may also have a fundal placenta, meaning that the placenta is located at the top of the uterus. This is very much like the posterior placenta in behavior.

The final option for positioning of the placenta is known as a placenta previa. This is where either part or all of the placenta covers the cervix, the opening of the uterus. It is very common to have this diagnosed through an ultrasound exam near the middle of your pregnancy. More than 95 percent of the time, this condition will resolve itself. This happens because the time of greatest growth for the uterine body is the second half of the pregnancy, meaning that as the uterus grows, the placenta is moved away from the opening of the cervix.

If you fall into the other 5 percent, you will be evaluated at the end of your pregnancy to see how much of the placenta is still covering or near the cervix. If there is only a tiny bit of the placenta near the cervix, which is called a marginal placenta previa, it may be that a vaginal birth is still the safest option for mother and baby. However, if the placenta is still mostly or completely covering the cervix, a Cesarean section will be done to protect the mother and baby because the cervix would open in labor, causing bleeding problems for both.

Many mothers do not experience symptoms with placenta previa. Bleeding can be a sign and bed rest may be prescribed, as can an early delivery via Cesarean. However, the majority of mothers will not need to worry about placenta previa at the end of their pregnancies because only about 1 in 200 pregnancies suffer from this type of placental placement. It is more common to have a placenta previa if you have had a previous Cesarean section or uterine surgery.

## HOT MAMA

Sometimes when your baby is growing, your belly button decides to pop out. This can happen fairly early in pregnancy, or it may happen at the end. The good news is that it goes away after the baby is born. As far as dealing with it in pregnancy, there are two schools of thought: deal with it or ignore it.

If you chose to deal with it, you could try hiding it with clothing. This may mean wearing longer shirts that cover the area. You might also choose pants that hit just in that spot to lessen the definition of the small bump. Other moms just want their belly buttons to disappear. They try taping their belly buttons down, with varied success, only to deal with skin irritation from the adhesive (though it doesn't harm the baby).

## COPING WITH BED REST

Bed rest is not something that women look forward to in pregnancy. While in theory we all may dream of a day when we don't have to get out of bed, in reality it's very difficult to maintain for a variety of reasons. Lying in bed with nothing to do for long stretches or time can get very boring, and it also can become physically painful. The lack in movement leads to a loss of muscle tone and mass, and, in extreme cases, problems such as bedsores.

However, when medically necessary and done properly, bed rest can help lower your blood pressure, lessen the pressure on your cervix, and increase blood flow to your baby.

During pregnancy, you may find yourself placed on bed rest for a multitude of issues, many surrounding the health of your baby. Some examples include the following:

- Bleeding
- Preterm contractions
- Early dilation of the cervix
- Multiple babies
- Maternal conditions, such as extremely high blood pressure

Bed rest comes in a couple of forms. The lightest is more of a strict resting policy. You may be allowed to go to work and stay in one place all day, but you are asked to curtail physical and sexual activity. A stricter form of bed rest requires you to be at home lying down most of the day. You may be allowed to move from the bedroom to the couch, to get up for meals, and to take bathroom breaks. The strict-est form of home bed rest requires that you only get up for bathroom breaks and trips to the doctor or midwife. And finally, hospital bed rest is available for very severe cases.

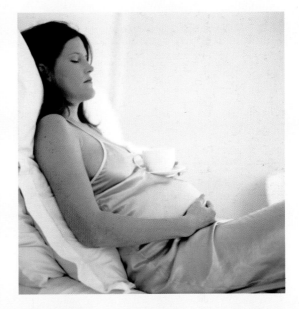

*Bed rest might sound like a good thing unless it happens to you. Be sure to tap into your support networks for help, both physical and emotional.*

Because many studies show that bed rest has potential drawbacks, it should only be used in cases where it is proven to be beneficial. For example, bleeding in early pregnancy is rarely helped with bed rest, but in later pregnancy it seems to make a difference. Some of the side effects of bed rest include the following:

- Loss of muscle mass and muscle tone
- Bedsores
- Emotional distress
- Family hardship

Talk to your doctor or midwife about support services available for moms-to-be on bed rest. For example, you might find that a physical therapist can help you with special exercises, and a postpartum doula might be available to prepare meals and do light housework.

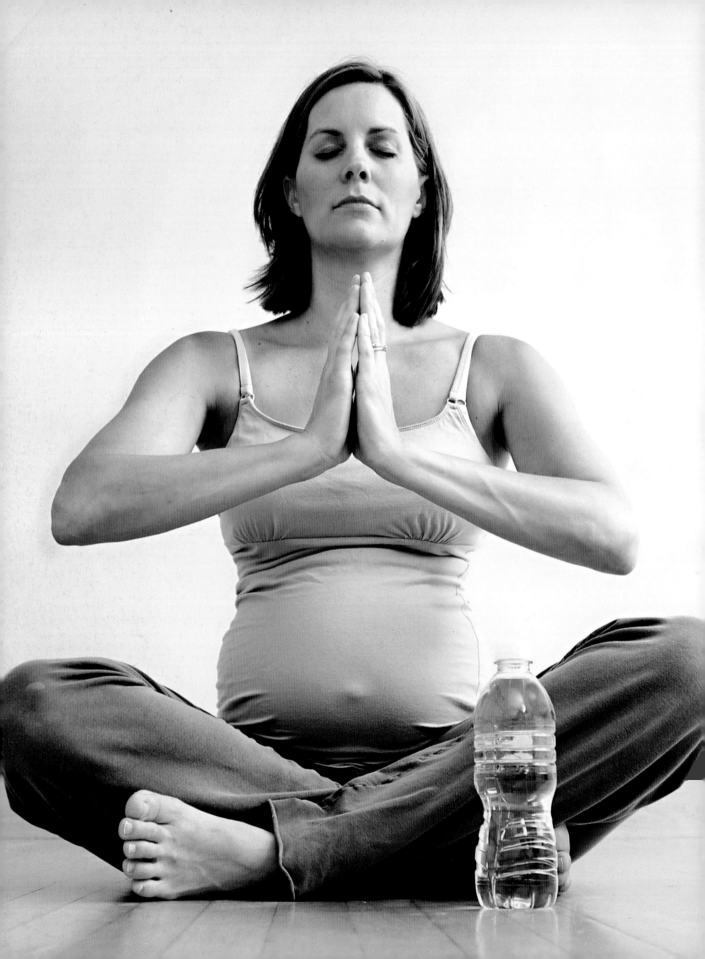

# WEEK 21

## ✏ CHECKLIST FOR WEEK 21

[ ] Order furniture on your list.
[ ] Plan a romantic getaway.
[ ] Know the signs of preterm labor.
[ ] Learn some yoga poses.

## 🔍 WHAT TO WATCH FOR THIS WEEK

**Swelling:** Watch for sudden swelling in the face or hand, which is a sign of pregnancy induced hypertension (PIH) or preeclampsia. Normal swelling in pregnancy does not come on suddenly, will dissipate after a period of rest, and is usually not severe.

### Double Check

**Headaches:** Severe headaches can point to problems with blood pressure that should be assessed by your practitioner. Sometimes a headache is the simple consequence of pregnancy hormones, or it may be part of a group of symptoms that make up PIH. You also need to rule out preeclampsia, a severe illness in pregnancy related to blood pressure, protein in your urine, and other complications.

**Blurred vision:** Blurred vision should be reported immediately to your practitioner as it is one of the signs of PIH and preeclampsia.

**Bleeding or spotting:** Bleeding or spotting at this point in pregnancy can happen after sexual intercourse, a vaginal exam, or vaginal ultrasound. In the absence of these activities, report any spotting to your practitioner, because it may be a sign of infection, premature dilation of the cervix, or issues related to your placenta.

**Back or abdominal pain:** Pain in your back or abdomen can be a sign of contractions or premature dilation of the cervix, a sign of potential preterm labor. **More than six contractions per hour.** This can be a sign of preterm labor. It can be normal to have contractions, just not at this frequency.

**Gush of fluid from the vagina:** This can be a sign that your water has broken prematurely. Your practitioner can determine if fluid leaking from your vagina is amniotic fluid or normal vaginal discharge.

*Report any strange or troublesome symptoms to your practitioner immediately.*

##  BODY BASICS

You are showing at least a bit and likely still feeling really good. You can move without feeling unencumbered, although some mornings you may wake up feeling stiff. Try doing some stretches before you get out of bed and right afterward. If you experience leg cramps, try doing calf stretches before bed and watch your diet for the right balance of nutrients, particularly calcium and potassium.

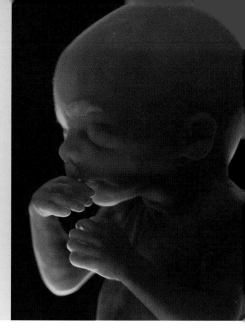

## BABY DATA

Your baby has been growing and growing. This week, your baby weighs in at about thirteen ounces (370 grams), just shy of a pound. Your pregnancy is halfway through, and your baby still has a lot of weight to gain, which will be his or her primary focus during the second half of your pregnancy.

Right now your baby is able to move throughout the uterus, flipping at will. Due to the increase in baby's weight, his or her movements will feel bigger, which can feel strange at times.

**PREGNANCY PARTICULARS**

## Order Furniture on Your List

If you have selected baby furniture that you want to order, it is wise to do so well in advance of when you think you will need it. Some retailers or manufacturers may say that your items will take between eight and twelve weeks to be delivered. If so, assume the outer end of the time frame, and you may be pleasantly surprised.

This means that if you order furniture this week, you can expect to receive the furniture around week 35 of your pregnancy. After this point, you're likely to be fairly tired, which will make the process of setting up new furniture a lot less fun.

When you order furniture, keep the following things in mind:

- Do you like the wood or material used?
- Does it match your other furniture?
- Is it safe for baby?
- Is the paint, if any, lead free and child safe?
- Are the slats on the crib at most 2⅜ inches apart?
- Did you choose a rocker or glider?
- Do you need a matching ottoman?
- Will this furniture grow with the baby?

- Do you need a changing table or does the top of the dresser have a changing table top with a safety strap?
- Is this furniture practical?
- Can you order similar furniture later if needed?

Among the biggest complaints from parents about nursery furniture is that they did not use all the stuff they purchased. Ask other parents what their must have items are and what they could have done without. This may save you from the unnecessary expense and hassle of buying more than you need.

## Plan a Romantic Getaway

It can be so easy to focus all your attention on your baby and the upcoming birth, but it is vitally important not to overlook your relationship. The two of you need to spend time together and focus on each other.

Many couples wait until very late in the pregnancy before planning a last-minute getaway. By then, however, the woman may not be feeling her best. It may also be a time when you'd rather not travel and would prefer to stay close to home, nest, and prepare for baby's arrival. Don't miss out on a fun trip with your honey. Plan something simple but special—just for the two of you.

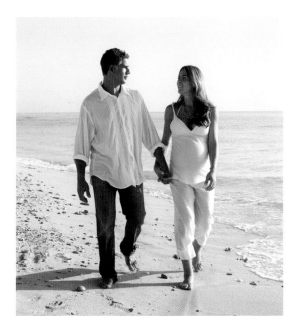

*A romantic getaway may be just what you need mid-pregnancy. Even if you can only get away for a night at a local B & B—go for it!*

## PREGNANCY AFFIRMATION FOR WEEK 21

# I am enjoying my pregnancy to the fullest.

special. Reserve a table at a new restaurant, see a movie, attend a play or concert, or make an appointment for a couples massage. When making the plans, keep in mind whatever physical limitations you may have at that point. For instance, sitting through a three-hour play in week 38 could be quite painful.

You might want to take a full-blown vacation, and that is terrific. Doctors usually don't place restrictions on travel until the very end of your pregnancy. And other than avoiding remote regions because of the vaccinations you'd need but shouldn't have, the choices are endless. Just plan the trip for a time in your pregnancy when you're feeling good enough to enjoy yourself.

Do not fall into the trap of thinking you can pull together something later. Life happens now, not later. Take any chance you get, whether it is a weekend or a week, to celebrate your happiness as a couple. Having a baby brings stress to every relationship, so you should renew yourselves while you have the chance.

You may even want to think ahead to your first getaway after the baby arrives. It may not happen for a while, but it's good to commit to doing it and have it to look forward to.

Spending time together does not have to involve a long vacation, which can be a problem if you're looking ahead to maternity and possibly paternity leave. It also does not have to cost an arm and a leg.

Try a local bed and breakfast. Stay in town and skip the long drives or air travel. Make a point of getting out and doing things in your own city that you haven't made the time for in the past.

Or spend the weekend in bed with a bunch of great movies. Without airport hassles or car traffic, you'll be amazed at how relaxing, romantic, and affordable a plan this is. Stay home, but tell everyone you're gone. This is the ultimate in inexpensive, quiet weekends. The trick is to resist answering your phone or doing housework. Instead, snuggle up, order in, and do whatever you want in the comfort of your own home.

Or if you can't swing a weekend away, set aside several nights over a month's time and plan dates. The planning is what matters if you want it to be

## Know the Signs of Preterm Labor

Preterm labor can be frightening, and it is on the rise. With a 20 percent increase since 1990, the latest data shows that nearly 13 percent of women will give birth before the thirty-seventh week of pregnancy.

The risks for babies born early include lengthy stays in the neonatal intensive care unit (NICU), breathing difficulties, permanent physical and mental handicaps, and a higher risk of death. It's a scary prospect for any parent, but the good news is that by watching for signs of preterm labor, you can help prevent preterm birth.

The signs of preterm labor include the following:

- More than six contractions in one hour
- Water breaking
- Increase in vaginal discharge
- Low back or abdominal pains, which may be like menstrual cramps
- Pelvic pressure

If you experience any of these signs prior to the 37th week of pregnancy, it is important that you report it immediately to your doctor or midwife. The sooner you report problems, the more likely it is that you practitioner will be able to stop labor.

You may be asked to try some simple things at home first, depending on your symptoms. For example, you may be asked to drink two large glasses of water or juice and to lie on your left side. Because some preterm labors are caused by dehydration, rehydrating the mother can be an easy fix. You will then be asked to report back after a certain period of time, such as after an hour.

You may also be asked to go to the hospital or your practitioner's office to be checked out or observed. They may try other treatments, including IV rehydration and medications administered orally, via IV, or intramuscularly to try to relax the uterus and stop contractions. You may be given a vaginal exam or an ultrasound exam to measure the internal portion of the cervix.

You should talk to your practitioner about preterm labor during one of your prenatal visits. The following women are at a higher risk of premature birth:

- Mothers carrying more than one baby
- Women with a history of preterm labor or birth
- Those who have had previous cervical surgery
- Women with vaginal infections

The best way to prevent preterm labor and birth is by keeping your prenatal appointments. This gives your practitioner a chance to look for subtle clues that you may be at risk for preterm labor. While it's not possible to prevent preterm labor and birth all of the time, screening is an effective way to reduce the numbers drastically.

**MEMORABLE MOMENTS**

"When I passed 20 weeks, I felt like I was on the downhill slide with my first pregnancy, like the hard part was over. With my next pregnancy, I knew better. I knew to save my energy and that the 'hard' part was to come. I knew I'd eventually stop feeling great and slowly descend into the end of pregnancy, where 'tired' ruled my day."

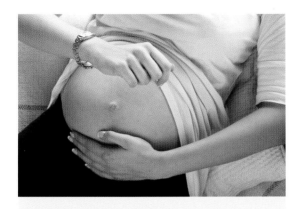

## HOW TO TIME CONTRACTIONS

Timing contractions is typically associated with later pregnancy and labor. But because one of the signs of preterm labor is contractions, it is important to have this information early in your pregnancy so that you can alert your doctor or midwife to any contractions you may be having.

The easiest way for some women to feel contractions is by placing their hands on their bellies. This may work best if you are sitting or lying while relaxing. If you are in a high-risk situation, such as carrying twins, your practitioner may have you do this once or twice a day just to monitor for contractions. You then note the start of a tightening, the time you notice when it starts and when the next one begins. The time from the beginning of a contraction to the end is how long your contraction lasts. The time from the beginning of one contraction to the beginning of the next is how far apart they are. If you are having contractions that are very far apart, you may be better able to say that you are having a certain number per hour.

Report contractions that occur more than six per hour to your practitioner immediately. This will give you both plenty of warning o try to stop preterm labor. If you can't get a hold of your practitioner, go to the emergency room with which your practitioner is associated.

# Learn Some Yoga Poses

Yoga is a great exercise for pregnancy. It helps to focus your body and also your mind. The nice thing is that even beginners can do some yoga poses in pregnancy. Here are some great poses for pregnancy. Depending on your experience level, hold the stretches anywhere from ten seconds to several minutes.

**Cat-Cow Pose:** This is a wonderful stretch for your back and belly and allows you to practice pelvic tilts.

Position yourself on your hands and knees, with your hands under your shoulders, with your palms down and fingers forward, and your knees aligned under your hips. (It's easier to do this on a yoga mat, which will relieve the pressure on your knees.) Try to keep your spine straight.

On your next breath, drop your gaze toward your belly and lengthen your spine upward, like a cat. This provides a great stretch of the upper back. Tuck your pelvis inward.

Next, slowly drop your belly down, which will simultaneously bring your tailbone up. Last, lift your gaze up to the sky.

**Cobbler's Pose:** This is a great stretch for your thighs and can be used in conjunction with relaxation or when you need to stretch.

Sit on the floor. Place the soles of your feet together and let your knees fall to the sides. You can rest your hands on your feet pressing inward. If you are a beginner or it is not comfortable, place yoga bricks under each knee to support them. If you don't have yoga bricks, you can improvise with cardboard boxes. (Even if you were able to do this without supports before, changes in your body, such as the production of Relaxin, can change how you move and feel in certain poses.)

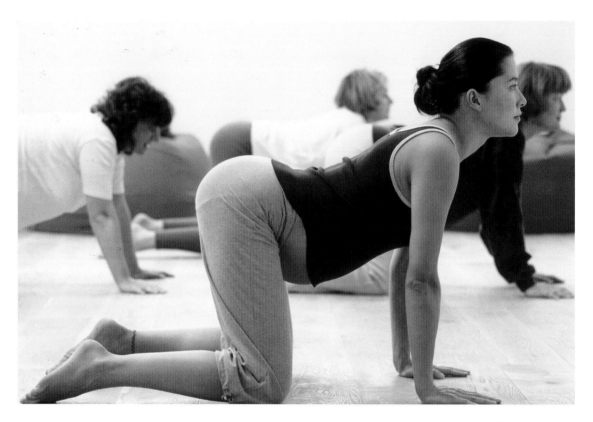

*Yoga can be a great way to connect with others as you learn to care for yourself in pregnancy. It's a great mind and body workout.*

**Pigeon Pose:** This pose stretches your upper and lower body.

Sit on the floor, as in Cobbler's Pose, with the soles of your feet together and your knees falling out to the sides. Next, extend one leg behind you with the sole of your foot facing up. Rest your hands forward on the floor on either side of your front leg. Stretch your chest open and forward, leaning your weight on your hands. Then switch legs.

**Child's Pose:** This pose is a great resting pose for relaxation or stretching. It can be done at any time in pregnancy. However, you may need to move your knees farther apart to accommodate your growing belly, and you may require a bolster or pillow to support your forehead.

Kneel on the floor and move your knees apart, making enough room for your belly. Try to keep your big toes touching behind you. Lean forward, moving your belly to the floor. Rest your forehead on the floor.

Your arms can lay on either side of you, palms facing upward, or lay your hands above your head with your palms facing downward.

## HOT MAMA

Because you will be pregnant for nine months, you will cycle through a few seasons of clothing. Will you need a maternity bathing suit or a winter coat? Either way, it's worth considering what you will need to keep up with changes in the weather—and your belly. Bathing suits are great for swimming year round, so you may want to invest in one early on. A heavy coat may be optional if you find that you're feeling really warm toward the end of your pregnancy. You might get away with wearing one of your nonpregnancy coats that you leave open.

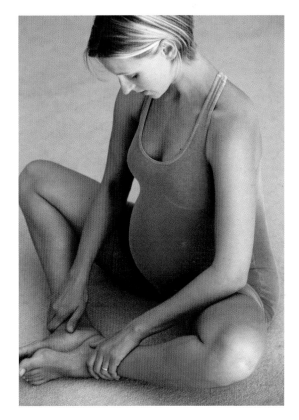

*Yoga at home can help alleviate certain pregnancy symptoms like back ache, cramps, and strains. It's also a great mental health break.*

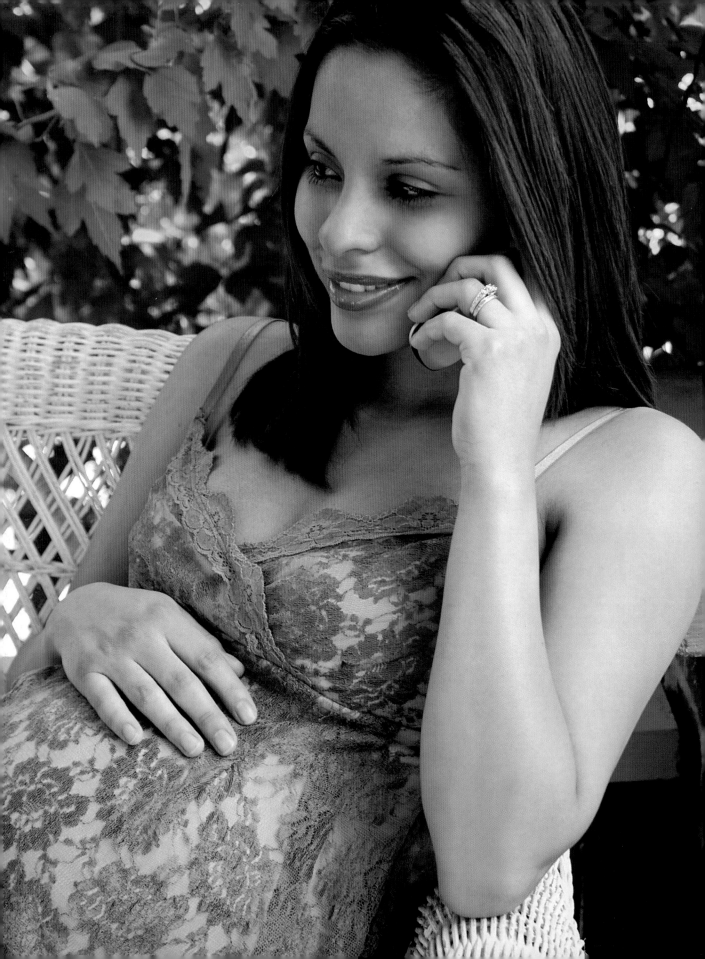

# WEEK 22

## ✎ CHECKLIST FOR WEEK 22

[ ] Begin to interview doulas.
[ ] Find out about domestic violence in pregnancy.
[ ] Ignore unsolicited advice from strangers.
[ ] Learn how to listen to a birth story.

## ⌕ WHAT TO WATCH FOR THIS WEEK

### Double Check

**Swelling:** Sudden swelling in the face or hands is an indication of pregnancy induced hypertension (PIH) or preeclampsia. Normal swelling in pregnancy does not come on suddenly, will go away after a period of rest, and is usually not severe.

**Headaches:** Headaches can be brought on by pregnancy hormones, but severe headaches can be a sign of issues with your blood pressure that your practitioner should examine. Moreover, a headache may be tied to PIH or even preeclampsia, which is a severe illness in pregnancy related to blood pressure, protein in your urine, and other complications.

**Blurred vision:** Blurred vision should be reported immediately to your practitioner, whether or not it is accompanied by a headache. It, too, can be a sign of PIH or preeclampsia.

**Bleeding or spotting:** Bleeding or spotting that is unconnected to sexual intercourse, a vaginal exam, or vaginal ultrasound should be reported immediately to your practitioner, because it may be a sign of infection, premature dilation of the cervix, or issues related to your placenta.

**Back or abdominal pain:** This type of pain can be a sign of contractions or premature dilation of the cervix, a sign of potential preterm labor.

**More than six contractions per hour:** Having contractions during the second trimester is not worrisome unless they happen too often. At this level of frequency, you might be having preterm labor and should consult your practitioner.

**Gush of fluid from the vagina:** Make an appointment to see your midwife or doctor to determine if the fluid leaking from your vagina is amniotic fluid or normal vaginal discharge.

*Report any strange or troublesome symptoms to your practitioner immediately.*

##  BODY BASICS

Your uterus is now growing past your belly button. As the lower part of your abdomen fills out, it becomes harder for you to hide the growing baby in your uterus. So if you haven't made the move to bigger clothes, you should get ready. And if there are people who stand to be hurt if the news of your pregnancy is delivered from another source, you had also better consider telling them before your burgeoning belly makes the announcement for you!

## 🛏 BABY DATA

It is hard to imagine that your baby who started out as two merging cells has grown so big. Your baby is practicing many of the skills that he or she will need after birth. This practice time is important to your baby. Your baby has been busy with reflexes, breathing, and even sucking.

This week, your baby weighs in at nearly a pound (450 grams). That is a huge gain from the beginning, when the weight was measured in terms of paper clips! Your baby is also nearly eleven inches (28 centimeters) long. Remember that your baby still has a lot of growing to do before birth.

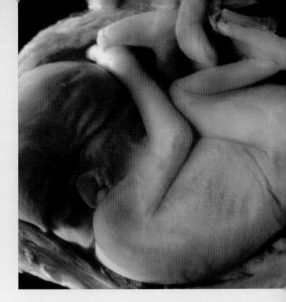

## Begin to Interview Doulas

A doula is a professional labor support person. Think of her as your private helper for your labor and birth. A doula is trained to help you find comfortable positions in labor and to use various techniques to stay comfortable—from back rubs and birth balls, to relaxation and even medications. Your doula can also help you address questions and understand language used during labor and birth, helping you to navigate the waters of your chosen birth place. A doula stays with you for the entire process; no shift changes or going off call as you might experience with hospital staff or even your primary care provider.

Studies show that using a doula can provide you with many, many benefits during labor and birth. It can help you have an easier, shorter, and more comfortable labor. A doula can help you reduce the likelihood of requiring certain interventions such as drugs to speed labor, an episiotomy (a surgical incision in the perineum), or a Cesarean section. And while the presence of a doula is linked to fewer requests for pain medications, most doulas will work with women who intend to use pain medications. Doulas are not only for women who want unmedicated births. Working alongside a doula also leads to positive postpartum outcomes, such as a decrease in postpartum depression and an increase in the length of breastfeeding.

If you're interested in hiring a doula, you should interview several to ensure that you have a good fit with the one you choose. Starting the interview process early can help you have more time to talk to your doula and to get to know her. When you interview doulas, you should be prepared to ask a series of questions, some of which may be generic and others that have specific importance to you, including the following:

- How much experience do you have?
- What is your training?
- Are you certified or working toward certification?
- Have you ever worked with my practitioner or at my place of birth?
- What is your fee?
- What does your fee cover?
- Do you have a back up in case you become unavailable? Can I meet her?
- Do you have any experience with (your method of childbirth education)?
- How do you see your role in my labor and birth?

- When will you join me in labor?
- How long will you stay with us after the birth?
- How will you include my partner and family?
- Can I call or email you with concerns or questions before the birth?
- How often will we meet before the birth?
- Will you meet with my practitioner if I desire?

You should try to talk to as many doulas as your can over the phone. When you have narrowed the list to two or three doulas, it's time to conduct personal interviews. During the interview, you should have a candid conversation about the type of birth you are looking for and how you intend to get it. Your final choice should be based on whom you felt the most comfortable with and how your questions were answered. Did you feel at ease? Did you feel listened to? How did your partner feel?

Once you have made your decision, it is time to look at the contract. Be sure that the contract has everything that you discussed, including a refund policy and payment arrangements. Doulas offer various prices across the United States and some include different services. Sometimes the fee is determined by the experience level of the doula.

Talk to your childbirth educator and your midwife or doctor about good doulas in the area. You should also ask friends who have used doulas in the past for recommendations. And finally, DONA International (formerly Doulas of North America) is a wonderful organization that you can contact for help gathering names in your area *www.dona.org*.

## Find Out about Domestic Violence in Pregnancy

Shocking as it may sound, domestic violence or intimate partner violence is more likely to start during pregnancy than at any other time in a woman's life. It is estimated that about in one in five women will be abused during pregnancy.

Signs of intimate partner violence can include the following:

PREGNANCY AFFIRMATION
FOR WEEK 22

# My body was designed to give birth.

- Bruises on the breasts or abdomen
- Delay in seeking prenatal care, or poor compliance with appointments
- Trouble sleeping
- Continued use of harmful substances in pregnancy (such as alcohol and tobacco)
- Psychosomatic illnesses

While all the major organizations of care practitioners for women recommend that every woman be screened for domestic violence, particularly in pregnancy, fewer than one-third of practitioners conduct the screening at the first prenatal visit, and even fewer screen at subsequent visits. Occasionally a woman may be asked random questions in the labor and birth units of many hospitals, but this is obviously very late in the game, and the woman's partner is typically present.

Violence in pregnancy has physical, mental, and emotional consequences. A woman may be physically hurt, and that damage extends to the developing baby. Moreover, women who are abused suffer complications such as abruption of the placenta (where the placenta prematurely separates from the uterus), leaking amniotic fluid, preterm labor, and hemorrhage. It is also a little known fact that homicide is the number one killer of pregnant women, even more so than car accidents and falls.

If you are having issues with domestic violence, or you know someone who is, it is critical that you seek support. It does not mean that you are weak

## WHAT ARE THESE STRAY BLACK HAIRS?

During your pregnancy, you may notice stray hairs growing in unexpected places. These hairs can be coarse and black, and they most often show up on your belly. It may not be a happy discovery, but nor is it a cause for concern. It is yet another symptom of the raging hormones in your body, and they usually show up right around now.

Do not believe old wives' tales that if you pull out one hair, two more will grow back in its place. Nor should you believe that the hairs can predict the sex of your baby. They are simply stray hairs that tend to vanish within a few months of giving birth.

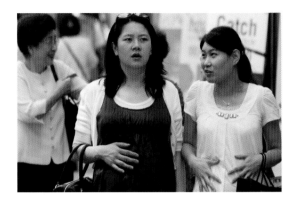

*Have a game plan in place to help you deal with unsolicited advice from strangers or people you know.*

or that something is wrong with you, despite what you may have been told. You can always go to your practitioner for support and help or seek support from a local resource, including your health department. The National Domestic Violence Hotline is 1-800-799-SAFE or *www.ndvh.org*.

## Ignore Unsolicited Advice from Strangers

The bigger your belly gets, the more strangers will be eager to talk to you. But unlike the advice you receive from people you know and trust, input from strangers can be difficult to accept. Well-intentioned people simply walk up to you, stroke your belly and dispense unwanted advice.

You could use any number of snarky replies to respond to these strangers, but most pregnant women tend to smile, stare blankly, and nod. How you respond depends on your personality and the particular situation. For example, the older woman who lives on your block might truly be concerned for your safety when she sees you carrying a lot of groceries, but the man on the subway who refuses to give up his seat because, "pregnant women need the exercise..." is just being rude.

The simple truth is that there is no shortage of free advice for pregnant women, and people feel more inclined to offer it as your abdomen grows larger. There may be only one point in your life when the amount of advice heaped on mothers tops that of late pregnancy: when you have a newborn baby.

You'd be smart to allow the proffered advice to go one ear and out the other. Don't get embroiled in a discussion by answering questions, even simple ones, like when are you due or is your baby a boy or a girl. Simply say or imply you're busy and have to rush off; then promptly leave. If you get caught—waiting in line, for instance—nod as if you're listening but don't do anything to feed their interest or the conversation. The goal is to move on as quickly as possible without being rude.

## Learn How to Listen to a Birth Story

There is a way to hear a birth story—and a way not to hear a birth story. For starters, virtually all women who have had babies—from your closest

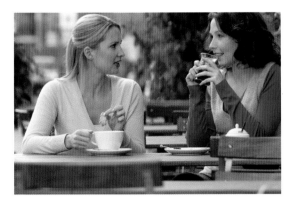

*Listening to other's birth stories can be a great way to learn about birth. But be sure to learn how to avoid the horror stories that can sometimes be offered.*

friends to complete strangers—love to tell their birth stories. It does not matter how traumatic or scary their stories are, they feel it is their public duty to tell you what they went through.

Now, hearing some birth stories is a good thing. It can give you an idea of how all the pieces of the pregnancy, labor, and birth puzzle go together. It can help give you a dose of reality. But it should never scare or unnerve you. The problem is that other people, especially people who don't know you, may have no clue what scares you.

Everyone has different fears when it comes to being pregnant or giving birth. One woman's ideal birth might be a short three-hour labor, and yet that might scare the mucous plug out of another woman. And regardless of where you fall on the scare meter, the fact is, you can't stop these stories from coming your way.

You can, however, put a damper on them. When someone begins to launch into a birth story, you can say a variety of things to stop them. Try the following on for size:

- I've already had my quota of birth stories today, thanks.
- My practitioner recommended I don't listen to birth stories because every birth is different.
- Excuse me, my bladder is calling.

- I can only agree to listen if you can promise it's not scary/bloody/worrisome (insert your requirements).
- I'd love to hear your story, but first I want to tell you about my first Pap smear.

Most birth stories are told for a reason. Sometimes the reason is altruistic — "I'm sorry I agreed to schedule an induction, my labor would have been much easier if I hadn't" or "If I had told my doctor about my symptoms sooner, perhaps we could have stopped labor." Other times it's nothing more than a woman eager to share an incredible moment in her life. Try to smile, ignore what you'd rather not hear, and take up the rest with your practitioner.

**HOT MAMA**

As you are shop for clothes, explore each store's return policy. Some stores have very strict policies with time limits as well as returns only for store credit. The same is true for online stores, which also sometimes charge return shipping fees and restocking fees. If you like to shop online, look for companies that accept returns at local brick-and-mortar stores.

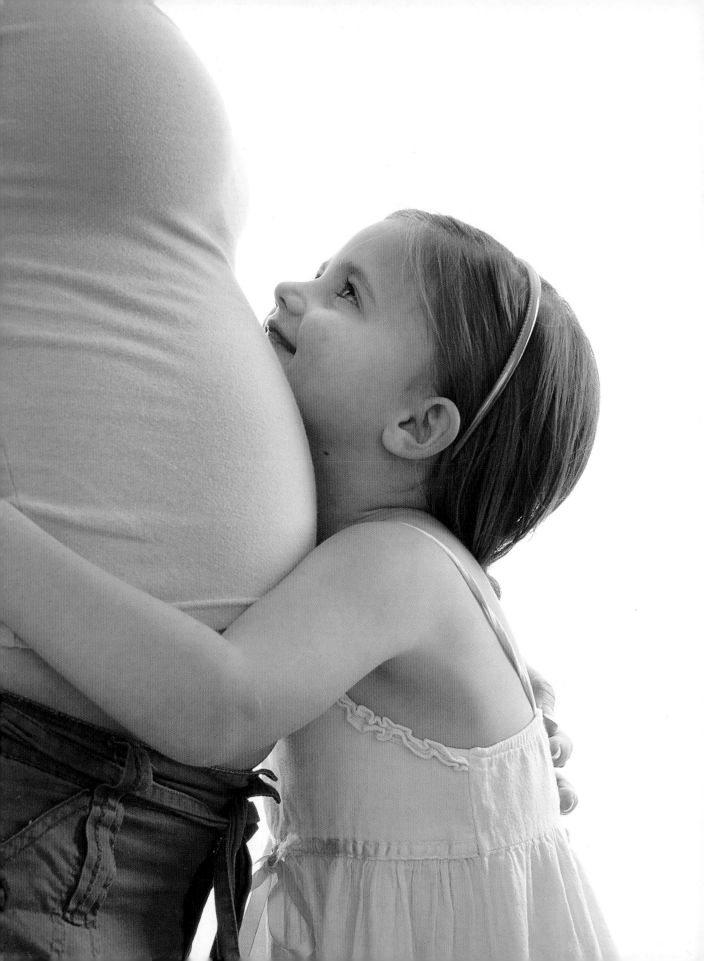

# WEEK 23

## ✎ CHECKLIST FOR WEEK 23

[ ] Check for stretch marks.
[ ] Learn about baby showers and other ceremonies.
[ ] Look for varicose veins.
[ ] Consider the shape of your belly.

## 🔍 WHAT TO WATCH FOR THIS WEEK

*Double Check*

**Swelling:** Swelling that develops suddenly in the face or hands is a sign of pregnancy induced hypertension (PIH) or preeclampsia. Swelling in pregnancy that is not worrisome develops gradually, goes away after a period of rest, and is not severe.

**Headaches:** When you suffer from severe headaches, it might be related to your blood pressure, and you should report the problem to your practitioner. It's possible that the headaches are nothing more than the result of pregnancy hormones, but you need to rule out PIH and preeclampsia, which is a severe illness in pregnancy related to blood pressure, protein in your urine, and other complications.

**Blurred vision:** If you find that your vision is blurry at times, contact your practitioner immediately because you might be suffering from PIH or preeclampsia.

**Bleeding or spotting:** Red or brown spotting at this point in pregnancy can happen after sexual intercourse, a vaginal exam, or vaginal ultrasound. You may be warned in advance of this possibility should you have this type of exam or activity. You should report bleeding or spotting unconnected to these activities immediately to your practitioner, because it may be a sign of infection, premature dilation of the cervix, or issues related to your placenta.

**Back or abdominal pain:** Pain in your back or abdomen can be a sign of contractions or premature dilation of the cervix, a sign of potential preterm labor.

**More than six contractions per hour:** This can be a sign of preterm labor. It can be normal to have contractions, just not at this frequency.

**Gush of fluid from the vagina:** This can be a sign that your amniotic sac has ruptured. Make an appointment to see your practitioner to determine if the fluid leaking from your vagina is amniotic fluid or normal vaginal discharge.

*Report any strange or troublesome symptoms to your practitioner immediately.*

##  BODY BASICS

You are becoming more comfortable with your pregnant body. You look good and very likely feel good, even though you find you are starting to tire more easily as the weeks go by. One helpful tip is to incorporate a short period of rest into every day, even if it's just a few minutes to lie down and read mail rather than running around preparing for dinner. If you have older kids, have them lie down with you and read together or go over homework. This small step can make you feel infinitely better.

## 🛒 BABY DATA

Your baby's intestines are lined with a thick, tarry substance known as meconium, which is your baby's first stool. It will normally not be seen until after birth and for the first few days of life. Occasionally your baby may leak a bit of stool just prior to birth into the amniotic fluid.

Lanugo, the fine hair on your baby, is darkening. (If your baby is born near or after his or her due date, the lanugo will mostly be gone.) The baby's fingernails are growing. By the time of birth, the nails may extend to the end of the finger tips, and some babies need their fingernails cut at birth. Your baby weighs in at just over a pound (450 grams)!

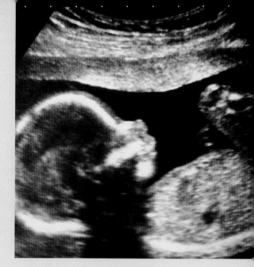

## Check for Stretch Marks

Stretch marks are something that many women worry about during pregnancy and sometimes even before pregnancy. The vast majority of pregnant women will get stretch marks on some part or parts of their bodies. Studies say that 50 to 90 percent of pregnant women will get them at some point in their pregnancy.

Stretch marks, which are also known as striae gravidarum, are the result of the collagen in your skin breaking down. This process isn't remotely painful; in fact, most mothers do not even notice it until they see the telltale red marks on their skin.

Stretch marks tend to appear on the abdomen, buttocks, breasts, and inner thighs and arms. While pregnancy is not the only time that people get stretch marks, it is among the most common. Stretch marks occur more frequently as the result of the following:

- Rapid growth or weight gain (such as in pregnancy and puberty)
- Family history of stretch marks
- Personal history of stretch marks
- Certain ethnicities that are more likely to get stretch marks
- Carrying more than one baby
- Having polyhydramnios (too much amniotic fluid)

Store shelves are full of lotions and creams promising to prevent or erase stretch marks. Plenty of women swear by products that help avoid stretch marks. The truth, however, is that very little can be done to prevent stretch marks, but every little bit counts.

First, eat a well-balanced diet and drink plenty of water. Healthy, well-nourished skin is more elastic and less apt to break down. You should also make an effort to gain weight slowly over the course of your pregnancy and avoid huge jumps in weight gain.

Try lotions that hydrate your skin and make it feel less itchy and raw as it expands. These products probably won't reduce the number or severity of stretch marks, but they will help you stay comfortable.

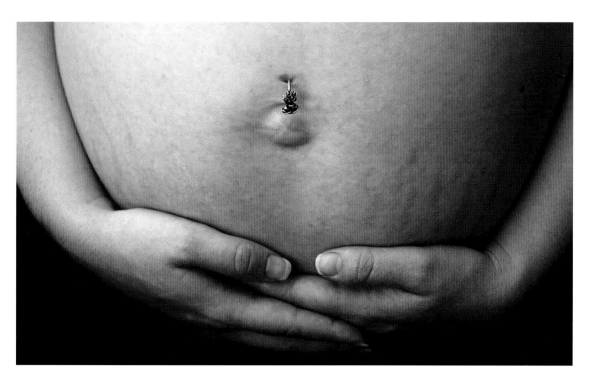

*Stretch marks may be in your future. Check your family history for the most reliable way to find out if that's what's in store for you, too.*

The good news is that while stretch marks may look bright red and angry in pregnancy, they are not destined to stay that way after you give birth. Over the course of the first few months postpartum, they will begin to fade to a silvery color.

There are some treatments to reduce stretch marks that you can use after giving birth, though most practitioners advise that you wait until you are completely done having children before embarking on expensive treatments that have varying levels of success.

## PREGNANCY AFFIRMATION FOR WEEK 23

## I am connected to my baby.

### Learn about Baby Showers and Other Ceremonies

Having a baby shower is a long-held tradition for first babies. Another ritual designed to help celebrate and welcome a new life is the mother blessing. Be sure to explore all of your options before deciding which celebration is right for you.

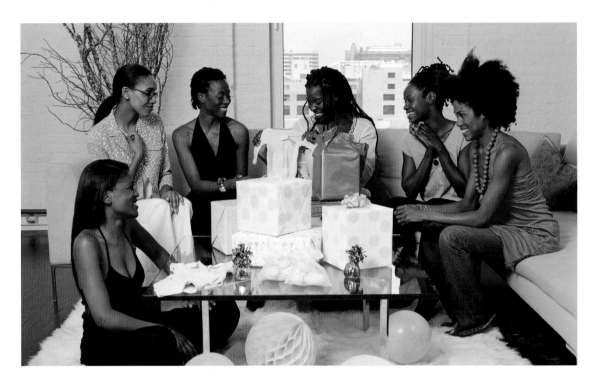

*Baby showers and other celebrations are a great way to pamper yourself as an expectant mother and share the joy of your upcoming arrival.*

## BABY SHOWERS

A traditional baby shower is typically very baby-centered with the expectant mother being showered with gifts for her newborn.

Baby showers are usually scheduled for the beginning of the third trimester, or as the needs of the pregnancy and family otherwise dictate. For instance, you might hold a baby shower earlier than the third trimester if the mother's family is in town for another event or holiday, or if the mother is expecting twins and prefers to have the shower sooner.

Baby shower food may depend on who is throwing the shower, what time of day or year the party takes place, and how many people are expected to attend. Whether it's a brunch or afternoon tea, there is almost always a baby shower cake and punch, and frequently baby-themed sweets and treats.

Baby shower games can be really fun or really silly, depending on your preference. There are baby shower games for almost every type of shower. Some bring a historical perspective, such as having guests bring baby pictures of themselves that get posted on a wall for all to guess who is who. Other games involve tasting baby foods or distributing diapers and guessing who has the "poopy" one.

Baby showers used to be for women only. This trend is changing as more and more couples decide that they want couples showers. Bringing men into the mix changes baby showers very little or a lot, again depending on the preferences of the guests of honor. Most likely, there will still be plenty of silly games, food, and piles of wrapped packages.

## MOTHER BLESSING

This type of celebration is very mother-centered. It comes from the Navajo tradition of a blessing way, blessing the journey a new mother will walk from labor and birth through early parenting. This celebration is a thoroughly positive event, with no horror stories or tales of seventy-two-hour labors; rather it is a chance for people to gather and give the mother-to-be special blessings and lavish her with attention.

Some mother blessings include prayer and scripture readings, while others may include belly casting (a plaster cast made of your belly), feet washing, or massage. Usually a gift that has been handmade communally is presented to the mother, such as a prayer flag with good wishes written by the attendees, a necklace with beads for labor, or even a quilt of blessings for the baby. Purchased gifts and games usually have no place at mother blessings.

To help attendees know what to expect, the invitation to a mother blessing should be quite specific about what will take place and what is asked of the invitees.

A mother blessing can be held at any point in pregnancy, though it is common to hold it fairly close to the birth. This allows the mother to take the good thoughts with her into labor and early parenting.

Although baby showers and mother blessings are the two most common types of baby celebrations that take place prior to a baby's arrival, you can have other types of celebrations, too. There can also be quiet dinner parties and other celebrations that are more family-focused or religious in nature. It's not unheard of to agree to more than one celebration, for example a family shower and a work celebration.

## BABY SHOWERS FOR SECOND BABIES

There is a controversy over whether or not second (or more) children deserve baby showers. The key to how you feel is probably rooted in how you see the purpose of a baby shower or party. If you feel that the primary purpose is for people to buy presents for a new baby, you will most likely think that having a shower for a second baby is inappropriate, unless the couple is having a baby of a different sex from their first, it's a second marriage and/or there have been number of years between children.

If, on the other hand, you tend to think of these celebrations as a way to celebrate the mom and her baby, having another shower is perfectly appropriate. Many second-time moms forgo presents at showers, because they already have everything they need, but they still want to gather with family and friends to celebrate a new life.

If gifts are welcome at a second baby shower, the invitation should reflect that and even suggest what type of gift guests should bring. Because the parents' needs have changed since having their first child, the following are the types of gifts that are popular at subsequent showers:

- Frozen meals
- Gifts to pamper the new mother
- Small gifts for the sibling-to-be

The choice as to what type of celebration you decide to have is personal, but the current wisdom is that every baby deserves to be celebrated in some manner. It is up to you to decide which celebration will make you feel special and supported by your friends and family.

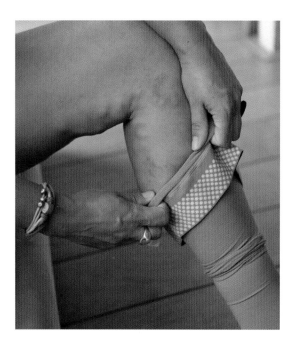

*While support hose are not typically a fashion statement you want to make, they can help you feel better and prevent blood clots. Talk to your practitioner.*

## Look for Varicose Veins

Varicose veins, which appear as bluish, bulgy squiggles on the legs, are veins that have lost some of their elasticity. They can develop during pregnancy due to hormones and the increased blood work load.

In pregnancy, a woman's blood volume increases to accommodate the baby. Your body works hard to circulate this blood through your entire system. However, it is more difficult for your legs to return the flow of blood, forcing your lower body to work harder as you gain weight. The strain, along with hormonal indications, can cause the veins to break down.

While you may not be able to prevent varicose veins, the following are some measures that you can take:

- Exercise regularly
- Prop your feet up while sitting down
- Do not stand for long periods of time, particularly in a stationary position
- Wear support hose as directed by your practitioner
- Do not gain excessive amounts of weight
- Move frequently throughout the day
- Lie with your feet higher than your head for about thirty minutes a day

Some practitioners may also recommend that you take vitamins to help you with vein elasticity, such as vitamin C. Be sure to talk to your practitioner before self-medicating with vitamins because it is possible to ingest too much of certain vitamins.

If you develop varicose veins, avoid massaging them, even if they tingle or are painful, because you can loosen blood clots. Use some or all of the suggestions above to minimize the appearance of varicose veins and the likelihood that new varicosities will form.

After pregnancy, you can have your veins treated, although most doctors request that you are done having children before fixing varicosities in your lower extremities.

## Consider the Shape of Your Belly

If you have not been documenting your pregnancy with photos, now is the perfect time to start. It's an amazing process to watch your belly develop and change shape over the course of your pregnancy. Now that your baby is bigger and your belly is bigger, your shape will change as your baby moves. One day your belly may look really small and a few hours later, it may look huge—all because your baby shifted his or her position in your uterus!

Try to enjoy these changes, even when they present a wardrobe issue because just this morning you still fit into your in-between clothes. Study the shape of your belly and try to guess the

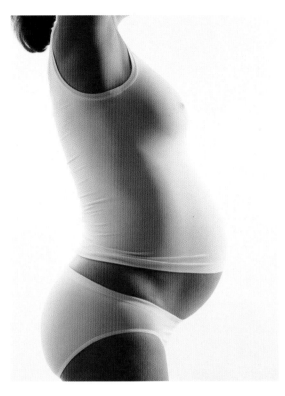

*The shape of your belly doesn't tell us the sex of your baby, but it's still fun to look at, to consider where your baby is, and how he or she is positioned.*

baby's exact position. Some couples use eyeliner to draw pictures on the belly to help them figure it out by tracing the baby as it moves and how each movement alters the shape of the belly.

At this stage of the game, your baby is doing lots of flips and turns, so his or her position can change rapidly and frequently. This will not be the case for long. Most babies begin to settle into a head-down position starting at about week 28. This will differ slightly if you have had a baby before or if you are having multiple babies.

## HOT MAMA

You may love your perfume or you may have grown tired of the scent. Pregnancy can be the perfect time to try a new, light scent. Find something that matches a cheerful, upbeat you and try it for a while. You might find that a new scent gives you a soothed or refreshed feeling you didn't even know you were missing. After your baby comes, you may find you want to return to your old perfume or stick with the new scent. The choice is yours.

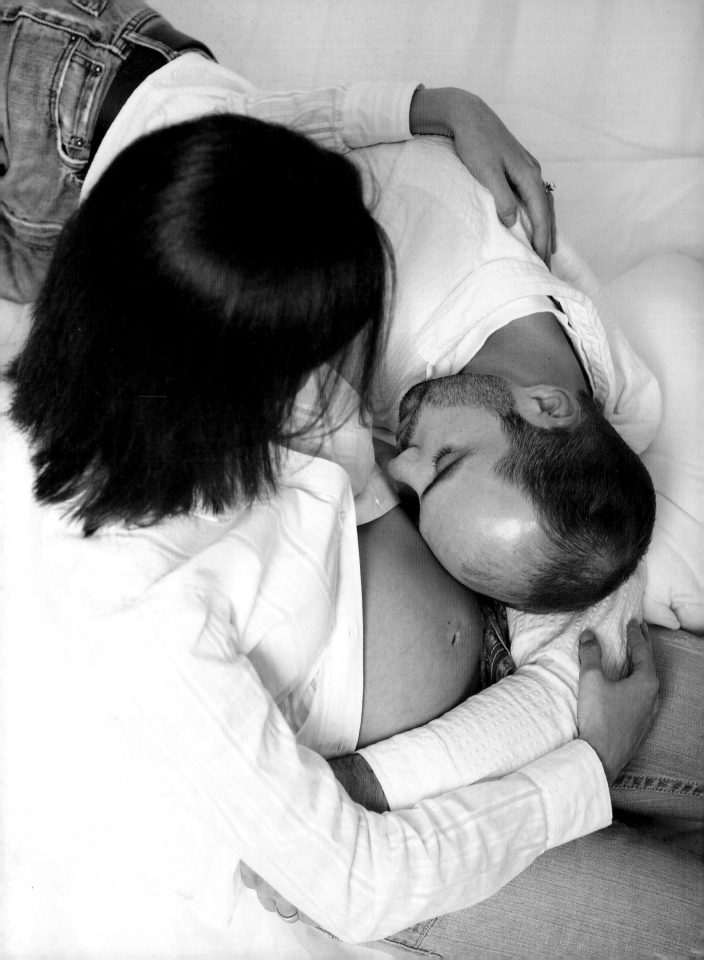

# Week 24

## CHECKLIST FOR WEEK 24

[ ]  Start fetal kick counts.
[ ]  Begin to interview pediatricians.
[ ]  Consider your belly button ring.
[ ]  Treat snoring and a stuffy nose.

## WHAT TO WATCH FOR THIS WEEK

*Double Check*

**Swelling:** If you notice a sudden swelling in your face or hands—signs of pregnancy induced hypertension (PIH) or preeclampsia—contact your practitioner. Normal swelling during pregnancy tends not to be severe or sudden and will go away following a period of rest.

**Headaches:** Severe headaches can be a sign of issues with your blood pressure that can be determined by your practitioner. Sometimes headaches are the product of pregnancy hormones, or they may be tied to other symptoms that together are known as PIH or even preeclampsia, which is a severe illness in pregnancy related to blood pressure, protein in your urine, and other complications.

**Blurred vision:** Report blurred vision to your practitioner right away. Like severe headaches, it can be a sign of PIH or preeclampsia.

**Bleeding or spotting:** Bleeding or spotting at this point in pregnancy is normal following sexual intercourse, a vaginal exam, or vaginal ultrasound. Bleeding or spotting that happens at other times should be reported immediately to your practitioner, because it may be a sign of infection, premature dilation of the cervix, or issues related to your placenta.

**Back or abdominal pain:** Pain in your back or abdomen can be a sign of contractions or premature dilation of the cervix, a sign of potential preterm labor.

**More than six contractions per hour:** Contractions that take place at this rate raise the possibility of preterm labor.

**Gush of fluid from the vagina:** Report this symptom to your doctor or midwife to determine if your water has broken prematurely or if the fluid leaking from your vagina is normal vaginal discharge.

*Report any strange or troublesome symptoms to your practitioner immediately.*

##  BODY BASICS

Your uterus measures about twenty-four centimeters from your pubic bone all the way to the top of the fundus. You can really feel your baby move, and you might even notice that your baby has sleep and wake cycles when he or she is active or at rest. Starting about now, others might be able to feel some of the baby's bigger kicks and punches.

## 🛒 BABY DATA

Week 24 has great significance for your baby. This is the week when neonatologists would give the baby a reasonable chance of survival if he or she were born early. Typically, babies born early don't go home until what would have been their original due dates, which is more than three months away at this point.

Your baby is busy working on maturing his or her lungs to prepare for life outside your uterus. He or she is also layering more brown fat to help regulate body temperature at birth.

This week your baby is nearly twelve inches long (30 centimeters) and weighs a bit over a pound (450 grams), inching toward that pound-and-a-half mark.

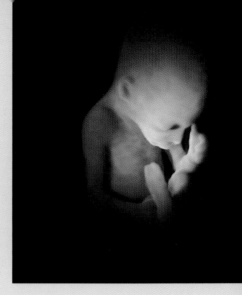

PREGNANCY PARTICULARS

## Start Fetal Kick Counts

You are your baby's best monitoring system. At various points in your pregnancy, your practitioner will recommend that you begin to monitor your baby's movements. This is done through what is called a fetal kick count.

Research has shown that fetal movement is one of the best indicators of your baby's health. Because you are the one through which all movements flow, you are also the best source of this information. The fetal kick counts are an organized way of keeping track of your baby's movements.

There are a few different ways to do fetal kick counts. The simplest is usually the easiest way to start or if you have a low-risk pregnancy. You simply pick a time of day that your baby tends to be very active and count how many movements you have during a thirty-minute period. A movement can be a kick, roll, punch, or flip

If your baby does ten of these movements before the thirty minutes are up, you are done until the next day. You should do this every day until your baby is born.

If after thirty minutes of counting, you have not recorded ten movements, it is normally recommended that you eat something and lie down on your left side and count for another thirty minutes. If after this time is up, you still do not feel ten movements, you should call your practitioner for advice.

It is recommended that you write down the fetal kick counts. It can be difficult to rely on your memory in pregnancy, particularly when it's something that you are doing on a daily basis. By keeping a small chart or list, you can easily refer back to your baby's history of movements to notice small changes.

Babies have sleep and wake cycles just like adults. Occasionally they will sleep while you are trying to do your fetal kick counts. Sometimes they are simply not moving as much and nothing is wrong, but further investigation is warranted to ensure the health of your baby.

Your midwife or doctor may suggest that you wait to start fetal kick counts until later in your pregnancy, such as week 28 or even 32. Your practitioner will help make the determination for you.

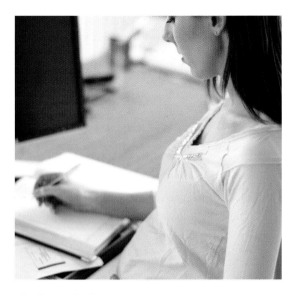

*The choice of pediatrician is an important one. Use your list of questions as you interview potential doctors.*

## Begin to Interview Pediatricians

A pediatrician is a physician trained to care for children from infancy to early adulthood. The vast majority of parents use a pediatrician for their baby's care, though you also have the option of a neonatologist (a specialist for premature and ill babies), a certified nurse midwife (trained in well baby care for the first year), or a family practitioner (trained to care for the family's general health at all ages). Whomever you pick to care for your baby is going to play a very important role in your life in the upcoming months and years.

It is important to start your pediatrician search early. This allows you a chance to meet your choices and to find one that is the best fit for your family.

Ask other new parents for recommendations. Find out whom your insurance covers and recommends. Then compile a list and begin making calls. Prepare a few questions to help you narrow your list on the phone. Some deal-breaking questions might include the following:

- Insurance issues
- Staff politeness
- Office hours and locations

## PREGNANCY AFFIRMATION FOR WEEK 24

✚

# I know my baby's movements.

Once you have narrowed your choices down to a handful of names, it is time to conduct the interviews. The vast majority of pediatricians will not charge you for an interview. Most will agree to meet with you in the office, so come prepared to be brief and focused. Some pediatricians hold new-parent meetings when you can meet the members of the practice. While this is a nice touch, be sure that there is time for you to speak privately to a physician or two. If this meeting is held in a location other than their office, ask to come in to see the office before making a final decision.

While there are lots of questions you will want to ask the candidates, be sure to trust your gut instinct. If you get a great vibe or an off feeling from someone, do not ignore it. Remember, you have to be comfortable calling this person at all hours of the day or night, even if you're not sure something is wrong with your baby. You want to find the practitioner who will help you without belittling you.

Consider the following:

- Office hours (be sure to ask about evenings and weekends)
- Office location
- Types of insurance acceptance
- Parenting philosophies
- Important health issues (such as vaccinations, antibiotic use, and breastfeeding)
- Number of practitioners in the practice
- Hospitals attended by the practitioner

## AROMATHERAPY

Aromatherapy is the art of using smell to help alter how you feel emotionally and even physically. Certain scents have been known for centuries to influence our feelings and our bodies. You have most likely used aromatherapy without even thinking about it, such as with room scents or perfume

The science behind aromatherapy is a bit more advanced than what's behind a room spray. Think about what how certain scents make you hungry or sleepy or happy. For example, lavender has long been known to help promote relaxation, which explains why so many relaxation aids are treated with the herb.

True aromatherapy uses essential oils, which are distilled from plants. These highly concentrated oils are normally diluted in lotions or in a bath before being used. A diffuser can also be used to spread a scent over a large room or other area.

Other common scents include peppermint for energy, chamomile for relaxation, and neroli for anxiety. You can visit any health food store or herb shop to learn more about essential oils and aromatherapy. Be sure that the practitioner knows that you are pregnant. It's unsafe to use certain oils in pregnancy, but they may be fine to use during labor.

- Tone of the office staff
- Cleanliness of the office

When you make a final choice, share your birth plan with him or her. If the plan is done when you

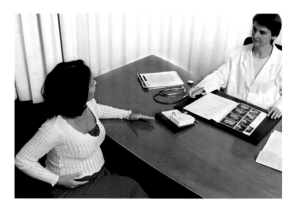

*A personal interview will go a long way to helping you select the right match.*

meet with them, feel free to bring it along. Once your baby is born, he or she becomes the responsibility of the pediatrician and not your practitioner any more. So the pediatrician will be the person to sign orders for things you may wish to have or not have for your baby in the nursery. If you don't have a birth plan ready, ask how to send it to them at a later date. Many will fax it back to you with a signature, acknowledging that they have read and approved it.

## Consider Your Belly Button Ring

If you have a belly button or navel ring, you are likely wondering what you need to do as the pregnancy progresses. The answer is there is no standard answer.

It is up to you whether you take it out or leave it in. In the past, the issue with leaving it in has been that belly button jewelry failed to expand far enough to be comfortable during pregnancy. Newer forms of belly jewelry have made it easier for pregnant women to maintain their piercings—and even get new piercings.

If you choose to take out your belly ring, you may want to consider how long ago you got the piercing and if there's a chance the hole will close up. Some women don't really care one way or the other, while others would rather not have to re-pierce.

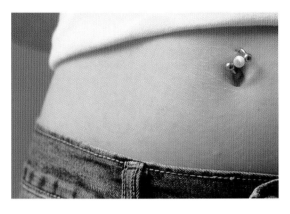

*Talking to your doctor or midwife about your belly button ring can save you some heartache down the line.*

## Treat Snoring and a Stuffy Nose

As you move further into your pregnancy, you may notice that you are experiencing nasal issues such as snoring and a stuffy nose. While these are fairly common occurrences in pregnancy, they can be quite annoying for you and those around you.

Snoring is about more than simply bothering your mate. Snoring can cause you to get poor or insufficient sleep, leaving you more tired than ever during waking hours. A chronic lack of sleep can have ill effects on you and your pregnancy, including a rise in your blood pressure.

Roughly half of all pregnant women snore, most commonly in the third trimester when the air passages begin to narrow. Some women find relief when they sleep in an upright or inclined position, while others rely on strips such as the Breathe Right strips to help prevent snoring and its associated consequences.

Stuffy noses can similarly lead to snoring at night and difficult breathing during the day. While it is not recommended that you use medicinal treatments on a regular basis, you can try other methods to help clear your sinuses. Some of these include using a humidifier, inhaling a saline solution, and other home remedies as approved by your practitioner.

**HOT MAMA**

Your feet might be in need of some loving kindness in the second half of your pregnancy. Be sure that you are wearing comfortable, well-fitting shoes. This may mean buying new shoes. Pick a store with helpful, knowledgeable salespeople who can assist you. Choose shoes that have low or no heels and that are comfortable for everyday wear. You may also wish to shop in the afternoon or evening because everyone's feet are bigger at that time of day, especially in pregnancy. Don't assume your old shoe size still applies. Some pregnant women say that their shoe sizes increased permanently during pregnancy.

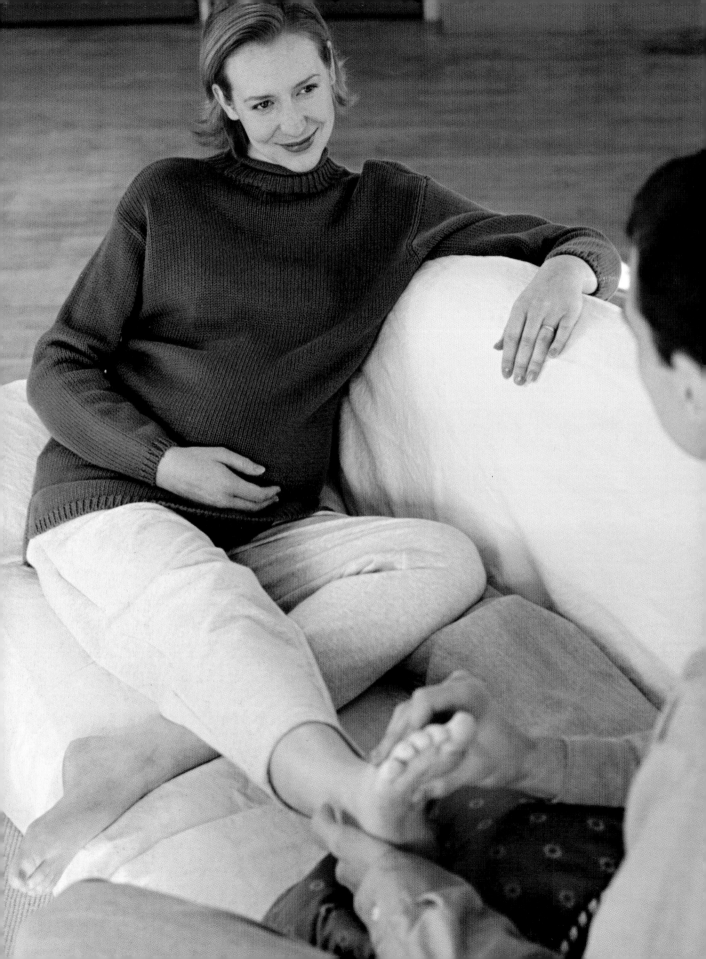

# WEEK 25

## ✏ CHECKLIST FOR WEEK 25

[ ] Talk to your baby.
[ ] Add to your pregnancy journal.
[ ] Learn about pelvic pressure.
[ ] Check for spider veins.
[ ] Discuss important topics with your practitioner.

## ○ WHAT TO WATCH FOR THIS WEEK

### Double Check

**Swelling:** Watch for sudden swelling in the face or hands, which are signs of pregnancy induced hypertension (PIH) or preeclampsia. During pregnancy, regular swelling develops slowly and will go away after a period of rest.

**Headaches:** Severe headaches can be a sign of potential problems with your blood pressure and should be discussed with your practitioner. They could be a side effect of pregnancy hormones, or they may be a symptom of something more serious, such as PIH or even preeclampsia, which is a severe illness in pregnancy related to blood pressure, protein in your urine, and other complications.

**Blurred vision:** Report blurred vision immediately to your practitioner, whether or not you also have been experiencing headaches. Vision problems are another sign of PIH and preeclampsia.

**Bleeding or spotting:** Bleeding or spotting (red or brown) that shows up at this point in pregnancy can result from sexual intercourse, a vaginal exam, or vaginal ultrasound. Typically, you are told before this type of exam that spotting may result. However, bleeding that has nothing to do with sex or vaginal exams should be reported immediately to your practitioner, because it may be a sign of infection, premature dilation of the cervix, or issues related to your placenta.

**Back or abdominal pain:** Pain in these regions can sometimes accompany contractions or be linked to premature dilation of the cervix, a sign of potential preterm labor.

**More than six contractions per hour:** This can be a sign of preterm labor. While it is normal to experience contractions at this stage of pregnancy, having them at this frequency is out of the ordinary, and you should contact your practitioner.

**Gush of fluid from the vagina:** It is possible that your water has broken prematurely, so call your doctor or midwife. He or she can determine if the fluid leaking from your vagina is amniotic fluid or normal vaginal discharge.

*Report any strange or troublesome symptoms to your practitioner immediately.*

##  BODY BASICS

Your body is slowly morphing into that of a very pregnant woman. Every week, you may notice gradual changes, or it may seem that your body changes overnight. These changes can be a bit alarming if you are not prepared for them. The good news is that it typically takes the full nine months to reach the point where you are tired of being pregnant. Try to remember that each stage of pregnancy offers something special, although sometimes you have to look hard to figure out what that is for you.

As easy as it can be sometimes, try not to wish your pregnancy would hurry up and move on to the next phase. Believe it or not, you will miss some things about pregnancy. If you are having a rough day, sit down and try to make a list of things you want to remember about being pregnant: Strangers offering you their seats on the subway or holding doors for you. Extra foot rubs from your husband. Or maybe you discover that grandma panties are much more comfortable than you ever imagined.

## BABY DATA

This week, your baby reopens his or her eyes, which have been closed since the eyelids fused around week 10. Your baby can now open and close his or her eyes at will. Your baby's bones are continuing to harden in a process called ossification; this will continue through the first years of life.

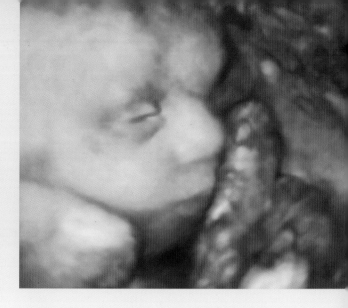

Your baby is continuing to grow, weighing in this week at just over a pound and a half (680 grams). The average birth weight for a baby is seven and a half pounds. That tells you that over the next fifteen weeks, your baby will put on the majority of his or her weight in preparation for birth.

## Talk to Your Baby

Talking to your baby is a great way to promote bonding before birth. Starting at this point in your pregnancy, your baby can hear your voice. The uterus is not a quiet place, and your baby has grown accustomed to hearing the sounds of your digestion, blood flow, and other bodily processes. The sound of your voice is a soothing and welcome addition.

You may wonder what you should say to your baby. The answer is whatever comes naturally. You could give an account of what you did that day. Or let your baby in on your hopes and dreams. What you say is much less important than the simple fact that your baby begins to hear and recognize your voice.

If you want to talk to your baby but really do not know where to start, sometimes reading a book works best. Read one of your favorite childhood stories or a passage from a book you are currently enjoying, whether or not it's baby related.

Books are also great ways for your partner to connect with the baby. Studies have shown that babies whose moms and dads read or sang to them in utero knew their voices after they were born. This is an incredible feeling, particularly for dads, when the baby turns toward them after recognizing their voices.

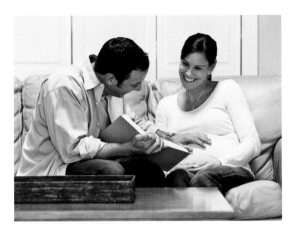

*If dad is too shy to talk to the baby, try having him read a book. It can be his favorite kid's book or his current favorite. Heck, even the newspaper works.*

## Add to Your Pregnancy Journal

If you have been neglecting your pregnancy journal, now is a great time to pick it up again. Be sure to record even the smallest, seemingly insignificant things you are doing or thinking during your pregnancy. You might include the following:

- Food cravings
- Thoughts, dreams, and desires
- How you feel about your body
- What you are doing to prepare for your baby
- What you are learning about childbirth and postpartum
- Photos of you pregnant

Some families write letters to their babies. These letters can incorporate the topics listed above or be completely different in nature. You can even create some artwork, whether it's a drawing, a collage of ads from stuff you are gathering for your baby, or a scrapbook.

## Learn about Pelvic Pressure

Pelvic pressure can be scary because the sensation almost feels like your baby is falling out. The reason many women feel pelvic pressure is due

### PREGNANCY AFFIRMATION FOR WEEK 25

### I accept my pregnancy for what it is.

to the increased weight of the uterus. The key is learning to distinguish between problematic pelvic pressure and pelvic pressure that is normal.

The best advice is not to take chances. Report any feeling of pelvic pressure to your practitioner. He or she will assess whether your pelvic pressure is due to a pregnancy complication or if it's normal intensity pelvic pressure.

It is not unusual to feel added pressure if this is not your first baby or if you are carrying more than one baby. Sometimes the sensation is actually pressure from your bladder. Doing Kegel exercises can be helpful in preventing or relieving the feeling of pressure. Your doctor or midwife might recommend that you do these exercises or wear a prenatal harness, such as the Prenatal Cradle, which helps distribute the weight elsewhere, such as your shoulders, hips, and back.

## Check for Spider Veins

Spider veins, also called spider nevi, are small blood vessels that can appear in pregnancy. They are the result of heredity, poor blood circulation, and increased blood flow in pregnancy. They appear as tiny reddish or purplish veins on the surface of the skin, and they are most commonly found on the face and legs but can appear nearly anywhere including the chest, arms, and neck. Spider veins are typically not painful.

Spider veins are more common in Caucasian women and in women who have a family history of them. The good news is that they will usually fade

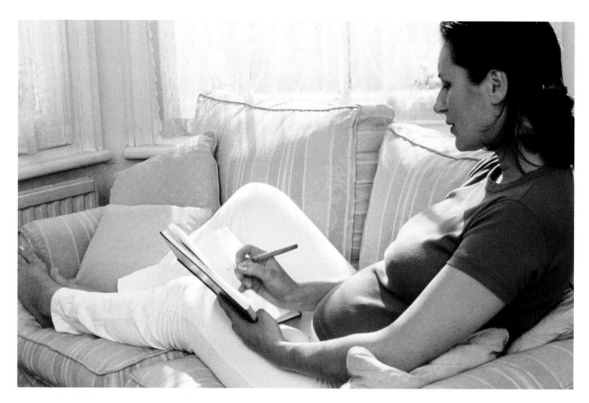

*Writing down questions and topics you want to discuss as you think of them between appointments, is a great way to ensure that you remember to have the conversation at your next prenatal visit.*

within three months of giving birth even without treatment. The bad news is that it's possible to develop varicose veins as well as spider veins.

To minimize your chances of getting spider veins, treat your legs well. Try not to stand for long periods of time. Rest with your legs up when you can during the day. Exercise and eat a well balanced diet.

## Discuss Important Topics with Your Practitioner

Talking to your practitioner should, by this point, feel natural and easy. By now you are likely to have a lot of questions, though the nature of these questions is beginning to change from questions you had earlier in your pregnancy.

Because your pregnancy is nearing the final months, you are probably starting to think about labor and birth. Here are some important topics to discuss with your practitioner.

WHEN TO COME TO THE PLACE OF BIRTH: Be sure to talk to your practitioner about when to head to the hospital or birth center. Explain whether you would prefer to hang out at home as long as possible or go in during active labor because that information may change their answer.

GENERAL POLICIES: Do they have a standard labor and birth policy for every patient? Can you get a copy of it? Is it negotiable? You should also ask about on-call schedules, to determine what your chances are of having your preferred doctor or midwife.

FETAL MONITORING: What type of fetal monitoring do they use? Do they go by the intermittent monitoring standards of the

American College of Obstetricians and Gynecologists? Will there be underwater or telemetry monitoring available?

INDUCTION POLICY: What is the practice's induction policy? At what point in pregnancy does the practice recommend induction? What percentage of the practice's births are induced?

EPISIOTOMY: Is there a policy on episiotomy? What practices can you employ before birth to prevent the need for an episiotomy or tear? What will your practitioner do at the time of birth to avoid an episiotomy or tear?

PAIN RELIEF IN LABOR: What forms of pain relief do they use? Will they order a transelectrical nerve stimulation (TENS) unit if you request it? Do they know about sterile water injections? (These are nonmedicinal injections to help relieve back pain, see 279.) Will they support you in having an unmedicated birth if that's what you wish? Do they have a policy on when an epidural (a medication injected through a catheter placed in your spine for continuous pain relief in labor) or other narcotics can be used in labor?

Remember that there is still plenty of time to discuss these and other topics, and your questions do not have to be resolved in one visit. And be sure to use positive communication skills when talking to your doctor or midwife. When you start a conversation, let them know that you value their opinions but that you also have ideas and desires. You should actively listen to what they have to say and expect the same from them. If they act like they do not have the time to listen, ask if there is a better time for you to schedule a lengthier discussion. This does not have to be during a prenatal visit.

## HOT MAMA

Some women may be tempted to hide their bellies—going so far as to actively try to avoid looking pregnant. Not only is this physically uncomfortable, but it usually leads to some emotional instability. Be proud of your belly. Talk to your midwife or doctor about your concerns. You might be afraid to tell someone you are expecting, or you may have unresolved body issues. These are normal feelings that you shouldn't try to conceal. In terms of being comfortable, however, it is best to work on these issues before you bust your seams.

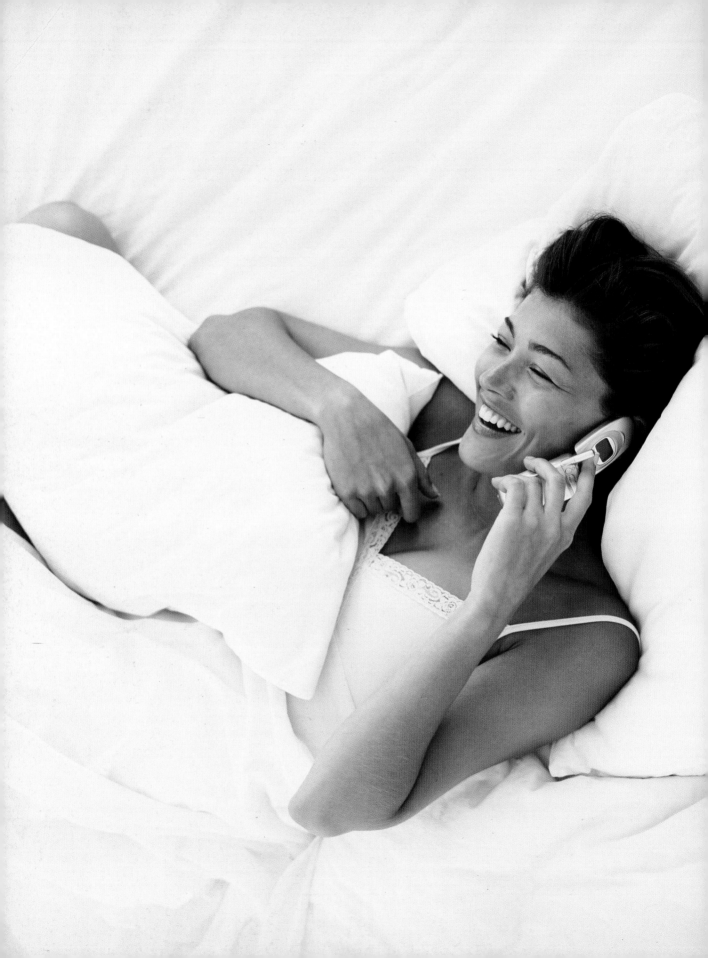

# WEEK 26

## ✎ CHECKLIST FOR WEEK 25

[ ] Check your newborn coverage with your insurance carrier.

[ ] Schedule your glucose tolerance test.

[ ] Resolve any conflicts with your practitioner.

[ ] Start thinking about baby names.

[ ] Buy a body pillow.

## ⚲ WHAT TO WATCH FOR THIS WEEK

**Swelling:** If you notice sudden swelling in the face or hands, it could be signs of pregnancy induced hypertension (PIH) or preeclampsia. It's not unusual for pregnant women to experience some swelling, but it's not severe, comes on gradually, and will go away after resting.

**Headaches:** Sometimes pregnancy hormones trigger headaches, but particularly severe headaches can be a sign of blood pressure abnormalities. Talk to your practitioner if you are concerned and to determine if you might have (PIH) or even preeclampsia, which is a severe illness in pregnancy related to blood pressure, protein in your urine, and other complications.

**Blurred vision:** Report blurred vision immediately to your practitioner; it can be a sign of PIH or preeclampsia.

**Bleeding or spotting:** Bleeding or spotting may be a sign of infection, premature dilation of the cervix, or issues related to your placenta. If, however, you've recently had sexual intercourse, a vaginal exam, or a vaginal ultrasound, spotting may be perfectly normal.

**Back or abdominal pain:** Pain in your back or abdomen can be a sign of contractions or premature dilation of the cervix, a sign of potential preterm labor.

**More than six contractions per hour:** A sign of preterm labor, contractions that happen this often should be reported to your doctor or midwife.

**Gush of fluid from the vagina:** It might be normal vaginal discharge, but you should discuss with your practitioner to make sure your amniotic sac has not broken prematurely.

*Report any strange or troublesome symptoms to your practitioner immediately.*

##  BODY BASICS

Are you getting used to your belly yet? Many moms find around this time that they occasionally bump into objects as they expand outward. You might find that other areas are extending outward as well, particularly toward the rear. You may also find bruises in places you didn't know you'd bumped. Don't worry; these incidents will stop as you adjust to your changing shape.

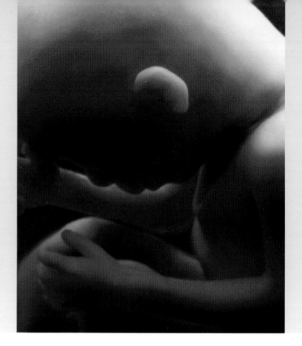

### BABY DATA

Your baby weighs nearly two pounds (900 grams). In addition to gaining weight, he or she is also busy preparing for birth. The skin on your baby is changing from transparent to more opaque. This means that you can no longer see your baby's veins clearly through the skin.

PREGNANCY PARTICULARS

## Check Your Newborn Coverage with Your Insurance Carrier

Now is a great time to call your insurance company to check on coverage for a newborn. Insurance companies vary widely in their coverage. This is particularly important if you have switched insurances or if you have been through open enrollment since you first discovered you were pregnant or since you last checked with them.

Ask what types of services they cover and where they cover them. (Some insurance companies will only cover certain procedures in certain facilities—for example, births only in hospital or birth center or circumcision only in a doctor's office.) The following are some of the major issues to think about:

- Will they cover the pediatricians you are considering?
- Will they cover the nursery in the hospital or birth center you are using?
- Do they cover routine newborn care or only care for ill newborns?
- Will they cover well baby care? What does that consist of?

- Which immunizations do they cover?
- Are lactation services covered? Breast pump parts or rental?
- Are procedures such as circumcision covered or is it considered cosmetic?
- Will they cover neonatal intensive care (NICU) if needed?
- At which hospitals will they cover NICU?
- Which neonatologists will they cover?

Some of these questions may seem obvious, but you would be surprised by what insurance companies will say or do. It is always wise to get answers in writing whenever possible. Make sure you have a copy of your policy or ask that they send you the information in writing. Having written proof can be enormously helpful if you are told something different at a later date.

If you are having more than one baby, alert your insurance company. Otherwise, they may deny claims they think are duplicates. This can be a huge headache that you have neither the time nor energy to deal with after the birth.

## Schedule Your Glucose Tolerance Test

This screening is done to see if you have developed gestational diabetes. Some practices only test women who are at higher risk for gestational diabetes. This category of women includes the following:

- Women who had gestational diabetes in a prior pregnancy

- Women who have a family history of diabetes

- Women who have had a baby larger than 8.8 pounds (4 kilograms)

- Women who are younger than twenty-five and overweight

- Women over a certain age

Other practices screen every pregnant woman in their practice, typically between 26 and 28 weeks.

Here's how the glucose tolerance test (GTT) is done. First, you eat a normal diet for the days preceding the test. The morning of the test, however, you are asked to skip breakfast before coming to the office or lab. Once there, you are given a drink called glucola. This sugar-packed drink is available in a couple of flavors, but not every practice carries every flavor. It tastes like flat soda, with more sugar. It is best to just drink it down and not sip it. Some women say that drinking it cold helps it go down, while others say the temperature didn't make any difference. Most women hate it, but every now and again, you'll meet one who loves the stuff!

You will be asked to stay at the office or lab for about an hour and then your blood is drawn. (Some practices will let you drink the glucola at home and then come in for the blood work.) If the results of the blood work are considered high (greater than 140 mg/dL), you will be asked to do another test, the three-hour challenge.

PREGNANCY AFFIRMATION
FOR WEEK 26

# My mind is open to the possibilities of labor and birth.

The test works the same way, in that you are given a drink of glucola, but this time it has even more sugar in it. Your blood will be drawn up to the following four times:

- After fasting

- One hour later

- Two hours later

- Three hours later

The numbers in the parentheses are the cut off levels for blood glucose at that particular timing. To pass the test and not be diagnosed with gestational diabetes, you must show a blood glucose level that is lower than the above scores for at least two of the times.

If you are given a diagnosis of gestational diabetes, you will likely meet with a nutritionist to discuss changes to your diet. This will include learning how to portion your food and to select foods that are healthy and have a good ratio of nutrients to help keep your blood sugar stable for the remainder of your pregnancy. You will also be given instructions on how to test and record your blood sugar at home via finger pricks.

The vast majority of mothers-to-be will be able to control their diabetes through diet and exercise alone, but some women will also require medication. Insulin can be taken orally or via injections, depending on how successful the least invasive method is at controlling your blood sugar levels. Uncontrolled blood sugar causes a greatest risk to your pregnancy, so that is the primary goal of whatever therapy you are given.

The risks of gestational diabetes include the following:

- Large baby due to uncontrolled blood sugar
- Breathing problems for the baby at birth
- Low blood sugar for the baby at birth
- High blood pressure for the mom
- Increased chance of needing an induction of labor or Cesarean section

Talk to your practitioner about how you can reduce your risks of these complications. You may also discuss the need for extra monitoring. With properly controlled blood sugar levels, many women go on to have full-term, healthy babies without complications.

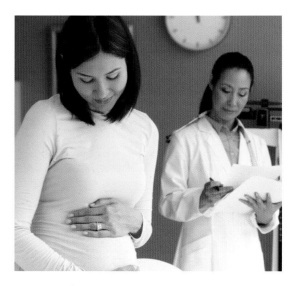

*A good relationship with your practitioner is imperative. Don't hesitate to discuss concerns you have before your labor.*

## Resolve Any Conflicts with Your Practitioner

Sometimes you and your practitioner may not see eye to eye, and this can be both confusing and stressful.

The first order of business is to make sure there really is a misunderstanding. Ask for clarification of the position that you feel is a problem. Then talk to your practitioner to see if there is any wiggle room. Restate your position and ask him or her to do the same. Request some literature on his or her position and offer to do the same. This should be an open discussion and one that your practitioner is receptive to having with you.

If you find that you and your practitioner cannot come to an agreement, you have a decision to make: Does the disagreement warrant changing

practices? The decision is entirely personal. For instance, some women might be willing to overlook rude behavior on the part of the practice's staff while others would view it as cause for switching. Red flags might be if you feel like you are constantly making excuses for the practice in general, worry about your care, find you don't trust their answers, or are constantly arguing. There might be a single deal breaker—for example, if your practitioner insists that all babies who they believe to be greater than eight pounds should be born via Cesarean.

If you're thinking of switching, go back to your original list of practitioners. Was there a close second? Have you found other names since making the list that you'd like to consider? Decide how many practitioners you'd like to interview and call to set up appointments.

Some practitioners have time limits on switching and won't accept new patients after a certain point in their pregnancies. If the practitioner you most want to see is not taking new patients, ask your childbirth educator or doula if she can provide you with an inside referral. She may have an established relationship with the practice or may simply know how to get past the receptionist who usually screens calls from patients looking to switch in, preventing the doctor or midwife from having a say in the decision.

Your insurance company should not have a problem with you switching practitioners. It will simply pay the old practitioner a flat fee for the care you have received up until the point you switch. Then they will pick up where you left off with the new practitioner. In the vast majority of cases, you will not have to pay your co-pay again.

Make certain that you have a new practitioner in place before informing your old practitioner that you're switching. To inform them, you simply need to ask the office to send a copy of your medical records to your new practitioner. This will have to be done in writing.

You are not required to provide an explanation for why you're leaving the practice, although many women choose to. You can either do so in person, explaining the reason for your departure, or you can write a note, thanking them for their care up until that point.

Once your medical records have been moved over, you will start seeing the new practitioner. You will have less time to get to know the new practitioner, so try to fit as much as you can into your appointments. Some practitioners may even give you an opportunity to have additional appointments to gather as much information as you'd like.

Once you have switched practitioners, you will likely go through an adjustment period. Most mothers-to-be who switch practices wind up being delighted with the new practice. So hang in there!

## GLUCOSE TOLERANCE TEST ALTERNATIVES

Many women strongly dislike the taste of the glucola drink that's most often used for the glucose tolerance test. Fortunately, there are alternatives!

Studies were conducted to see if eighteen Brach's jelly beans provided enough sugar for the test, and the answer was yes. Then women were tested to see if the test was affected in any way by using jelly beans instead of glucola. The researchers found that it was perfectly acceptable to use jelly beans in place of glucola. The only catch was that the candy had to be consumed rather rapidly. Turns out the jelly beans prevented much of the nausea and vomiting women experienced with glucola, and they certainly rated more highly for taste. Free to ask about eating jelly beans instead of drinking glucola, but many practitioners still insist on glucola.

Another option is to eat a special breakfast purchased from a fast food restaurant. This one is less common than the others but is used, so talk to your doctor or midwife for specifics. The important goal is to ingest the same amount of sugar as the glucola provides.

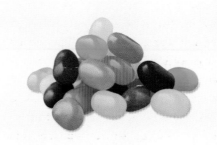

## Start Thinking about Baby Names

Your baby's name is probably something you started thinking about even before you got pregnant. Because your baby's name is a very important decision, you will want to take your time and give it a lot of thought.

To begin, you and your husband could each write a list of girl's and boy's names that you love. Then compare lists and circle any names that appear on both lists, because these are obviously the front-runners.

You may find that your lists are incredibly short, and you wish you had more names to consider. That's where baby name books and websites can be helpful. These resources can be arranged any number of ways, from alphabetical to country of origin, but they all offer an abundance of options and supply the meanings and origins of each name. If the thought of scanning through 50,000 baby names is not your idea of a fun evening (or multiple evenings), choose a book that breaks the names down to manageable pieces—for example, the most popular names by decade and celebrity baby names.

If you already know that you are having a girl or a boy, your search will naturally be more focused because you only need to compile one list of names. Looking only at one sex's names, however, doesn't make the name selection necessarily any easier or faster.

As you look through the lists and add to and delete from your core group of candidates, you will be working toward the names that mean the most to you. This process takes awhile and should not be rushed. The name you ultimately select will become a part of your family for a very long time.

As you narrow your list, ask yourself the following questions:

- Do you like the name's nicknames? (For example, you may love the name Robert, but dislike Robbie or Bob.)

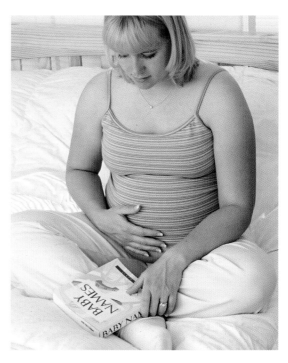

*Baby names can be a big source of conflict in pregnancy. Try to enjoy the selection process rather than force it.*

- How does the name sound with your last name?
- Do the initials spell anything rude? (Annie Sue Smith, Clara Owen White, Braden Uriah Thomlin)
- Is the name easy to spell and pronounce?
- Does it mesh with the rest of your family's names? (Sue might feel strange with siblings Anastasia and Kennsington.)
- How does the name sound when you say it ten times out loud?
- Can you scream the name out the back door without cringing?

Once you have your list of favorite names, it's time to sit with them for a while. Don't look at the list for several days and then come back and see how you feel. Practice saying the names and imagine how they would look on backpacks, schoolwork, and camp rosters. Certain names may fall off the list while other new ones will occur to you. Keep your mind open and flexible and see where it leads you.

## Buy a Body Pillow

A body pillow is designed to help keep you comfortable while you sleep. You can choose from a ton of different types of body pillows, and you may be reluctant to spend money on one only to find that it doesn't work well for you.

Start by asking yourself where you need support in bed. Do you sleep with a pillow between your legs? What about behind your back or to prop up your belly? These are the most common spots for pregnant women looking for additional support.

Then take a look at what is available. See what you can find that covers the areas you most need to support. Check the firmness of the pillow. Is it what you would normally choose? It may be wise to choose something that's firmer than what you put under your head at night because the body parts you're looking to support are heavier than your head, and a soft pillow will squish instead of support. Next consider is the pillow washable? Does it have a cover? Is that washable?

Some mothers avoid buying a body pillow because they think it will be too large. But the truth of the matter is that by the time you add up a few regular pillows, a body pillow actually takes up less space. Plus, anything that helps you sleep is worth it!

**HOT MAMA**

Sleepwear isn't something that gets much attention during the first half of pregnancy. By now, however, you may find that you're increasingly mobile at night, shifting to get comfortable and getting in and out of bed more frequently. You may also find that you are warmer or even sweating during the night. For these reasons, what you choose to sleep in should be comfortable and lightweight. Look for nightgowns or large T-shirts that don't cling to your skin or restrict your movements.

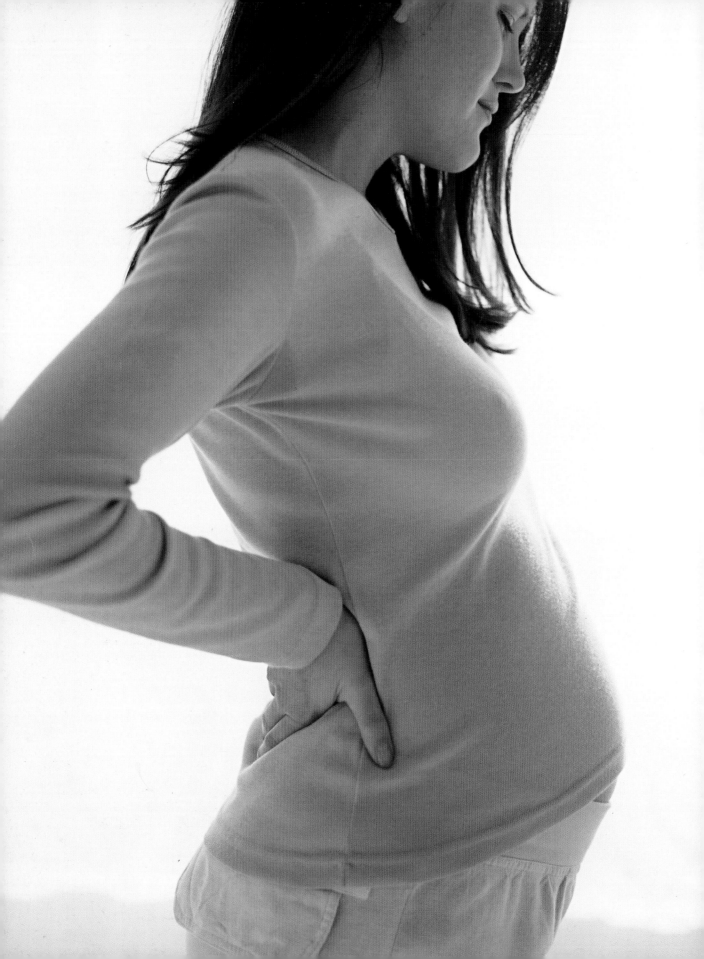

# WEEK 27

## CHECKLIST FOR WEEK 27

[ ]  Take another tour of your hospital or birth center.
[ ]  Watch out for preterm labor.
[ ]  Deal with insomnia.
[ ]  Choose baby clothes.
[ ]  Be tested for anemia.

## WHAT TO WATCH FOR THIS WEEK

*Double Check*

**Headaches:** Severe headaches can be a sign of issues with your blood pressure that should be assessed by your practitioner. Sometimes headaches are merely the result of pregnancy hormones, or they may be tied to other symptoms that together are called pregnancy induced hypertension (PIH), or even preeclampsia, which is a severe illness in pregnancy related to blood pressure, protein in your urine, and other complications.

**Swelling:** The key here is sudden swelling in the face or hands as opposed to the normal swelling pregnant women experience. Sudden swelling is linked to PIH or even preeclampsia, whereas normal swelling develops slowly and should go away after a period of rest.

**Blurred vision:** Another sign of PIH or preeclampsia, report blurry vision immediately to your practitioner.

**Bleeding or spotting:** Bleeding or spotting, either red or brown in color, can happen after sexual intercourse, a vaginal exam, or vaginal ultrasound. If bleeding or spotting occurs at other times, report it to your practitioner immediately.

**Back or abdominal pain:** This type of pain can be a sign of contractions or premature dilation of the cervix, a sign of potential preterm labor.

**More than six contractions per hour:** This can be a sign of preterm labor. It can be normal to have contractions, just not at this frequency.

**Gush of fluid from the vagina:** This can be a sign that your water has broken prematurely. Your practitioner can determine if the fluid leaking from your vagina is amniotic fluid or normal vaginal discharge.

*Report any strange or troublesome symptoms to your practitioner immediately.*

## BODY BASICS

Your baby is now large enough that his or her movements can be felt by others. This is such an exciting time for families as they get to share in these movements with mom. That said, all too often, the moment you tell someone that the baby is moving, the baby seems to sense this and stop. This can lead to some giggles.

As the weeks pass, you may begin to experience more symptoms related to the end of pregnancy, such as backache, leg cramps, heartburn, and hip pain. The more you keep active and exercise, and the healthier your diet, the less you will be plagued by end-of-pregnancy symptoms and miseries.

## 🛒 BABY DATA

Your baby continues to grow and gain weight. The eyelids are able to open and close again. Your baby's skin is still very thin and wrinkled from living in the amniotic fluid, making it possible to see the veins underneath. As your baby grows and deposits more fat under the skin, the veins will become less visible and your baby's body will fill out.

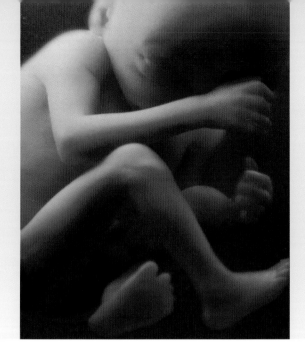

PREGNANCY PARTICULARS

## Take Another Tour of Your Hospital or Birth Center

While you probably took a tour of the hospital or birth center earlier in your pregnancy, you are much further along and wiser. Now your questions will have a completely different thought process behind them, because the idea of giving birth is becoming more real to you and your family.

A good plan of action is to take your birth plan with you on the tour, even if it is not finished. Use it as a cheat sheet for your questions. You will want to talk about policies for many different items and situations, including the following:

- Fetal monitoring
- Food and drink in labor
- Equipment available for use (such as birth balls and squat bars)
- Visitation policy in labor and postpartum
- Rooming in policies (keeping your baby in your postpartum room after birth)
- Medications
- Pre-registration information

These are just some of the policies that you will want to discuss. Add other topics that are important to you. Now is the time to find out if a policy conflicts with something you'd like to do or try for your birth.

If you discover that there is a conflict, ask who sets the policy and who can override it. Sometimes it is a practitioner preference. This means that your midwife or doctor has the ability to approve whatever it is you'd like to do. But other times, the policy is hospital-wide, and you will have to go through the administration to be granted an exception. While this can take time, you have that time if you act now, and it's worth putting in the effort to gain approval for something that's important to you.

Many hospitals and birth centers offer tours at pre-arranged times. If you or your partner cannot go at that time, ask about scheduling a tour for a different date or time. Typically this request can be easily accommodated.

## Watch Out for Preterm Labor

Preterm labor is labor that starts prior to 37 weeks. If any of the following applies to you, you may be an increased risk of having preterm labor:

- Having had a previous preterm labor
- Carrying more than one baby
- Being a smoker
- Having had certain cervical or uterine surgeries
- Having certain infections, such as bacterial vaginosis

It is important to watch for signs of preterm labor, because if treated early enough, it can usually be stopped, thus preventing the preterm birth of your baby. You can learn the signs of preterm labor from your childbirth class or from your practitioner, but it is helpful to remind yourself and those around you of the signs so that they can be rapidly identified and stopped. These signs include the following:

- Dull backache
- Pelvic pressure
- Fluid leaking from the vagina
- More than six contractions per hour
- Bleeding from the vagina
- Difficulty urinating

If you experience any of these symptoms, you should call your practitioner immediately. While you are waiting for a call back, drink water and lie down. One of the first treatments for preterm labor is ensuring that the mother is hydrated. Typically this is done at the hospital with an IV line, but starting orally can't hurt.

If preterm labor is suspected, you will probably be asked to come in for a period of fetal monitoring, during which your contractions and your baby are monitored. In addition, you will most likely be given IV hydration and a vaginal exam to check for cervical changes.

If your contractions are adequately controlled, you will probably be sent home. Sometimes it is necessary to administer medication such as Procardia or Terbutaline. These help relax the uterus, but they can make you feel warm, short of breath, and even a bit dizzy. There are even more powerful drugs like Magnesium Sulfate to help stop labor. It's possible that you will meet with a neonatologist to discuss your baby and the use of steroids to mature the lungs more quickly if the labor cannot be stopped.

This process can be extremely frightening. Call someone to accompany you to the hospital and stay with you, even if you are there for only a few

## PREGNANCY AFFIRMATION FOR WEEK 27

# My baby is happy and growing well inside my body.

hours. While preterm labor is serious, early intervention can help dramatically to improve the length of your gestation.

## Deal with Insomnia

Insomnia is the inability to fall asleep or the inability to get back to sleep once you wake up. During pregnancy it is possible to suffer from either or both of these sleep disturbances.

Insomnia can be caused by a host of things, including the following:

- Being overly tired
- Exercising too close to bedtime
- Excessive napping
- Constant activity of the mind
- Stress
- Physical aches and pains

Obviously some of these are easier to address than others. For example, if having caffeine late in the day keeps you up at night, put away the after-dinner chocolates and drink warm milk instead of black tea before bed. Finish your exercise routine by early evening to prevent exercise-induced insomnia. Be judicious about napping. If you are napping for long stretches of time, try to shorten these periods to contribute to a better night's sleep.

Stress and an overactive mind can be a bit trickier to deal with, particularly the pregnancy variety. Let's face it, when you are pregnant, your mind is constantly in motion, and that causes a great deal of stress. You can do things to help turn off or tone down your mind. First of all, try to avoid conversations that could be upsetting or require intense thought before bed. The same goes for watching disturbing television shows and movies and reading disturbing books. Anything that could upset or provoke you should not be part of your prebedtime routine.

If your mind naturally starts to compile mental checklists when you get into bed, resist the urge. One strategy used by many women is to keep a notebook and pen on the night table. When a thought crops up, write it down and let it go.

Using relaxation tools such as breathing, meditation, aromatherapy, and listening to a sound machine that mimics natural sounds—such as rain, ocean waves, and a babbling brook—can also help calm your mind before bed.

If it's not your mind but your body that is keeping you awake, you must try to identify what is going on. Is it a backache? Leg cramps? Address each issue as you would normally, but remember that prevention is the best approach. For example, try to stretch the affected areas before bed. Add a body pillow and do pelvic tilts to prevent backache from developing while you sleep.

## Choose Baby Clothes

Baby clothes are irresistibly cute! The only thing better than baby clothes is your baby in baby clothes.

In fact, most mothers report that the first thing that they purchased for their babies was baby clothes. The question to ask is will these clothes actually be helpful when the baby arrives? Here are some things to keep in mind.

STYLE: Even if you know whether your baby is a boy or a girl, styles change, and your tastes may differ from that of your family. So be careful not to buy too much of a single style until your baby is around to prove that it works for him or her.

PRACTICALITY: Whether you want to admit it or not, the super cute baby clothes are not always the most practical. Does the garment have

openings in the bottom so you can quickly access the diaper? Does the top open wide enough to fit easily over baby's head?

BABY'S COMFORT: Pay attention to comfort when choosing clothes for your baby. For example, lots of buttons or bows will hurt if your baby has to sit or lie on them. Watch for these on both the front and back of garments.

MATERIALS: Is your baby's clothing made out of materials that you like or that feel soft? Some families look for 100 percent cotton, or even organic cotton, while others don't care as much. What should matter is that the fabric feels nice on baby's sensitive skin.

SEASON: Hand-me-downs are great, but will they work for the particular season you need them? This also goes for clothes that you buy ahead of time. You often can't predict how fast your baby will grow, making it difficult and inadvisable to buy too far ahead.

SAFETY: Choose clothing that is safe for baby to wear. For example, some sleepwear is covered with flame retardant while some is not. Fire safety also dictates that night clothes fit snugly. Ribbons and other decorations can be choking and strangling hazards.

As you receive baby clothes as gifts and hand-me-downs, organize them so you can figure out what pieces are missing and should be purchased. Even though your baby will wear the smallest sizes for a short period of time, it is nice to have some clothes that fit well rather than hang on baby like a sack of potatoes.

And remember that babies should be dressed in one layer more than you would wear. Stock up on one-piece body suits, which are great for layering in the winter and make the perfect summer outfit.

Once you identify the gaps in your baby's wardrobe, you can register for those items. Remember to include baby socks and sleepers on your gift registry. These are popular gifts and even more popular with new parents.

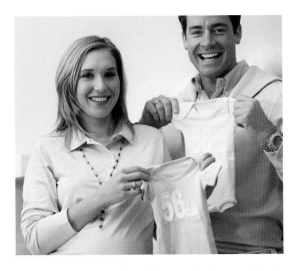

*Consider only buying a few select items before your baby's arrival. Birth weight, length, and other factors may make some clothing decisions for you.*

## Be Tested for Anemia

Toward the beginning of the third trimester, many practitioners will test you for anemia, or low iron levels. If you suffer from anemia, you may experience greater fatigue than is normal for this stage of pregnancy. This is because low iron can interfere with the delivery of oxygen to your cells. Having anemia can also make you more likely to have a problem with blood loss at birth and prevent you from being able to take certain forms of medication in labor and birth. (Many hospitals have epidurals on the no-no list if you're very anemic, if your platelets are low, or if you're on blood thinner.) Your practitioner will explain how best to prevent and treat anemia, including the following:

- Eat a diet filled with iron. Load up on leafy greens, beans, whole grains, liver, and meat.
- Avoid things that prevent absorption. Caffeine and calcium block iron absorption, so they should be avoided when taking iron supplements or eating iron-rich foods. Wait a few hours to allow the iron to be properly absorbed before eating or drinking these products.

- Sneak iron in. You can sneak iron into your diet by cooking with cast-iron skillets or tossing a handful of spinach into your spaghetti sauce or soup.
- Consider liquid supplementation. While your diet is the best way to get iron into your diet to combat anemia, supplements can be useful. Some women have trouble taking iron pills because of stomach upset or constipation. Liquids tend to perform better in this category.

Your practitioner may want to recheck your iron levels after a few weeks to see if the approach is working. It is also possible during this time frame to be given a reading of false anemia because it takes your red blood cells a while to catch up with the huge expanse in your blood volume. So do not panic.

**HOT MAMA**

Getting a tan while pregnant is not recommended, whether you use the sun or a tanning bed. Instead, you can fake a tan with makeup or spray-on bronzers. Check with your practitioner before using a spray, however, because some contain chemicals that you don't want on your skin while pregnant.

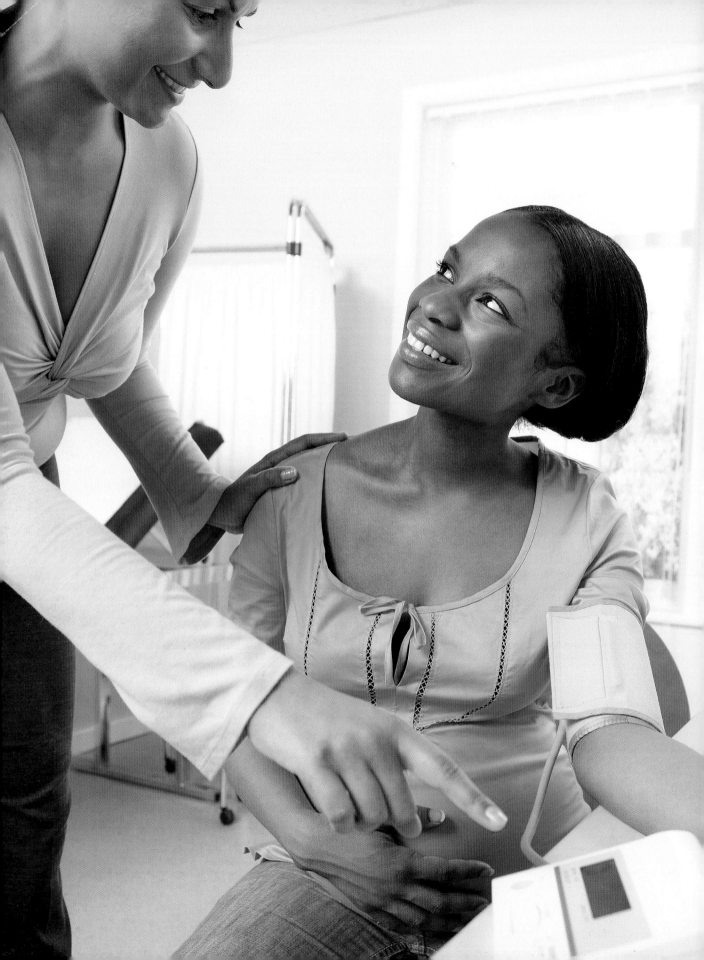

# WEEK 28

## ✎ CHECKLIST FOR WEEK 28

[ ] Make prenatal appointments for every two weeks.
[ ] Hire your doula.
[ ] Schedule your Rhogam shot if you are Rh negative.
[ ] Watch out for preeclampsia.

## ⌕ WHAT TO WATCH FOR THIS WEEK

### Double Check

**Swelling:** Watch for sudden swelling in the face or hands. These are signs of pregnancy induced hypertension (PIH) or preeclampsia. By contrast, normal swelling in pregnancy will go away after a period of rest, not arise suddenly, and is usually not severe.

**Headaches:** Severe headaches can indicate potential problems with your blood pressure that should be discussed with your practitioner. When headaches are the result of more than pregnancy hormones, they may be tied to PIH or even preeclampsia, which is a severe illness in pregnancy related to blood pressure, protein in your urine, and other complications.

**Blurred vision:** Report blurred or troubled vision to your practitioner right away. Alone or accompanied by a headache, it can be a sign of PIH or preeclampsia.

**Bleeding or spotting:** Red or brown spotting, when it doesn't follow sexual intercourse, a vaginal exam, or vaginal ultrasound, could be a sign of infection, premature dilation of the cervix, or issues related to your placenta.

**Back or abdominal pain:** If you experience pain in your back or abdomen, it might be a sign of contractions or premature dilation of the cervix, a sign of potential preterm labor.

**More than six contractions per hour:** Contractions that occur this frequently can be a sign of preterm labor.

**Gush of fluid from the vagina:** Contact your practitioner to determine if the fluid leaking from your vagina is amniotic fluid, meaning your water has broken, or normal vaginal discharge.

*Report any strange or troublesome symptoms to your practitioner immediately.*

##  BODY BASICS

Your uterus measures about twenty-eight centimeters from your pubic bone, well above your umbilicus, or belly button. A mother carrying twins is likely to have a uterus that is already forty centimeters, the size of a full-term mother, at this point in gestation. When you think about it in terms of centimeters, it doesn't always sound so bad, but the reality is that it can be a big strain on your body to carry a baby in your uterus, let alone more than one baby.

Doing what you can to watch your posture, exercising, stretching often, and eating well will help eliminate some of the pregnancy symptoms associated with the third trimester. And while these tactics may not prevent every problem or uneasy feeling, they can help reduce their intensity and make them much more manageable.

## 👶 BABY DATA

At 28 weeks, your baby is growing toward maturity. Weighing more than two pounds (1 kilogram), and possibly reaching two and a half pounds (1.1 kilograms). Much of this added weight comes from more layers of brown fat.

This week is considered a huge milestone for babies that are born or threatening to be born early. If your baby were born from this week forward, the chance of survival is very, very high. Though your uterus is still the ultimate in incubators, it is reassuring for many mothers-to-be to know that should preterm labor happen, the outcome is a long road but one that most likely will have a happy ending.

Your baby is busy growing eyelashes this week to match the body hair. Babies born before now have no eyelashes, which is a fact that surprises many parents. If you are having a boy, his testicles may start to come down from his

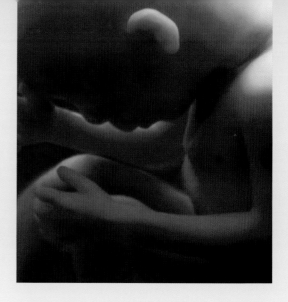

abdomen, called descending. Most of the time both testicles will descend before birth, although in a few cases, it will take a couple of months after birth for both to descend fully. This is screened for at birth and, should your son not have descended testicles, followed by your baby's pediatrician.

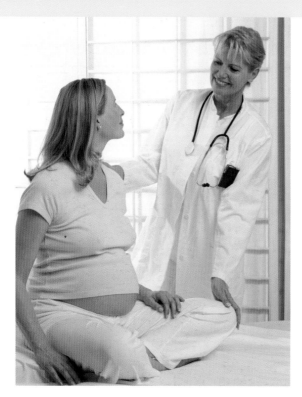

## Make Prenatal Appointments for Every Two Weeks

Now that you are in the third trimester, your practitioner will want to see you more frequently. This is to monitor you and the baby and also to help facilitate a relationship between you and the person who is likely to attend the birth of your baby.

During weeks 28 through 36, you will most likely see your doctor or midwife every two weeks. This schedule may vary, depending on your health and the health of your baby. For example, a mother expecting twins may already be seeing her practitioner every two weeks. Or if your practitioner has

*Prenatal appointments are your chance to ask questions and prepare for your baby's birth. The two-week schedule allows more time for that interaction.*

identified a complication in your pregnancy, you may be asked to come in more often.

For some women, the realization that they are having prenatal appointments every two weeks can be a wake-up call that the pregnancy is coming to an end. Soon they will be holding their babies. This can lead to some frantic last-minute planning.

Being seen every two weeks can cause problems for women who work. Taking time off once a month may have been inconvenient, but leaving every two weeks, and later every week, can be a major hassle, even if your boss knows why you are leaving. You might try the following to minimize problems at work:

- Call ahead to see if your practitioner is running on time. If not, stay at the office for a bit longer.

- Schedule appointments early in the day or late in the afternoon to minimize wait times at the doctor's office and time away from work.

- Schedule several appointments ahead to be sure that you get the appointment times that work best for you.

- Consider seeing the nurse practitioner or physician's assistant, if available, every other visit if that will reduce wait times.

- Ask about alternative scheduling such as weekend or evening appointments. These may occasionally be available.

These tips may not work for every appointment, but they may be helpful sometimes. If wait times become a huge problem, you should consider talking to your practitioner. Your time is just as valuable as his or hers, and you might even be able to offer some suggestions for how to improve the situation.

## Hire Your Doula

The time has come to decide on a doula if you have not already done so. If you have spent the past few weeks coming up with a list of potential doulas, the task should be fairly easy. If you have not yet

## PREGNANCY AFFIRMATION FOR WEEK 28

✛

## Relaxation helps me prepare for the birth of my baby.

compiled a list and started your initial interviews, you should begin to do so now.

Once you have your list of doulas narrowed to two or three candidates, it is time for face-to-face interviews. This is a chance for you to see the doulas and assess your ability to work with each of them. It is also their chance to decide if you are a good fit for their doula practices. In addition to the list of interview questions on pages 146–147, keep the following in mind:

- What services does the doula provide?

- How do her services compare to other doulas on the list?

- What is her fee?

- Is it in line with the others?

- Is she certified? Does this confer special benefits such as insurance reimbursement for you?

- How far does she live from you?

- Will she spend time with you at your home in early labor?

- How well does she know your practitioner and the place you've chosen to give birth?

- Does her personality mesh with yours and your husband's?

It is very difficult for some women to pick a doula; for others the right choice is obvious. If the right doula is not obvious to you, do not panic. Talk to your husband, and review all the answers given by each doula. Ask which doula seemed like

## DEALING WITH WHITE COAT HYPERTENSION

White coat hypertension is a problem for some mothers-to-be who get nervous during prenatal visits. The anxiety could be due to unrelated life issues, or a generalized fear of doctors or it could result from seeing a particular member of the practice who makes them upset. But the end product is a blood pressure reading that is higher than normal.

This might not sound like a big deal, because in a regular appointment, you could come back for a later screening before being labeled as hypertensive. When you are pregnant, however, every blood pressure reading that is above normal is flagged. It can be difficult to tell the difference between hypertension in pregnancy and white coat hypertension. If you have one stray reading and you are feeling upset, angry, or nervous, speak up. Ask to come back before your next prenatal appointment just to have your blood pressure checked. Chances are if you are not showing other signs such as protein in your urine or swelling, the reading will be normal.

You also have the choice to do home blood pressure monitoring. Many drug stores sell inexpensive blood pressure units to monitor your blood pressure at home. By having your blood pressure screened away from your practitioner's office or away from your regularly scheduled appointment, you may be able to show that you do not suffer from hypertension.

A study in the *Journal of the American Medical Association* showed that white coat hypertension led to an increase in interventions in pregnancy and birth, despite the fact that the pregnant women did not actually suffer from high blood pressure. Share your concerns with your practitioner to avoid some of these issues.

the best fit and why. If you do not agree right away, keep talking until you reach an agreement. Some mothers allow the dad to pick the doula because the doula's job is to support him during labor in an effort to help him help his wife. Other mothers-to-be want complete control. How you work it out is between the two of you.

Some families find that they prefer a team approach and hire two doulas. Or if you have two that you really like, hire one and ask if the other can be the back-up doula should the need arise.

Once you have decided on a doula, call her right away because doula calendars fill up. Just as your doctor or midwife only takes so many clients, so does your doula. Ask her about a contract or fees to secure her services. Then relax and enjoy the process of preparing for your baby's birth, knowing you have added a wonderful member to your birth team.

## Schedule Your Rhogam Shot If You Are Rh Negative

Early on in your pregnancy, your doctor or midwife ran blood tests to screen for a variety of issues. One of the things they screened for was your blood type and Rhesus factor (Rh), which is listed as positive (present) or negative (absent). (This is why your blood type is given as a letter and positive or negative sign, such as A+ or O−.) If you have a negative Rhesus factor, such as O−, you may need to have a shot of Rhogam.

You and the baby have separate blood systems even though there may be times when your blood mixes with the baby's blood. To prevent an Rh negative mother from getting Rh antibodies in her blood, she is given a shot of RHIg (Rh immunoglobulin), called Rhogam. A shot of Rhogam is typically given to all Rh negative mothers at the following times:

- 28 weeks

- Following a miscarriage

- Following an amniocentesis

- 72 hours after the birth
- After postpartum sterilization

If an Rh negative mother gets Rh antibodies in her blood, it's called becoming "sensitized." This is not a problem in the first pregnancy when the sensitization occurs. However, subsequent pregnancies may face problems such as anemia in the baby and preterm labor. In other words, if you are Rh negative but are carrying a baby who is Rh positive, your blood might become contaminated by the positive blood, meaning you have become sensitized. The result is that your body will attack any future pregnancies where the baby is Rh positive, causing potentially serious problems. To prevent this from happening, a sensitized mother will have blood transfusions done to the baby before and after birth in the most severe cases. Only about 5,000 cases of Rh sensitization occur each year. And they can be easily prevented with the simple Rhogam shot.

If both you and your partner have the negative Rh factor, you may not require Rhogam. Your doctor or midwife will most likely not take your word for your partner's blood type. They will want records of medical screenings or may insist on doing the lab work themselves.

## Watch Out for Preeclampsia

Sometimes high blood pressure or pregnancy induced hypertension (PIH) goes beyond simple high blood pressure. If you have additional symptoms, such as swelling and/or protein in the urine, high blood pressure turns into something called preeclampsia.

This is a much more serious complication of pregnancy than simple high blood pressure. Symptoms of preeclampsia include the following:

- Blurred vision or seeing spots
- Sudden or rapid weight gain
- Severe headaches

- Pain in the abdomen
- Decrease in the amount of urine produced

Report any of these symptoms right away to your practitioner. Typically bed rest and medication can help lessen some of the symptoms. If treatment fails to reduce the symptoms, the only option is to have the mother give birth to prevent more serious complications such as seizures and renal failure. This is true even if the baby will be born prematurely.

Some studies show preeclampsia and its more severe form, eclampsia, can lead to problems later in life, such as coronary artery disease and diabetes. If you suffer from preeclampsia or eclampsia in pregnancy, you should be screened later in life, too.

While preeclampsia occurs most often with first-time mothers, it can reoccur in subsequent pregnancies. It can also show up for the first time in later pregnancies, even after a number of uncomplicated pregnancies.

**HOT MAMA**

One can never have too many earrings, the perfect accessory. They don't have to be wild or expensive, but changing your earrings can really change your overall outfit and drawing attention away from your belly.

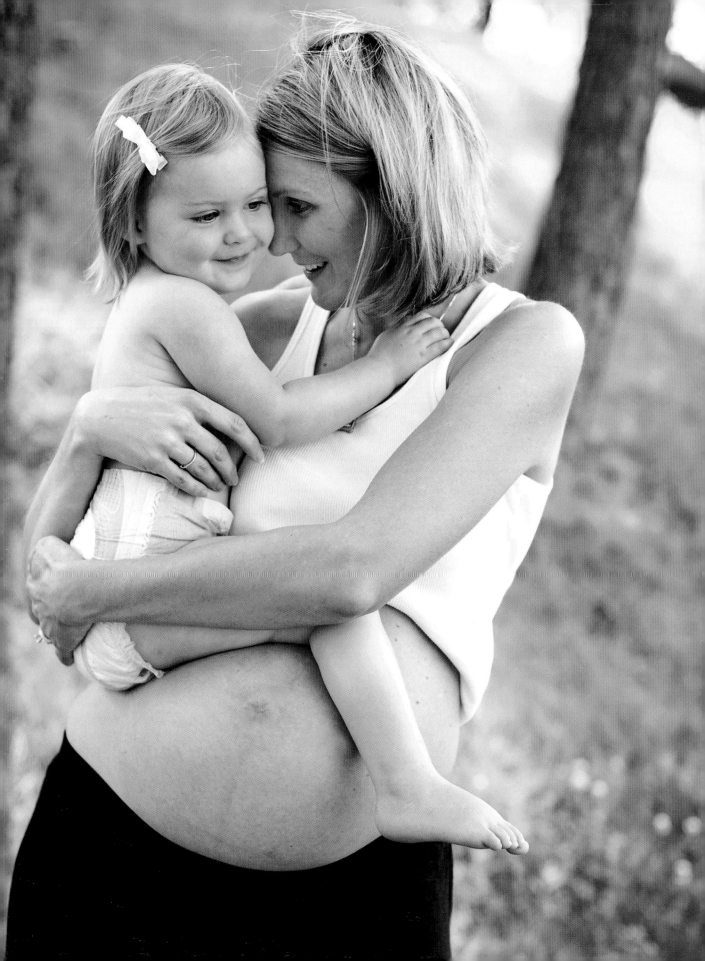

# WEEK 29

## ✎ CHECKLIST FOR WEEK 29

[ ] Research your childcare options.
[ ] Schedule a sibling class.
[ ] Register for baby items.
[ ] Learn about Braxton-Hicks contractions.

## ♀ WHAT TO WATCH FOR THIS WEEK

*Double Check*

**Swelling:** Swelling that develops suddenly in the face or hands can be an indicator of pregnancy induced hypertension (PIH) or preeclampsia. Normal swelling in pregnancy develops slowly and should go away following a period of rest.

**Headaches:** Headaches that are severe, more severe than the headaches brought on by pregnancy hormones, can be a sign of issues with your blood pressure. Talk with your practitioner to see whether or not your headache is tied to other symptoms associated with PIH or even preeclampsia, which is a severe illness in pregnancy related to blood pressure, protein in your urine, and other complications.

**Blurred vision:** Report blurred vision immediately to your doctor or midwife because it, too, can be a sign of PIH or preeclampsia.

**Bleeding or spotting:** Bleeding or spotting (red or brown) at this point in pregnancy can happen after sexual intercourse, a vaginal exam, or vaginal ultrasound. Other types of spotting should be reported immediately to your practitioner, because it may be a sign of infection, premature dilation of the cervix, or issues related to your placenta.

**Back or abdominal pain:** Pain in your back or abdomen can be a sign of contractions or premature dilation of the cervix, a sign of potential preterm labor.

**More than six contractions per hour:** It is normal to experience contractions during the third trimester, just not at this frequency. When they occur this often, it can be a sign of preterm labor.

**Gush of fluid from the vagina:** This can be a sign that your water has broken prematurely. Your practitioner can determine if the leaking fluid is amniotic fluid or normal vaginal discharge.

*Report any strange or troublesome symptoms to your practitioner immediately.*

## ♀ BODY BASICS

At 29 weeks, your breasts may begin to leak colostrum, if they have not done so already. This premilk substance is rich in antibodies and the perfect starter food for your baby. If the leaking becomes a problem, you can wear disposable or washable breast pads in your bra. If you do not notice any colostrum, that's perfectly fine and does not mean you will be unable to breastfeed.

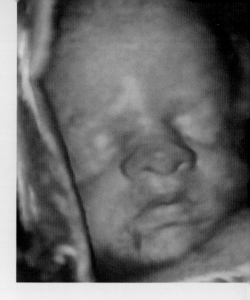

## BABY DATA

Your baby weighs more than two and a half pounds (1.1 kilograms) at this point. You may begin to notice that the big kicks and rolls that you felt earlier take on a different quality. Because your baby is more likely to be head down with every passing week, you may also notice that you feel more action at the top of your uterus from the movement of tiny feet.

Your baby is busy producing about 36 ounces (half a liter) of urine per day, which is partially what makes up the amniotic fluid. You can even see babies urinate on ultrasound if you catch them at the right moment. Your baby is also producing his or her own red blood cells, which come from the bone marrow.

# Research Your Child Care Options

Choosing child care is not a simple or an easy choice for most families. The decision to leave your child under the care of another person, no matter how wonderful and caring, is difficult. You may also find that you have more options than you originally thought, which tends to complicate the decision. Or, conversely, you may find that you have fewer childcare options than you would like. Either way, this is an enormously important process that requires time and effort for you to feel good about the decision you ultimately make.

The first step is determining what type of childcare you want for your baby. There are the following options:

- Traditional day care, on- or off-site from your work

- In-home day care with other children, in the provider's home

- A nanny who comes to your home for set hours each week

- An au pair or nanny who lives in your home full time

To make this decision, you need to figure out what is available to you geographically, monetarily, and philosophically. For example, you may live in an area where there are very few in-home day cares. Perhaps your house is too small to accommodate an au pair, or the cost of a live-in nanny may be prohibitive.

Each type of child care offers advantages and disadvantages. For example, if you and your partner work odd hours, a traditional day care might not be helpful to you, unless it is on-site at your office and caters to the working hours of the employees. Another advantage of traditional day care is that there will likely be same or similar-aged children for your baby to play with as he or she gets older.

Ask yourself and potential providers the following questions about choosing a day care:

- How much does it cost?

- Do the hours of the facility mesh well with your work schedule?

- Are the teachers or workers certified or licensed in first aid?
- Is the location easy for you and your husband to reach?
- What is the sick child policy?
- Are there set vacation days or days when the center is closed?
- What happens if a care provider becomes ill? Is there a back up?
- What are the age ranges of the children?
- Does the center follow a particular philosophy of care?
- What protection measures are in place for emergencies such as fire and hurricane?
- What is the staff education policy?
- Are there openings for when you anticipate needing one?
- Are there fees for holding a spot open?
- Will the fee be reimbursed if you change your mind?
- How are staff/caregivers chosen?
- Can you speak to parents who are currently using or have used the day care in the past?
- Is the center bonded or insured?

Begin by making an initial list of day care facilities, nanny/au pair agencies, and programs. You can gather names from friends and work colleagues who have children. You can also ask your neighbors, your practitioner, mothers at the playground, and pediatricians as you interview them. These are great recommendations, but do not fear if you don't have a bunch of them pouring in. You can also look at the yellow pages and on the Internet. Many cities will provide listings of in-home day cares that are licensed and other day care type facilities.

Once you have your list and narrowed it down according to basics such as location and hours of operation, you can begin to call the facilities for more information. Sometimes what you learn

# PREGNANCY AFFIRMATION FOR WEEK 29

## My baby is growing and preparing to be born.

over the phone will chisel your list further, and with that shorter list, you are ready to begin interviews in person.

These in-person interviews give you a chance to see the facilities, meet directors, watch the care providers in action, and get a sense of how the children are treated and cared for. Ask yourself the following questions:

- Does the staff seem friendly and nurturing?
- Is the director knowledgeable and responsive to your questions?
- Do the children seem happy?
- Do they seem well cared for?
- If any children are crying, are they being comforted?
- What are the nap policies?
- Does the facility look clean?
- What are the diaper changing policies?
- Do the toys look new and clean?
- Are the toys age appropriate?
- What are the policies on breast milk and cloth diapers?
- How do you feel being there?

When you think you have chosen a day care facility, make a surprise visit. Just show up without making an appointment to see if the facility looks the same as it did when you first visited. This can either cement your decision or convince you to keep looking. It is also helpful if both parents evaluate and select a facility even if only one of you will be the person dropping off and picking up your child.

If you are looking into nannies or au pairs, you will also want to investigate their credentials and talk to their previous employers. Many placement agencies have very strict rules about what you need to have a live-in au pair or nanny, such as her own room and health insurance. Be sure to get this information up front. The rules will be different and less stringent for day-time nannies. You should also inquire about an agency fee for matching you with a nanny or au pair.

If once you have your baby you find that the facility or provider is not meeting your needs, speak up. You are likely to find a workable solution if you discuss your concerns. If not, you can switch facilities or providers to better suit you and your baby's needs.

*Your older children need to be prepared, too. Tailor what you say to their age and skill level.*

## Schedule a Sibling Class

If you have older children or step-children, taking them to a sibling class at a local hospital, birth center, or education center is a great idea. At the class, they'll likely hear age-appropriate stories and get a tour to help them understand what will happen when you go there to have your baby.

The class may be geared toward a particular age group, so be sure it's a good fit for your child. Depending on the age of your child, you may need to sit with him or her during the class.

Before signing up, ask for the class agenda to make sure that the contents are appropriate for your child. You should also determine if it is appropriate for your belief systems. For example, will they show a three-year-old how to diaper a newborn? Will they offer only bottles, not mentioning breastfeeding, when discussing how to feed a baby? If you hear something that concerns you, speak up. If you don't find out until after class,

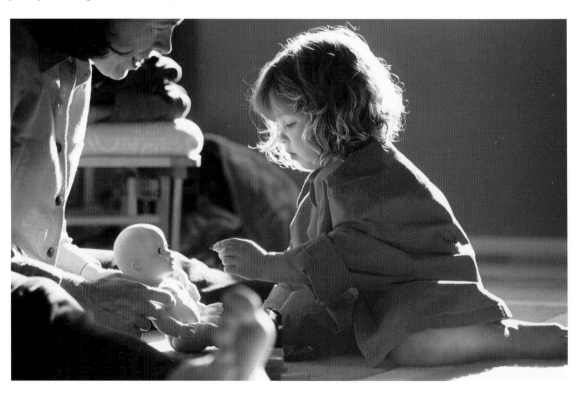

simply explain to your child that some families do that but not your family.

If the class is a match for your children, prepare them ahead of time for what they will be doing. Ask if they have questions and be sure to leave plenty of time after the class to answer questions that came up. You might have your children bring dolls or favorite books about new babies with them.

If you are planning a home birth, you can ask your practitioner if they offer a class or what they suggest. A home birth practitioner may simply ask you to bring your older kids to a prenatal appointment and will conduct a mini-class there for them. This arrangement is sure to be age- and child-appropriate and will most likely mirror your beliefs about birth and baby care. However, some families choose to go to a local hospital and pay a small fee for the class.

If your child is reluctant to go to a group class, or if there is no local class that works for you, take the time to teach your child at home. In fact, even if your child goes to a class, this can be a lovely supplement to it. Some topics to cover include the following:

- What newborns look like
- How newborns behave
- The fact that babies are not playmates
- An explanation of acceptable behavior around the baby
- Daily baby care, such as feeding and diapering
- An explanation of why and how much babies cry

## Register for Baby Items

Registering for baby items is a great way to let people know what baby items you need or want. However, these stores can be overwhelming, and as new parents you might not know what you need or want for your baby. The advertising can make it difficult to tell what's truly necessary and what's merely frivolous.

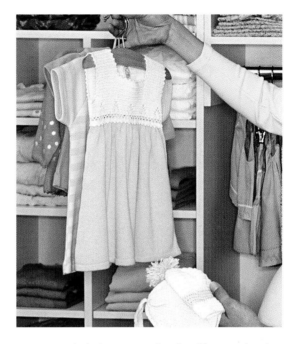

*Registering for baby items can be a lot of fun. Do a bit of research online and then go a bit wild. You can do this in person or online.*

Most baby stores will give you a list of recommended baby items to outfit a nursery. Take the list home and go over it with friends who already have kids. Or talk with parents with similar views to yours when it comes to babies and parenting and create your own list before you to go register. You can also take an experienced parent with you to register for items in the stores.

Ask yourself the following questions before registering:

- Can you access the registry online?
- Is the store local or national?
- Will the store ship to other locations, such as the location of the baby shower, without revealing your address to others?
- Can you add or delete items from your list in person and online?

- Can you add extra information to your list, such as nursery theme or color, sex of your baby, or other information you feel is important?
- What is the store's return policy?

It is important to remember that not everyone who wants to give you a gift will use your registry or shop at that store. You may decide to register at multiple stores, which is perfectly appropriate. And because you're apt to receive some duplicate gifts, knowing the store's return policy is important.

**MEMORABLE MOMENTS**

"I had been feeling the baby move for quite awhile, but one night I laid down and got a real wallop of a kick as I was reading a book. The book jumped off my lap, and my husband happened to catch the whole thing. It was quite the sight. I never got caught quite like that again, and it was a great chance to start talking to my husband about the baby. It was like the baby knew I needed an opening line."

## PLAN FOR OUT-OF-TOWN BABY SHOWERS

If you live far away from your family and friends, someone is bound to offer to throw you an out-of-town baby shower. This can be the perfect excuse to make the trek back to your old neighborhood to visit family or friends you rarely get a chance to see.

As nice as it is, though, having a baby shower out of town can be tricky. The main stumbling blocks are timing the shower and finding an easy way to get the gifts home.

As far as timing goes, be sure you are far enough along to show off your belly but not so far along that travel would be difficult or dangerous. Most moms who are planning a far-away baby shower recommend scheduling it for early in the third trimester.

As for shipping gifts home, there are many creative ways to do it. If you live close enough to drive, you could take your car and haul the presents home. If you are flying to the shower, you need a different solution. Some hostesses ask that guests bring a photo or written description of the gift and mail their gift to the mother's home. This is easy to do if you have registered online for baby shower presents.

Remember that the point of a baby shower is not to furnish your baby's nursery or clothe your baby for the first year. The point is to celebrate the new life inside you and to celebrate your impending parenthood. Try to enjoy your trip and catching up with people you do not see often, but remember that you are pregnant and shouldn't overdo it.

## Learn about Braxton-Hicks Contractions

Braxton Hicks contractions are painless contractions that are felt at any point in pregnancy, though usually after the first trimester. They were named for the obstetrician who first described them in the nineteenth century. These contractions do no dilate the cervix and are not a part of labor. They are believed to tone the uterus in preparation for labor.

While these contractions are often described as being painless, some women would disagree. Due to the position of the baby or some other physical characteristic, it's possible to feel uncomfortable. Typically these contractions are ten to twenty minutes apart, and they do not often occur over a long period of time.

First-time mothers are likely not to notice these contractions, leading them to believe that they are not experiencing them, even if they are. Some mothers do not notice them until the very end of pregnancy, or they will accidentally notice that their uteruses feel hard by touching their abdomens at the right time.

If this is not your first baby, you are more likely to notice Braxton-Hicks contractions because you have felt contractions before either in pregnancy or during labor. If you have questions about Braxton-Hicks contractions, raise them with your midwife or doctor.

**HOT MAMA**

It's a fashion truism that horizontal stripes and plaids are not flattering on overweight bodies. The same is true of pregnancy. When your lower body is expanding on a daily basis, does it seem smart to cover it with eye-grabbing plaids and stripes? The smarter move is to steer clear of small prints and maybe even prints all together. Save those for cute tops.

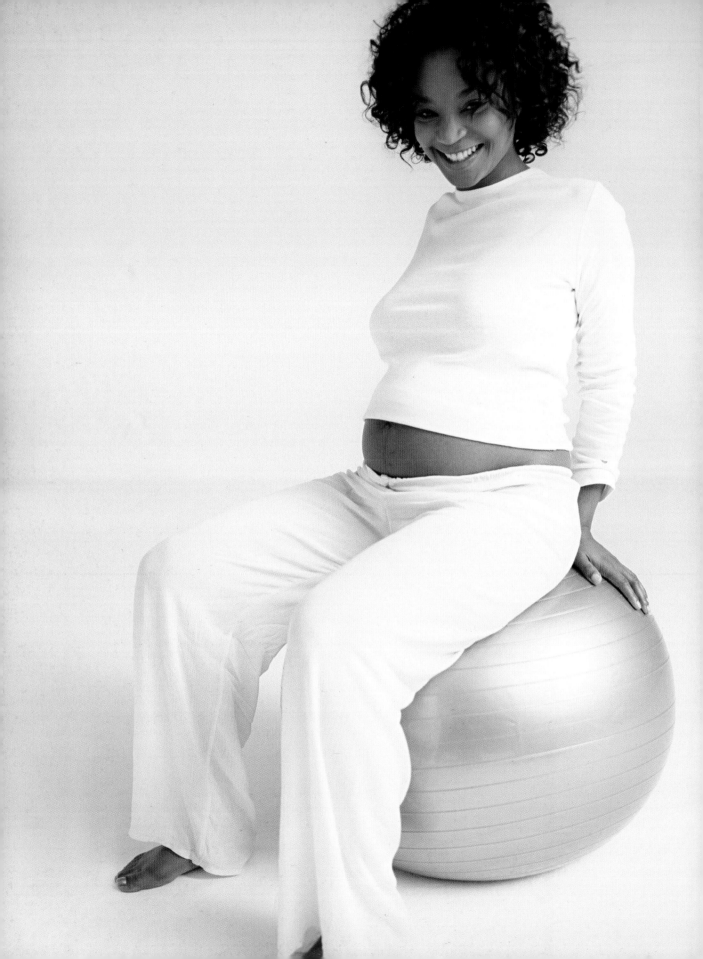

# WEEK 30

## CHECKLIST FOR WEEK 30

[ ] Order your home birth kit.
[ ] Deal with an aching back.
[ ] Choose a breast pump.
[ ] Learn about sex in the last trimester.

## WHAT TO WATCH FOR THIS WEEK

**Decrease in fetal movement:** A reduction in fetal movement, either fewer kick counts than normal or fewer than the required number of movements, may be a sign of problems with your baby. Bring it up with your midwife or doctor immediately. It may be an issue of you not noticing changing habits or a different kind of movement due to limited space, but your practitioner can help analyze the situation.

*Double Check*

**Swelling:** If you experience a sudden swelling in the face or hands, mention it to your practitioner. Unlike normal pregnancy swelling that develops gradually and goes away after resting, this type of swelling can be a sign of pregnancy induced hypertension (PIH) or preeclampsia.

**Headaches:** Severe headaches can be a sign of issues with your blood pressure, and your practitioner should be called to evaluate. Regular headaches can be caused by fluctuating pregnancy hormones, but severe headaches are associated with PIH or even preeclampsia, which is a severe illness in pregnancy related to blood pressure, protein in your urine, and other complications.

**Blurred vision:** Whether or not you've been suffering from headaches, report problems with vision immediately to your practitioner because they are another sign of PIH or preeclampsia.

**Bleeding or spotting:** Bleeding or spotting that is not connected to vaginal exams or sexual relations should be reported immediately to your practitioner. You may have an infection, premature dilation of the cervix, or issues related to your placenta.

**Back or abdominal pain:** A sign of potential preterm labor, pain in your back or abdomen can be a sign of contractions or premature dilation of the cervix.

**More than six contractions per hour:** Another sign of preterm labor, report contractions that take place this often to your practitioner.

**Gush of fluid from the vagina:** This can be a sign that your amniotic sac has been leaking. Your practitioner will evaluate to decide if the liquid leaking from your vagina is amniotic fluid or normal vaginal discharge.

*Report any strange or troublesome symptoms to your practitioner immediately.*

##  BODY BASICS

Your belly is shifting as your baby gets bigger. As your baby turns head down, you may notice a shift in how your belly looks. Do not panic. You may also notice more stretch marks or the appearance of your first stretch marks. If your belly is itching, try rubbing it with a good moisturizer. This relieves your skin, and the massage is nice too.

## 🛒 BABY DATA

This week, your baby is three pounds (1.4 kilograms) and fifteen inches (38 centimeters) and still growing. While your baby is no longer developing new organs or anything terribly exotic, he or she is still busy preparing to be born. Lung development is one of the last things that the baby works really hard to complete. Your baby's eyes are open, and the eyelashes are lengthening.

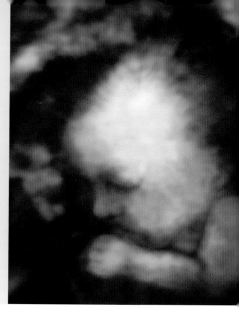

## Order Your Home Birth Kit

If you are planning a home birth, you should discuss with your midwife or doctor what things you will need to have on hand. The majority of practitioners will have you order a birth kit.

Different practitioners may recommend a birth kit containing different things. Birth kits typically include the following:

- Appropriately sized gloves for your practitioner
- Waterproof pads
- Umbilical cord clamps
- Oil for massaging the perineum
- Betadine or other medical grade cleanser
- Warm baby hats

Your practitioner will tell you where to purchase your birth kit. You'll order it under your practitioner's name so it contains the particular supplies he or she needs. The items are then shipped to your house. It can take a few weeks for the kit to arrive, so be sure to plan ahead. You should plan to have your home birth kit no later than the 35th week of pregnancy so you can fix any errors that may have occurred or plan for back-ordered items.

A birth kit is not terribly expensive, averaging between $30 and $50. You may find that your insurance or flexible spending program will cover the cost, so don't forget to ask.

In addition to ordering the birth kit, your home birth practitioner will ask you to have other items on hand. Some of these things will be for your comfort—such as foods and drink for labor—and others will be for medical purposes—such as a bowl to catch the placenta and plastic sheets for the bed. Your practitioner will give you specific instructions on how to prepare the items so that they are on hand and easily located in time for the birth.

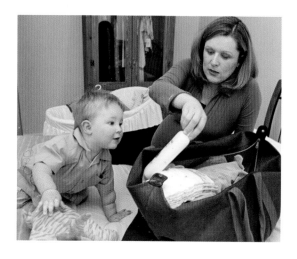

*Your birth kit should be kept in a place where it can be easily accessed. Consider also packing a small bag for the hospital should transport be needed.*

# PREGNANCY AFFIRMATION FOR WEEK 30

✛

## My pregnant body is beautiful.

## Choose a Breast Pump

Choosing a breast pump depends on how you intend to use it. If you plan to pump each day, you should buy a high-quality breast pump. You should also consider a breast pump that does double pumping (pumping both breasts at the same time) to reduce the time you spend pumping.

If you think you'll only do casual or relatively infrequent breast pumping, you can use either a battery or hand pump. They require a bit of work on your part and do not have the same power as electric breast pumps. Some of these are also only single pumps, meaning that you can only pump one breast at a time. This can take a bit longer, but it works well for an occasional bottle of expressed breast milk when you are away from your baby. The cost is much lower, as low as $30 compared to $200 for the fancier models.

If you have issues such as a premature or sick infant or trouble with your milk supply, your pediatrician or lactation consultant is likely to recommend that you rent a hospital grade pump. These are multi-user pumps, meaning that they are closed systems so that breast milk cannot get into the motor and contaminate it. A sterile kit will provide you with the breast shields and bottles to pump with. These can be used on a short- or long-term basis. These are considered the best breast pumps available.

A breast pump can make a great baby shower gift, and because the cost can be high, it is perfect for a group gift. If you do not receive a breast pump at your shower, it is well worth the cost to purchase your own.

## USED BREAST PUMPS

Electric breast pumps that are not hospital grade are not meant to be passed from person to person. They are considered single-user pumps. The risks of passing contaminants from mother to mother are small but it is possible.

Contaminants from a mother's breast milk can travel through the air and lodge in the motor of a breast pump. Even sterilizing the breast pump and purchasing a new sterile kit will not prevent this from happening. Contaminants such as HIV, hepatitis, and Candida can be transmitted this way. So while you may like the idea of saving money by getting a used breast pump, you are risking contaminants as well as an older motor that is less likely to work efficiently.

The FDA has warned against reusing breast pumps between different people. The only breast pump that is designed to be used by multiple people has a closed system to ensure that there is no breast milk contamination. These would be hospital grade pumps sold or rented by hospitals or breast pump rental stations, such as the Medela Symphony, Lactina, and Ameda Elite.

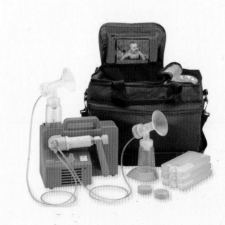

## WILL SEX BRING ON LABOR?

Sex in the final weeks of pregnancy is often discussed as a means for bringing on labor. Many studies have been done to see if it was true. The results have varied, with some studies finding that sex at the end of pregnancy did tend to help labor along while other studies showed that it did not matter one bit.

Of the studies that showed labor and last trimester sex were related, it was not an immediate thing. It seems that sex in the last few weeks tends to correlate with fewer women being induced and fewer women going past 41 weeks gestation. It is believed that sex can help labor because semen contains prostaglandins, which helps to ripen the cervix. Moreover, nipple stimulation and female orgasm can help a woman's body produce oxytocin, which is a hormone that is associated with labor and contractions.

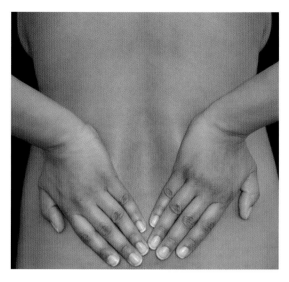

*Backaches are really not a lot of fun. Have an arsenal ready to attack, like massage, warm compresses, yoga moves, and stretching.*

Here's a news flash: While women may feel unattractive during the last trimester, men are usually very turned on by their bodies.

While you may need to make adjustments to your sex life at the end of pregnancy, sexual relations do not have to stop unless you have problems associated with pregnancy including the following:

- Preterm labor
- Premature rupture of membranes
- Active sexually transmitted disease

You can enjoy an active sex life with your partner for the duration of pregnancy, ending only when your labor gets underway or your water has broken. Creative positioning using woman-on-top positions, side-lying positions, and standing positions can be helpful. Some women will experience contractions after sex or having an orgasm, but the contractions usually last less than an hour.

The key to a happy sex life in the third trimester is communication. Talk to your partner about your feelings, physical issues, and libido. These discussions can help you both stay in touch with how the other is feeling and clear up any notion that there is something wrong with either of you.

## Learn about Sex in the Third Trimester

Sex in the last trimester is something that few people want to talk about because it brings up issues such as body image, creative positioning, and desire (or lack thereof).

Many women have issues with body image when it comes to sex and being naked, particularly as the pregnancy progresses. Some women describe themselves as looking like a whale or an elephant or even an obstacle course. It is hard for a very pregnant woman to move, and the circumference of her waist can make her feel unattractive.

## Deal with an Aching Back

Backache has become synonymous with the end of pregnancy. The reason that your back hurts is usually from the extra weight of pregnancy and the changing center of gravity. How you respond to these changes affects how you feel. In other words, unlike many other aspects of pregnancy, you can control back pain and make yourself more comfortable.

Improving your posture is the number one way to combat back pain in pregnancy. As your abdomen grows, the natural tendency is to slouch or sag, resulting in more strain on your back. Many people do not realize the power of the abdominals to help sustain the lower back, and in pregnancy that system is naturally compromised.

To improve your posture, particularly when seated, you should replace your normal work chair at home or the office with a birth ball. The ball, because it moves, forces you to sit upright, or else you would fall over. This subtle balancing act keeps your abdominal muscles engaged and in proper alignment, thereby helping your back.

In addition to ensuring proper posture, exercise—both in general and specific moves designed for the back—can prevent and alleviate back pain. Numerous studies have shown that women who exercise, even lightly, during pregnancy experience far fewer aches and pain, particularly at the end of pregnancy. Something as simple as yoga, walking, or swimming can help you keep your back stretched and less susceptible to pain.

Sometimes the shoes you wear can influence how your back feels. Wearing low heels or flat shoes can be very helpful in dealing with back pain. Higher heels may be sexier, but they tend to give you more leg and back pain.

If you are suffering from backaches, try a series of exercises to stretch your back, starting with the Cat-Cow yoga poses described on page 141. Pelvic tilts in any position (standing, kneeling, or sitting) also work to stretch out the lower back. Furthermore, apply hot and cold compresses to the region that's sore, and treat yourself to plenty of warm baths, showers, and massage.

**HOT MAMA**

While there are petite maternity fashion lines for small-sized pregnant women, it can be hard to find them. These lines have been developed in the past few years, but they are still not widely available. Try searching for online stores, especially on upscale maternity websites. Some petite women resort to having clothes made for their small frames.

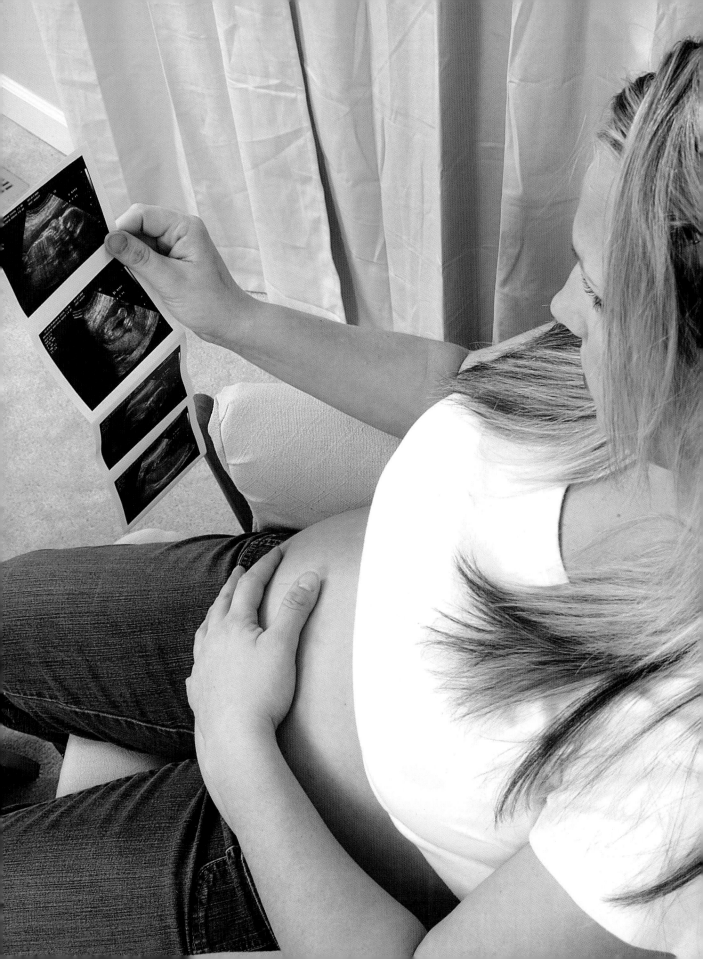

# WEEK 31

## ✎ CHECKLIST FOR WEEK 31

[ ]  Take a breastfeeding class.
[ ]  Buy a breastfeeding book.
[ ]  Eat, even if you're not hungry.
[ ]  Deal with breathing difficulties.

## ⌕ WHAT TO WATCH FOR THIS WEEK
### Double Check

**Decrease in fetal movement:** If you notice a decrease in your fetal kick counts, they take longer to perform, or your baby fails to complete the required number of movements, tell your practitioner. Sometimes this is just a matter of perception, but you should get input from your midwife or doctor immediately.

**Swelling:** Look for sudden swelling in the face or hands, which are signs of pregnancy induced hypertension (PIH) or preeclampsia. Normal swelling in pregnancy does not develop suddenly, will go away after a period of rest, and is usually not severe.

**Headaches:** Severe headaches can be a sign of issues with your blood pressure that can be determined by your practitioner. Sometimes headaches are linked only to pregnancy hormones, but at other times, they, along with other symptoms, point to PIH or even preeclampsia.

**Blurred vision:** Blurred vision can also be a sign of PIH or preeclampsia and should therefore be reported immediately to your practitioner.

**Bleeding or spotting:** Unless you've recently had sexual intercourse, a vaginal exam, or vaginal ultrasound (all of which can cause light bleeding), you are advised to report incidents of red or brown spotting to your practitioner.

**Back or abdominal pain:** Pain in your back or abdomen can be a sign of contractions or premature dilation of the cervix, a sign of potential preterm labor.

**More than six contractions per hour:** This can be a sign of preterm labor. It can be normal to have contractions, just not at this frequency.

**Gush of fluid from the vagina:** This can be a sign that your water has broken prematurely. Visit your practitioner to determine if fluid leaking from your vagina is amniotic fluid or normal vaginal discharge.

*Report any strange or troublesome symptoms to your practitioner immediately.*

##  BODY BASICS

Early in pregnancy, you probably spent your time counting how many weeks you had completed. Right around now, you start to count down how many weeks you have left before giving birth. This can provoke feelings of excitement and anxiety all at the same time.

If you have been coasting along and feeling great, you are quite aware by now that you are pregnant, but you might still feel pretty swell. For the remainder of your pregnancy, you will hopefully pick up a few tricks to keep yourself feeling as comfortable as possible.

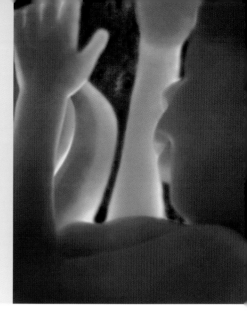

## BABY DATA

Your baby now weighs more than three pounds (1.4 kilograms). The brown fat that has been deposited over the past few weeks has changed the look of your baby's skin from a reddish color to a pink blush. Your baby is growing fingernails, just in time to be trimmed at birth. Be sure to pack a pair of baby fingernail clippers in the bag you plan to bring to the hospital or birthing center.

# Take a Breastfeeding Class

Breastfeeding is natural, but it is also a learned skill for both you and your baby. A great breastfeeding class will be helpful in teaching you the basics of nursing your baby. You can expect to learn the following:

- Benefits of breastfeeding
- Mechanics of breastfeeding
- Positioning your baby correctly
- Identifying a good latch for baby
- How to start breastfeeding
- How to tell if your baby is getting enough breast milk
- Possible problems and interventions
- When and where to seek support for breastfeeding

Classes may include other topics, including the following:

- Choosing a breast pump
- Nursing in public
- Breast milk storage
- Pumping issues
- Breastfeeding and going back to work
- Starting solid foods

Your best bet for finding a breastfeeding class is to contact your local hospital, birth center, or La Leche League chapter. La Leche League is a nonprofit organization that offers breastfeeding education and support, and their services and support groups are free of charge. In seeking out a class that's right for you, keep the following questions in mind:

- Who teaches the class?
- Is the instructor a lactation consultant, breastfeeding counselor, or peer counselor?
- How many students will be in the class? Who is invited? Is it moms only? Can you bring the baby's grandparents?
- When is the class held?
- When should you sign up?
- Will there be videos?

A breastfeeding class should be small enough so you can ask questions, sometimes very personal questions. Hopefully it will include time to practice the various breastfeeding positions using dolls. You should also have time to talk to other moms-to-be and watch instructional videos.

A good class should give you a realistic expectation of what breastfeeding is all about, from how to do it, to how often. You should bring along your husband, your partner, or another support person so they also understand what's

## WHAT TO DO IF YOUR CLASS ISN'T SO GREAT

If you take a breastfeeding class only to discover that you know more than the instructor or if you feel like the advice that you were given contradicted other information that you were told or learned on your own, what should you do?

First, you need to find a class that will meet your needs. Repeat the steps for choosing a breastfeeding class and take a different class. You might even want to interview the instructor before committing to the class.

Once you have lined up or completed a class that fulfills your expectations, consider writing to the facility that hosted the class that you found disappointing. Explain your concerns and provide constructive criticism in your letter. You can also recommend ways to improve the class, such as reeducating or replacing the teacher or revising the agenda to include overlooked topics.

involved in breastfeeding. You will need their encouragement and support once you being to breastfeed your baby, particularly in the early postpartum period.

## Buy a Breastfeeding Book

A good breastfeeding book is a must for every new mother. It is smart to purchase one before you have your baby so that you can read it more leisurely. This allows you to ask questions and to learn what you need to know before your baby is handed to you on birth day.

There are a lot of breast feeding books out there, but they are not all the same or equally beneficial.

## PREGNANCY AFFIRMATION FOR WEEK 31

✚

# My pregnant body is beautiful.

In fact, a book with bad or outdated advice can be detrimental to you, your baby, and your breastfeeding experience. So it is important to choose wisely.

First, seek advice from friends who are successfully nursing their babies. Ask them to recommend books they found particularly helpful or insightful. Ask the same of your lactation consultant, breastfeeding teacher, practitioner, and pediatrician. Take the list of recommended titles to a bookstore and browse through them.

Once you decide which book or books you would like to rely on for breastfeeding advice, ask around. You might find a used copy from a friend who doesn't need it anymore. You can also include these books on your baby gift registry. Finally, visit secondhand or consignment parenting and maternity stores and yard sales. These can be great places to find gently used books when you know precisely what you're looking for.

If you don't have a specific title in mind, you can still find helpful books on the topic. Consider the following:

- Is the book written by a lactation consultant?
- Does it contain medical information?
- Has it been reviewed favorably by professionals?
- Does it have clear pictures of breastfeeding positions and latches?
- Is the writing easy to understand?

Remember that the book you purchase will become your middle-of-the-night friend when it comes to breastfeeding issues. Familiarize yourself with the parts of the book that are most likely to be helpful. And keep it close at hand for times when you have a question or need a quick refresher.

## Eat, Even If You're not Hungry

As your uterus grows, you can sometimes feel too full to eat. You do not have much of an appetite, or you might even forget to eat. Normally, you would listen to your body's cues, but in this case, you and your baby need good nutrition to continue to grow.

If you are the forgetting-to-eat type, you can try a couple of things. Setting an alarm for a meal or a snack can certainly work, or you can make dates to eat with other people. For example, make a regular date with a coworker to have lunch together every Monday or meet a friend for breakfast every Friday. Dining with other people can help you eat, even if it is just a small portion.

If you remember to eat but just aren't hungry, you have a tougher issue. Instead of sticking to set mealtimes, let yourself eat whenever you feel like it. You might also give yourself the freedom to eat whatever you desire, just to get the calories.

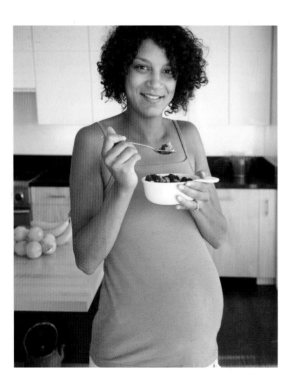

Switching from a few large meals to smaller, more frequent meals is a common way to cope with eating issues in pregnancy. If you can, carry small snacks with you at all times. That way, snacks such as fresh fruit, nuts, and other treats will be ready to grab when you feel like eating. Sometimes just seeing something tasty in your purse will encourage you to take a few bites. Add up enough bites, and you've succeeded in feeding yourself and your baby.

## Deal with Breathing Difficulties

As your baby gets bigger, your uterus expands upward. This means that something has to give, namely your internal organs and ribs. Your ribs can actually expand slightly to give your uterus and displaced organs a place to be housed during the final months of your pregnancy.

As your organs begin to move upward, you might experience difficulty breathing because your lungs do not have as much room to expand as they did before. You may feel short of breath toward the end of your pregnancy.

Certain things can exacerbate this problem. One is sleeping or lying down. This puts even more pressure on your lungs, which will make it difficult to breathe or sleep. In this situation, your best bet is to elevate your upper body. You can accomplish this by adding a pillow or two under your head. Some women also find that bed chairs work really well for this purpose.

Mothers who are carrying more than one baby or who suffer from polyhydramnios (too much amniotic fluid) are particularly susceptible to breathing difficulties. Some will run into the problem earlier or to a greater degree than mothers of singletons. If you find yourself short of breath, talk to your practitioner to ensure that the source of the problem is not another medical condition.

*Fixing comfort food to encourage you to eat when you maybe don't feel like eating can be one tactic to increase your calories.*

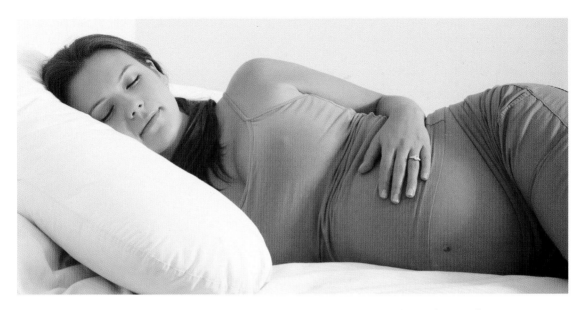

*Sleep before your baby gets here! With insomnia as a potential challenge, consider a daily nap as a necessity and not a stolen pleasure.*

## HOT MAMA

You might be considering a new haircut at this point in your pregnancy. Maybe you're bored with an old style, or you're in the mood to experiment. Just a bit of advice about haircuts at this juncture: Don't do anything drastic. Evidence suggests that when very pregnant women make dramatic changes to their appearance, they're responding to hormones and not necessarily careful thought. Before you regret doing something that can't be undone, choose a style that makes sense for a new mom—something that is low maintenance but flattering all the same.

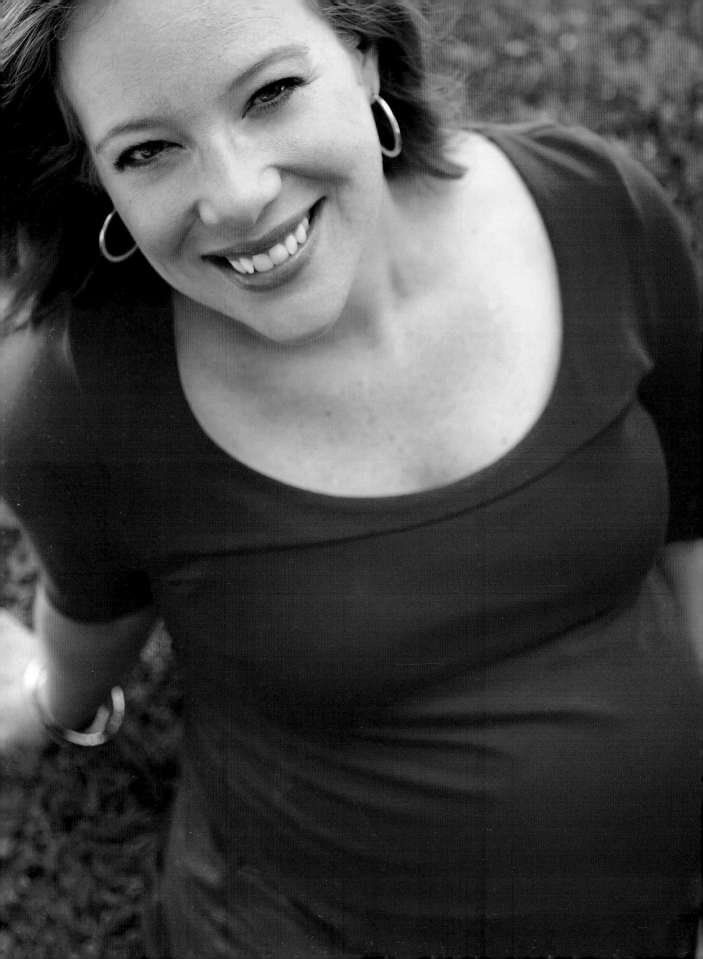

# WEEK 32

## ✎ CHECKLIST FOR WEEK 32

[ ] Deal with leg cramps.
[ ] Refresh yourself on how to time contractions.
[ ] Choose your final list of baby names.
[ ] Learn about late-pregnancy ultrasounds.
[ ] Prepare a place for your baby to sleep.

## ⌕ WHAT TO WATCH FOR THIS WEEK

### Double Check

**Decrease in fetal movement:** Decreased fetal movement may be a sign of problems with your baby. Sometimes it's a matter of perception, but contact your practitioner if you notice a decrease in your fetal kick counts, or if they take longer to perform or your baby is not completing the required number of movements.

**Swelling:** Normal swelling in pregnancy tends to develop slowly and diminishes if you allow yourself to rest. Sudden swelling in the face or hands, however, can signal pregnancy induced hypertension (PIH) or preeclampsia.

**Headaches:** A sign of potential trouble with your blood pressure, discuss severe headaches with your practitioner.

**Blurred vision:** Blurred vision is also considered a sign of PIH or preeclampsia. Report it immediately to your practitioner.

**Bleeding or spotting:** Bleeding or spotting (red or brown) at this point in pregnancy can happen naturally after sexual intercourse, a vaginal exam, or vaginal ultrasound. If you notice bleeding or spotting at other times, tell your midwife or doctor so he or she can examine you for signs of infection, premature dilation of the cervix, or issues related to your placenta.

**Back or abdominal pain:** Pain in your back or abdomen can be a sign of contractions or premature dilation of the cervix, a sign of potential preterm labor.

**More than six contractions per hour:** Another sign of preterm labor, bring contractions that number six or more per hour to the attention of your practitioner.

**Gush of fluid from the vagina:** It could be normal vaginal discharge, but in case your water has broken prematurely, you should report this to your practitioner right away.

*Report any strange or troublesome symptoms to your practitioner immediately.*

##  BODY BASICS

With roughly eight weeks left in the countdown, you are probably feeling a mixture of relief that the end is in sight and trepidation over how your life is about to change. The key is to not panic. Learn enough so that you can do what you need to and trust your instincts and common sense for those times you'll need to wing it. Whether you believe it or not, this is enough to get you started as a parent. It's often joked that we are better parents before we have kids. This is maybe not so funny when you are handed your little one, but it is comforting to think that not every parent knows what he or she is doing, and most of us turn out just fine.

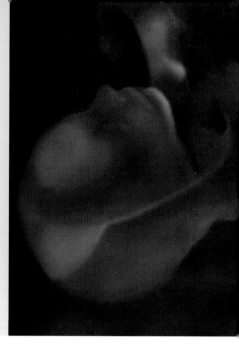

## BABY DATA

At nearly four pounds (1.8 kilograms) and fifteen inches (38 centimeters), your baby is beginning to fill out. For the next few weeks, your baby will really be putting on the weight in preparation for birth. If you looked at your baby's face via ultrasound earlier, it probably looked very skeletal, but not anymore. A lot of lung development has been taking place over the past few weeks to prepare the baby to breathe. The nervous system functions have also been maturing.

PREGNANCY PARTICULARS

## Deal with Leg Cramps

Leg cramps, or Charlie horses, can be very annoying toward the end of pregnancy. Most women will experience these cramps in their calves in the evenings or while they are sleeping. Some women are in such pain that they wake up screaming and awaken their husbands. The pain can be a result of vitamin and mineral deficiencies, lack of exercise, increased pressure on your legs from the weight gain of pregnancy, or even changes to the blood flow in the area.

A nutritionist will tell you that potassium and calcium are important for your overall health, but they may not mention that they also play a part in cramping muscles. One recommendation is to increase your intake of foods rich in potassium and calcium, such as bananas and dairy products, to see if that helps reduce or eliminate the cramps.

You can also add stretching to your pre-bedtime routine. Even the following few simple exercises that stretch your calf muscles can drastically reduce the amount of cramping.

First, stand with about a foot or more space between you and a wall. Place your hands on the wall at shoulder height. Step backward with your right foot, trying to place your foot flat on the floor.

You should feel the stretch in your calf. Hold for ten seconds. Switch legs and hold for ten seconds. Repeat three to five times on each side.

Second, place a phone book or other large book on the floor. Stand with both feet on the book and allow your heels to drop off the edge of the book, touching the floor if possible. Hold the stretch for ten seconds. If necessary, use a wall or chair for balance.

If you continue to wake up during the night because of leg cramps, do not panic. First, reassure your partner that you are not having the baby or dying. Then try flexing your foot upward, extending the heel of your foot and lengthening the muscle that's cramping. You should also try wiggling your toes—don't point them—to help alleviate the pain.

## Refresh Yourself on How to Time Contractions

Timing contractions is a simple process. All you need is a watch with a second hand, paper, and a pen.

Note the time you begin to feel a contraction, when the contraction ends, and when the next contraction begins. The time between the start of the first contraction and the beginning of the second contraction is the distance between contractions, known as how far apart the contractions are coming. The time between the beginning and ending of a contraction is called the length of a contraction.

During labor, your contractions will come at an amazingly regular pace. By timing a few contractions here and there, you can get a sense of where you are in labor. That said, it is possible to have a baby without timing a single contraction.

## Choose Your Final List of Baby Names

Now that you and your spouse have spent many weeks mulling over your baby name list, it is time to narrow down the contenders. While some families feel comfortable having only one name each for a boy or girl, others are reluctant to limit themselves to this extent. Either way is fine if it works for your family, but here's a word to the wise: Looking at your baby can be the final determining factor in choosing the best name. You don't want to find yourself with one name that simply has nothing to do with the baby you meet on his or her birth day.

If you find that you are having trouble narrowing down the list to a manageable size, about two or three names per sex, you will need to have lengthier discussions. Some families allow each partner one free "strike" to remove a name from the other partner's list, with no questions asked. This is a quick way to shorten the list.

You might also consider a deal. Some families allow moms to name girls and dads to name boys, or mom gets to name the first baby, dad the second, etc. Some even grant naming rights to the grandparents, which is a frightening prospect perhaps.

Don't feel panicked about going into labor without names picked out; this happens more often than you might think. Most states have very flexible baby naming laws that do not require you to choose a name in the first day or even a week

*Finally choosing a name for your baby can feel great. Consider celebrating!*

### PREGNANCY AFFIRMATION FOR WEEK 32

## My baby can sense the calm that I feel.

after the baby is born. Some states allow parents a month or more to name their babies. Some hospitals get a bit anxious because their paperwork—such as the birth certificate—needs to sit until you make that decision, but birth centers and home births are more flexible, allowing you time to get to know your baby before settling on a name.

Sometimes seeing the baby is all it takes, and one of the names on the list pops up as the clear choice. No matter how it happens, rest assured, it will happen.

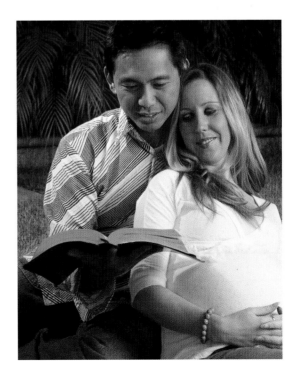

## Learn about Late-Pregnancy Ultrasounds

Late-pregnancy ultrasounds can be used for multiple purposes, including the following:

- Show the position of the baby
- Show the position of the placenta
- Report on the amount of amniotic fluid
- Give the condition of the placenta
- Report on fetal activity such as breathing and movement
- Give a fetal weight estimate
- Measure comparative growth for twins
- View fetal organ systems

After 20 weeks of gestation, the use of ultrasound to determine a due date is often off by more than the average correction with your period dates (plus or minus two weeks). An ultrasound done prior to 12 weeks gestation is preferred for dating purposes because there is less variation for genetically large versus smaller parents and because babies are more likely to be roughly the same size at this stage, but it is not at all a standard practice.

Ultrasound has also been used to try to guess the weight of the baby in utero. This has been shown to be off by up to 10 percent in either direction. Strictly speaking, the weight of the baby is not as big a deal as it may seem. The ultrasound cannot predict how your pelvis will open during labor, nor can it predict how your baby's head will mold and fit into your pelvis. Still, many mothers are eager to know their babies weight estimates. If you have an ultrasound, and it gives you a predicted weight, write it down and start taking bets!

Many women have had their labor induced for a suspected large baby, even though the American College of Obstetricians and Gynecologists says that a large baby is not a reason for induction. Many of these women have undergone additional risk

from the induction or other interventions, including the increased risk of Cesarean section, only to find that their babies were not as large as predicted.

If your practitioner would like to do an ultrasound at the end of pregnancy, ask questions, starting with why he or she feels it is necessary.

## Prepare a Place for Your Baby to Sleep

New parents spend a lot of time deciding where their baby will sleep. With all of the advice out there, it's no surprise that you may feel confused and conflicted about the best place for your baby.

The American Academy of Pediatrics recommends that your baby sleep very close to you, particularly in the beginning. They recommend that you place a bassinet or crib in your bedroom, but a co-sleeper works just as well. A co-sleeper safely attaches to your bed, giving you a small criblike space with an opening to allow your baby to be held close but in his or her own bed. They are available at most larger baby stores and online. They believe this is the safest sleeping arrangement for your baby. What's more, studies show that sleeping in close proximity to your baby is the best way for you to increase the amount of sleep you get each night.

The reason that sharing a room helps mother and baby sleep so well is that you are close enough to respond quickly when your baby needs you. Whether that response is a fresh diaper or food, your baby does not have to be in full awake and alert mode to get your attention.

This arrangement works well for most families for the first few months of baby's life. As your baby grows older and requires less attention in the middle of the night, you can move him or her into a different room and/or bed.

Remember that where your baby sleeps for the few weeks or months should follow stringent rules bearing from the manufacturer on his or her

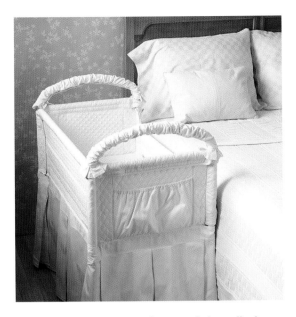

*A co-sleeper is a great way to have your baby really close to you without sharing your bed.*

weight and range of movement (such as rolling over and sitting up). Be sure to check and adhere to these guidelines.

Also consider the following when it comes to where your baby will sleep:

- Where is your room compared to baby's room?
- Can you get to baby's room quickly and easily?
- Can you hear your baby well?
- Will your baby be sharing a room with anyone?
- Do you have pets?
- Will baby's room be too noisy or sunny?

Answers to these questions will help you make the best choice for your baby and your family. There is more than one solution: the best advice is to be open to all of the possibilities and then figure out what feels right for you.

## WHAT ABOUT CO-SLEEPING?

Co-sleeping, or the term "family bed," refers to parents who choose to sleep with their babies in their beds. Although there have been numerous warnings about the dangers of co-sleeping, most studies find that the risks are from parental issues such as taking medication, drinking, or using unsafe bedding—and not the practice of co-sleeping itself.

Take the decision to sleep in the same bed as your baby seriously. Many moms do not intend to co-sleep, but in the middle of a weary night, they find themselves falling asleep with the baby beside them. This is when co-sleeping can be dangerous, because it was unplanned. There are strict rules that must be followed when sleeping with your baby in your bed. These include the following. Do not sleep with your baby:

- If you take medications such as pain killers or sedatives that may make your sleep too soundly and roll over onto the baby.
- If you smoke.
- If you have large comforters or heavy blankets.
- On a waterbed or a couch.
- If you are severely overweight.
- In a bed shared by adults who are not the baby's parent.

In his book, *Sleeping with Your Baby*, Dr. James McKenna, a sleep researcher from Notre Dame, has compiled a wealth of examples of safe co-sleeping practices and products to assist families. His work shows that there are many benefits to co-sleeping, including lower rates of SIDS and higher amounts of sleep for both parent and baby. If you choose to co-sleep, this book is a mustread.

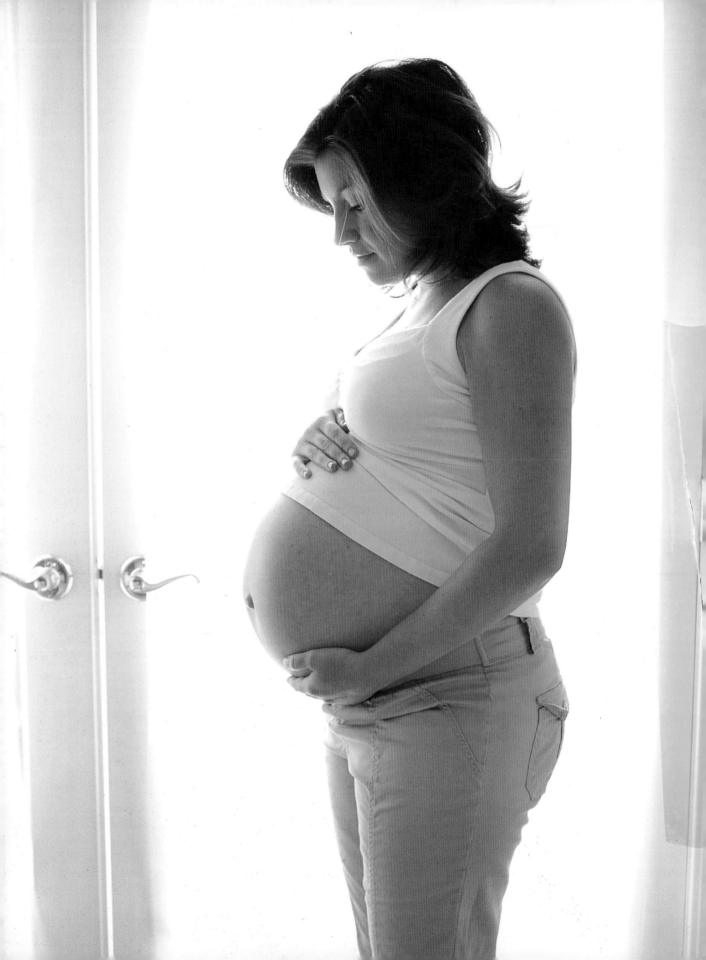

# WEEK 33

## CHECKLIST FOR WEEK 33

[ ] Learn about relaxation for labor.
[ ] Buy a breastfeeding bra.
[ ] Deal with comments on your belly size and shape.
[ ] Combat end-of-pregnancy worries.

## WHAT TO WATCH FOR THIS WEEK

*Double Check*

**Decrease in fetal movement:** If you notice your baby doing fewer fetal kick counts, taking longer to perform them, or not completing the required number of movements, tell your practitioner immediately. It may be that you haven't noticed your baby's changing habits or a different kind of movement in a constrained space, and your practitioner can help you make sense of it.

**Swelling:** Should you experience a sudden swelling in your face or hands, it could be related to pregnancy induced hypertension (PIH) or preeclampsia. Unlike normal swelling in pregnancy that usually goes away after a period of rest, this type of severe swelling should be reported to your doctor or midwife.

**Headaches:** Severe headaches can be a sign of trouble with your blood pressure. Less severe headaches can be caused by pregnancy hormones, but when a bad headache is accompanied by other symptoms, it can be the result of PIH or even preeclampsia.

**Blurred vision:** Report this immediately to your practitioner, with or without a headache, because it can also be a sign of PIH or preeclampsia.

**Bleeding or spotting:** Bleeding or spotting can be a natural side effect of having sexual intercourse, a vaginal exam, or vaginal ultrasound. If, however, none of these has happened, report bleeding or spotting immediately to your practitioner, because it may be a sign of infection, premature dilation of the cervix, or issues related to your placenta.

**Back or abdominal pain:** Pain in these areas raises the possibility of contractions or premature dilation of the cervix, a sign of potential preterm labor.

**More than six contractions per hour:** This is a sign of preterm labor and should be discussed with your practitioner.

**Gush of fluid from the vagina:** To determine if the fluid is a normal vaginal discharge or a sign that your water has broken prematurely, contact your practitioner right away.

*Report any strange or troublesome symptoms to your practitioner immediately.*

##  BODY BASICS

Your baby is growing, and so are you. You may wake up one morning and think that your baby has doubled in size over night. It is fun to watch how your belly changes. One day you look larger than the previous day only to look smaller the next day. Thank your acrobatic baby. He or she is busy doing turns and switching positions, making you change shape on a daily basis. All this movement and activity means that some of your clothes fit nicely some of the time.

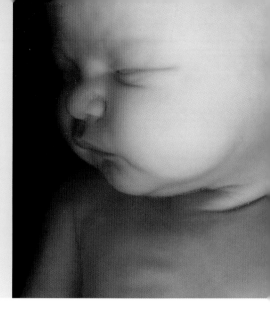

## 🛒 BABY DATA

Your baby is growing a lot. Lung development takes the forefront toward the end of pregnancy, and your baby's body is producing something called surfactant. This detergent-like substance helps your baby's lungs stay open once they inflate with his or her first cry. Premature infants are given artificial surfactant if they are born too early.

# Learn about Relaxation for Labor

Relaxation can take many forms: mental, physical, or emotional. Many childbirth classes teach relaxation as a way to cope with and ease labor.

You can approach relation in numerous ways. Some people start with a simple mind and body exercise such as tense and release, in which you

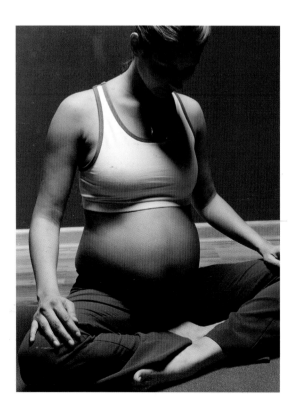

assume a restful position and then you or your partner think of or call out a body part that you first tense and then relax. Your job is to notice the difference between the tense and the released, or relaxed, feeling. Your partner can assist by noticing the differences visually and by touch.

You can change the script and use a relaxing image or mental vacation. Some people use the following questions as prompts:

- Describe your favorite vacation.
- Think of your most romantic moment.
- Imagine your ideal safe place.
- Visualize your ideal birth.

These questions are starters for visualizations that can be used to help induce relaxation. If you like, you can combine this mental and emotional relaxation with soothing touches, stroking, or massage. And feel free to move during relaxation or change positions that cease being comfortable.

It is important to note that what feels great in pregnancy and during your practice sessions may not have the same effect for labor. Go with the flow and see what works. When you're in labor, you might need to alter your approach as you need to ensure maximal comfort.

*Not only is relaxation great for labor, but also has many pregnancy and lifelong benefits. Get the most out of your newly found skills by practicing often.*

There are many, many ways to do relaxation. If you learned other methods in a childbirth or yoga class, or if you prefer your own relaxation or meditation exercises, feel free to bring them into your pregnancy and birth experience.

## Buy a Breastfeeding Bra

You may have heard conflicting advice about buying a bra specifically designed for breastfeeding: Should you buy underwire bras? How do you go about choosing the right size? Even if women differ on how they answer these and other questions, it is recommended that every expectant mother buy one or two nursing bras prior to the baby being born. If you do, you'll have a leg up on feeding your new baby, without having to fight around your bra.

A breastfeeding bra is specially constructed. It's designed to give your breasts support and protection from bouncing, and it also has easily accessible flaps that make it easy to nurse your baby. These flaps can pull down, snap down, or clip down from the bra strap. Choose a design that works easily for you and you can open using only one hand.

Now for the size to choose. Once the first week postpartum has passed, very few women need a larger bra than what they needed toward the end of the third trimester. So buy a bra or two that fits your current size at 32 weeks. If you are one of the few women who needs a bigger bra, buy it after your baby is born. In the meantime, the bras you purchase now will get you through until then.

Remember to pack a nursing bra in your labor bag. You might also want to break them in by wearing them during the final stage of your pregnancy.

It is typically recommended that breastfeeding moms avoid underwire bras because they can

*A good breastfeeding bra is a must. You can make this purchase during pregnancy.*

## PREGNANCY AFFIRMATION FOR WEEK 33

✚

# My baby's head fits snugly into my pelvis as we prepare for birth.

block milk ducts, causing pain and even mastitis, which is a serious breast infection. If you have large breasts and prefer underwire bras, talk to a knowledgeable salesperson at a store with a good inventory of nursing bras.

You can also buy other specialty bras for new mothers. These include hands-free breast pump bras for women who pump frequently and want the use of their hands while pumping and bras that are

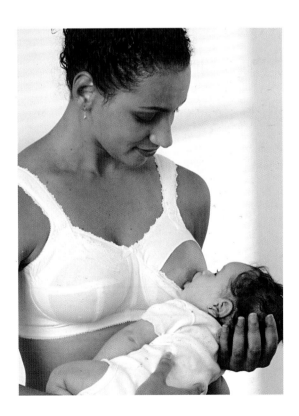

worn at night or for sleep. You may or may not feel the need to have support for your breasts at night. If you do, a bra is helpful, though it doesn't have to be a fancy or expensive bra. Many moms wear something as simple as a sports bra at night.

## Deal with Comments on Your Belly Size and Shape

You are soooo big! You are too small. Are you having twins? Are you due very soon? These are all typical questions and comments that pregnant women hear toward the end of their pregnancies.

The comments aren't mean or hurtful, but they can be a problem if you begin to internalize them. If every third person tells you how small or big your belly is, eventually you begin to believe them. You find yourself starting to worry even when you can't recall why you are worried. These seemingly benign comments become harmful if they undermine your faith in your body's normal, natural process.

The best strategy is to have comments of your own at the ready. Be direct: "My practitioner says that the baby and I are measuring just fine. Thank you very much."

This reminds the person and you that someone is looking out for your well being and your baby's welfare. It also restores your confidence that you have been checked out and that you and your baby are growing properly and according to guidelines.

If annoying comments continue to bug you and raise questions in your mind, it never hurts to discuss them at your next appointment or to call your practitioner and leave a nonurgent message seeking reassurance.

You may also find yourself on the receiving end of other types of comments such as the following:

- Your face doesn't look pregnant.
- You can't tell you're pregnant from behind.
- It looks like you swallowed a basketball.
- You must be having a _____ because you're carrying _____.

While these types of comments are perfectly innocent and are intended to be complimentary, you may not always hear them that way. It can also stop being funny when you hear a comment for the tenth time that afternoon. Try not to overreact and offer a smile instead.

## Combat End-of-Pregnancy Worries

Along with everything else you have going on, it's sometimes impossible to keep your mind from worrying. This is a common malady in pregnancy, particularly at the end. No matter what you tell yourself, the worries creep up, usually at night when you can do precious little except lose sleep.

You can employ some tricks to help prevent these worries from intruding and becoming unbearable. One is to ask your practitioner during your visits how everything is going. Even if you know that everything is fine, it is always reassuring to get confirmation and hear the words, "You and the baby are doing great!"

The second trick is to voice your concerns. This is true even if you know that your fear is unfounded. The person that you confide in does not have to be your practitioner. It can be your partner, your best friend, your Internet due date buddy—whoever has a knack for reassuring and comforting you.

If something crops up between prenatal appointments and is a reasonable request or question, feel free to call your practitioner for advice. This is part of his or her job. Getting answers from someone you trust will help you feel secure, relax, and enjoy the rest of your pregnancy.

**HOT MAMA**

Chances are you've reached the point where you feel like you are wearing the same two to three outfits over and over again. If your maternity clothes are getting tired and boring, it might be time to splurge on a new outfit or two. Even a new top can change your attitude about how you feel about your clothes—and yourself. We all know that looking good is connected to feeling good, so freshen up your wardrobe and see what it does for your outlook.

## WHAT TO DO WHEN WORRY STRIKES AT NIGHT

Late-night worries and even nightmares can strike toward the end of pregnancy, making you lose precious sleep. When this happens, you need to combat your fears in whatever way works for you.

Will relaxation help? Put on soft music, take a warm bath, and try some mental relaxation until you have forgotten about whatever woke you or was keeping you up.

You might try writing down your worries. This tells your mind that you are not ignoring what's going on, just shelving it until the morning hours. This strategy can also work for dreams and to do list items that come to you at 2 A.M.

Another approach is to talk it out. This might mean waking your honey up from a deep sleep, but sometimes nothing else works. If you'd rather not disturb him, you could try posting on your favorite Internet chat group or forum to get it off your chest. If you prefer to combat fear with information, keep a pregnancy book by your bed to answer questions that pop up in the middle of the night.

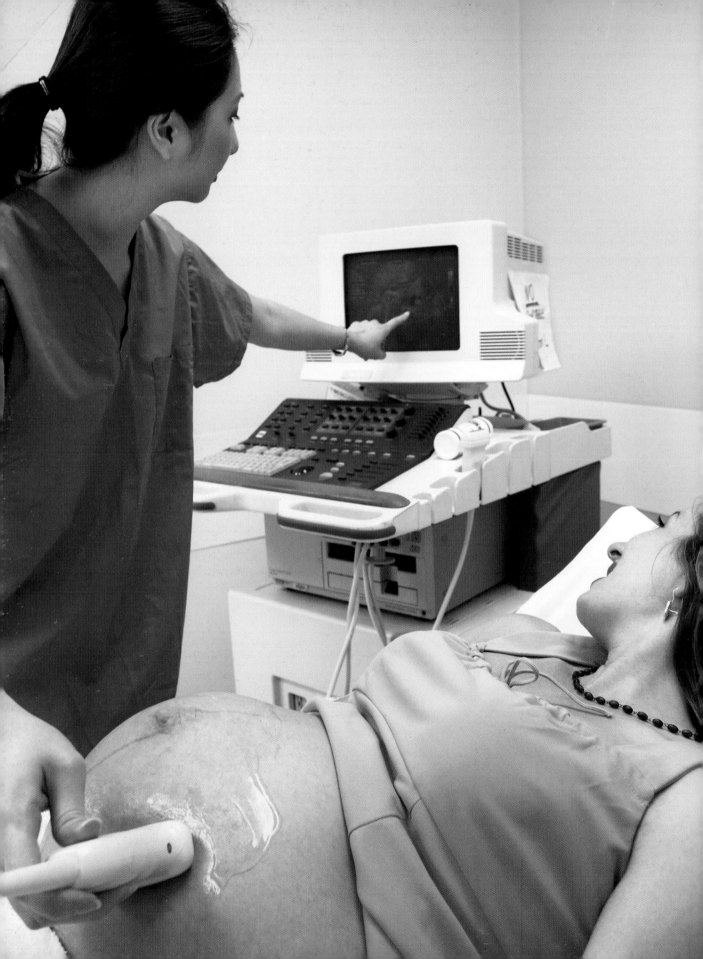

# WEEK 34

## ✏ CHECKLIST FOR WEEK 34

[ ] Prepare for nausea to return.
[ ] Schedule your group B strep screening.
[ ] Purchase nursing tops.
[ ] Choose your music for labor.
[ ] Learn about amniotic fluid.

## 🔍 WHAT TO WATCH FOR THIS WEEK

### Double Check

**Decrease in fetal movement:** A reduction in fetal movement can be a sign of problems, or it might be simply a matter of perception. Either way, report it to your midwife or doctor immediately. With his or her help, you may discover that your baby's kicking habits have changed or the movement is different because of limited space.

**Swelling:** Normal swelling in pregnancy will go away after a period of rest, but sudden, severe swelling in the face or hands is a sign of pregnancy induced hypertension (PIH) or preeclampsia.

**Headaches:** PIH and preeclampsia both involve severe headaches. When a headache is mild and results from normal pregnancy hormone fluctuations, you needn't worry. Your practitioner should evaluate severe headaches, however.

**Blurred vision:** Report blurred vision immediately to your practitioner, with or without the presence of a headache, because it can also be a sign of PIH or preeclampsia.

**Bleeding or spotting:** Bleeding or spotting may be normal if it follows sexual intercourse, a vaginal exam, or vaginal ultrasound. Without these triggers, however, you should tell your midwife or doctor about spotting because it could be a sign of infection, premature dilation of the cervix, or issues related to your placenta.

**Back or abdominal pain:** Pain in your back or abdomen can be a sign of contractions or premature dilation of the cervix, a sign of potential preterm labor.

**More than six contractions per hour:** It is unsurprising to experience contractions at this stage of pregnancy, but if they occur this frequently, it could mean preterm labor, and you should alert your practitioner.

**Gush of fluid from the vagina:** The fluid could be coming from the amniotic sac or be a normal discharge. Only your practitioner can make the determination and conclude if your water has broken prematurely.

*Report any strange or troublesome symptoms to your practitioner immediately.*

##  BODY BASICS

Hopefully you are managing to enjoy the end of your pregnancy. It can be easy to get caught up in the not-so-fun aspects of pregnancy, but try to maintain a positive attitude, knowing that you have but a few short weeks left. You may even be starting to think that having your baby will be easier than pregnancy, but many a mom will tell you that what you imagine will be better or easier is often just different.

## 🛒 BABY DATA

At week 34, the average baby weight is four and a half pounds (2205 kilograms). Your baby is still growing heavier and getting longer too. He or she measures approximately seventeen inches (43 centimeters), and you are sure to feel plenty of baby tucked into your uterus. As your baby moves, you are less likely to feel large movements because there's less room in which to move around. You will, however, feel the baby stretching and wiggling. You might catch glimpses of feet, knees, and elbows as they poke outward as your baby settles in to be born.

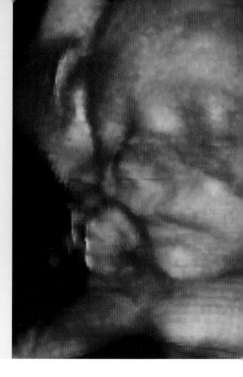

## Prepare for Nausea to Return

It's possible that as your pregnancy nears its end, you will experience a return to nausea, even vomiting. Being prepared can help you deal more effectively should nausea strike again.

You may find that you feel queasy just before mealtimes. This could be a signal from your body to eat smaller, more frequent meals, which help keep your blood sugar stable and ward off some types of nausea.

If the feeling is reminiscent of how you felt at the start of your pregnancy, the good news is that whatever worked then should be helpful now. Try to recall all of the tricks you used in the first trimester, and hopefully they'll be just as effective in combating your nausea now.

Late-stage nausea is caused primarily by fluctuating hormones as you prepare for birth, but it is also important to remember that nutrition plays a role. Eating well and staying hydrated can mitigate some of the discomfort you are feeling. Exercise can also help stem a problem with nausea.

## Schedule Your Group B Strep Screening

Group B strep, beta strep, and GBS are three names for the same thing: a bacteria that about 25 percent of all women carry. Between weeks 34 and 36, you will get screened for this bacteria through a procedure that's similar to a Pap smear in which samples are taken from your vagina and rectum.

Group B strep is not a sexually transmitted infection. It is a normal bacteria that about a fourth of all pregnant women have in their bodies that poses no harm to them or their sexual partners. However, there is risk at birth to your baby. If your baby contracts group B strep from you or the hospital personnel, he or she can get an active infection that can lead to the need for antibiotics after birth, swelling in the brain, spinal cord, and other locations and even die from the infection.

If you are found to have group B strep, you will be treated during labor with intravenous antibiotics. This drastically reduces the likelihood that your baby will become infected with the bacteria. The antibiotics should not interfere with your mobility in labor or delivery. They are given every four to six hours and take about twenty minutes to go in, at which point the tubing can be removed from the catheter, giving you more freedom to move.

By administering antibiotics during labor, the number of babies who contract group B strep is very small: Fewer than 1 to 2 percent of babies whose mothers received treatment in labor are affected. You may also be treated with antibiotics if the following circumstances occur:

- You are having your baby prior to 37 weeks, even if you were not tested or tested negative.
- Your water has been broken for longer than eighteen hours.
- You develop a fever in labor of 100.4 or higher.

If you test positive for group B strep, you may have questions. Perhaps you're wondering if a Cesarean can prevent a baby from contracting group B strep. The answer is no, a Cesarean section does not prevent the bacteria from being transmitted. If you'd like to know if it's possible to breastfeed with group B strep, the answer is yes; your baby is not at any increased risk.

You will be given a new test for group B strep during every pregnancy, no matter if you tested negative or positive in prior pregnancies. The Centers for Disease Control and Prevention recommend that you be treated if you receive positive test results in a current pregnancy or you gave birth to a baby who suffered from group B strep.

## Purchase Nursing Tops

Nursing wear makes your life so much easier when you are trying to breastfeed. A few simple tops can go a long way to making your wardrobe breastfeeding friendly. These tops have special openings to allow you to nurse your baby without showing your breasts or skin.

Nursing tops are designed with several different types of opening. To decide which is right for you, try on the tops while wearing your nursing bra. Can you easily reach each breast with one hand? Can you move your breast to the opening easily? For example, a nursing top with a single, center slit

PREGNANCY AFFIRMATION
FOR WEEK 34

+

My mind is open to my
labor and birth.

might not work well for a mother with small breasts. The opening is too far away from where her breast needs to be to function appropriately.

Once you find a style that suits you, remember the brand and size so you can buy more tops as needed. You might start by purchasing several T-shirts and a nice top in case you go to a party or restaurant. You can always buy more later.

If you have friends or relatives who aren't using their nursing clothes anymore, consider borrowing them. You may not have the ability to choose the styles or types of opening, but it is always good to have a few extra tops, particularly when babies tend to spit up. Borrowing from other mothers can also help you decide how many shirts you need and what types of shirts you like best.

Once you get used to breastfeeding, you can wear your regular, nonnursing tops with more frequency. As you and the baby become pros at nursing, you will be able to maneuver regular tops by unbuttoning from the bottom or figuring out how to keep yourself covered while breastfeeding.

## Choose Your Music for Labor

Music can be a powerful way to soothe your mind and body in labor. Music has long been known to affect our moods. Studies have shown that listening to music that you like can raise your endorphin levels and improve your mood.

It is therefore essential that you select music for labor that you enjoy. It's a good idea to choose

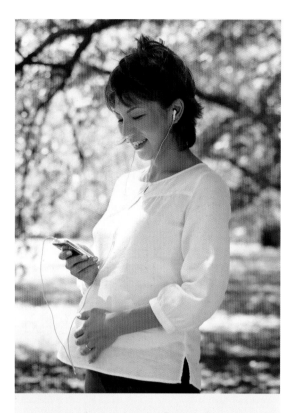

## LOAD YOUR MP3S FOR LABOR

Once you've compiled a long list of music that you want to have available during your labor, carting along all the compact disks seems like a hassle. This is where an iPod or MP3 player is a wonderful addition to the labor bag. It gives you a convenient way to carry all of your music, and it is sorted nicely as well.

If you plan to bring your iPod, be sure that it is loaded up with a specific play list for labor. This can be a great early project in the last few weeks of your pregnancy, maybe one night when you are having trouble sleeping. Make sure that you pack something to charge your iPod and both speakers and head phones so you can listen to the music in multiple ways.

music of various speeds and to include a bunch of different songs. You want lots of variety in your music choices because you simply do not know what you will feel like hearing during labor. That said, there tend to be some general guidelines when it comes to music for labor.

For early labor, if you are in the mood to relax, you will want music that is slow and gentle, such as classical or other instrumental music, love songs, easy listening, and relaxation specific music. If you are more in the mood to get up and move, choose your favorite dance music.

As you shift into the active portion of labor, you will most likely be moving around to help push your baby down into your pelvis. Dance music is appropriate here as well because it is upbeat, gives you a rhythm, and encourages you to get up and move your body.

For the later stages of labor and pushing, tastes in music vary greatly. Some women choose to stop listening to music altogether, while others change the music to match their mood. Mellow, relaxing music or even guided imagery can be beneficial for some, while others insist on rock and roll or forceful orchestral music when it's time to really push.

## Learn about Amniotic Fluid

The amniotic fluid that your baby floats in is relatively constant. Your baby drinks small amounts and urinates back into the water. Your body acts as a filter and replenishes the fluid every three hours or so.

Sometimes there are problems with the amount of fluid in your uterus. Too little amniotic fluid is known as oligohydramnios, and too much fluid is known as polyhydramnios. Most of the time, a

*A good playlist for labor should be chosen by you for the most benefit. Remember, your tastes may be different then, so pick a variety.*

problem is discovered when your doctor or midwife notices a discrepancy in your fundal height or via ultrasound.

To determine the amount of amniotic fluid, an ultrasound exam is used to measure the fluid pockets around the baby. This is called an amniotic fluid index (AFI). Measuring these pockets of fluid gives your practitioner an idea of how much fluid is there, but it is only an educated guess.

When the fluid level is off, it could be related to maternal hydration or caused by problems with the pregnancy. Your medical team will provide you with information if you are diagnosed with either condition.

## OLIGOHYDRAMNIOS

Oligohydramnios, or low fluid volume, is defined as an AFI of 5 centimeters or less. This can be caused from a prolonged rupture of the membranes, fetal kidney problems, intrauterine growth restriction, or other problems.

The risks associated with oligohydramnios include the baby being born with a physical deformity, such as a club foot. This happens because the baby has too little space in which to move, restricting growth. Because low fluid volume can sometimes also be a sign of fetal distress, it must be taken seriously by watching and intervening only when necessary. Treatment for oligohydramnios might involve maternal hydration (oral or IV) or even induction of labor.

## POLYHYDRAMNIOS

Polyhydramnios is defined as having more than 68 ounces (2 liters) of amniotic fluid. It occurs in less than 1 percent of women at the end of pregnancy. It is more likely to occur in pregnancies where there is the following:

- Multiple babies
- Maternal diabetes
- Congenital malformations

Ultrasound is also used to diagnose an excess of amniotic fluid. Some practitioners treat the condition by withdrawing amniotic fluid from the uterus with a needle, similar to an amniocentesis. During the birth process, there can be higher risks associated with polyhydramnios. The baby might be in a less favorable position for birth or frequently change positions, the umbilical cord could prolapse (come down before the baby), or the mother could be at risk for a postpartum hemorrhage due to the distention of her uterus.

If you are diagnosed with amniotic fluid issues, your practitioner will discuss the various treatment options with you so the risks and benefits associated with each course of action are clear.

**HOT MAMA**

As your pregnancy progresses and your baby and belly grow, you may notice your abdomen has developed dry skin and is frequently itchy. Splurge on a moisturizing body lotion that smells great and feels luxurious. It's a small thing that can help you feel fabulous while relieving the itching.

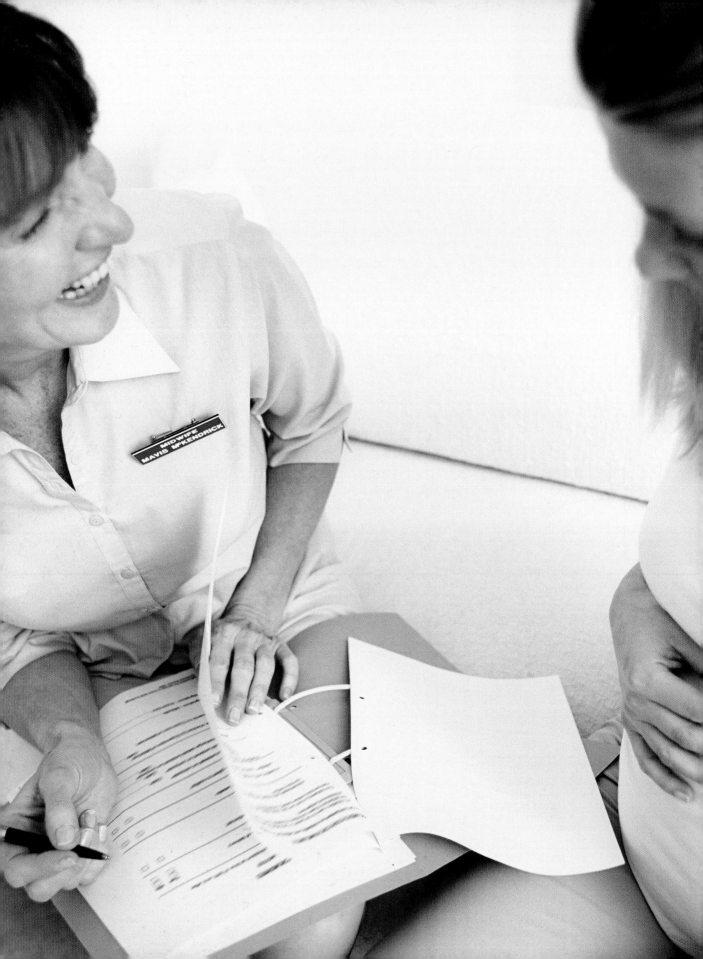

# WEEK 35

## ✏ CHECKLIST FOR WEEK 35

[ ] Finalize your birth plan.
[ ] Visit a breastfeeding group or new mothers' group.
[ ] Learn about breech babies.
[ ] Prepare your pet for the new baby.

## 🔍 WHAT TO WATCH FOR THIS WEEK

*Double Check*

**Decrease in fetal movement:** Contact your practitioner should you notice any of the following: decrease in your fetal kick counts, taking longer to perform the kicks, or not completing the required number of movements. It may be a simple question of your baby changing movement habits or doing a different kind of movement due to limited space, but your practitioner can help you figure this out.

**Swelling:** Signs of pregnancy induced hypertension (PIH) or preeclampsia can be found in the sudden swelling in the face or hands. You can recognize normal swelling in pregnancy because it doesn't pop up suddenly and will decrease following a period of rest.

**Headaches:** Severe headaches raise concerns with your blood pressure and should be reported to your practitioner. Sometimes headaches are triggered by pregnancy hormones, but when they become severe, the possibility of PIH or even preeclampsia needs to be discussed.

**Blurred vision:** Tell your midwife or doctor if you experience blurred vision, especially if you are also having headaches. Vision trouble, like severe headaches, is a sign of PIH and preeclampsia.

**Bleeding or spotting:** Bleeding or spotting that doesn't follow vaginal exams or sexual intercourse may be a sign of infection, premature dilation of the cervix, or issues related to your placenta and should be reported to your practitioner.

**Back or abdominal pain:** If you've noticed pain in your back or abdomen, tell your practitioner because it is a sign of potential preterm labor.

**More than six contractions per hour:** This, too, is a sign of preterm labor. Having fewer contractions is quite normal but at this frequency, you should consult your practitioner.

**Gush of fluid from the vagina:** This can be a sign that your water has broken prematurely. Your practitioner can determine if fluid leaking from your vagina is amniotic fluid or normal discharge. *Report any strange or troublesome symptoms to your practitioner immediately.*

##  BODY BASICS

If you have not been in a swimming pool lately, now is the time to try it, even if the weather means going to an indoor pool. The feeling of being nearly weightless in the water is a blessing at this stage of the game, even if you have not gained a lot of weight. You are no doubt tired and sore from carrying your baby all day. Exercising in water, even a few light strokes, has been shown to make pregnant women feel amazing. So dig out that swimsuit!

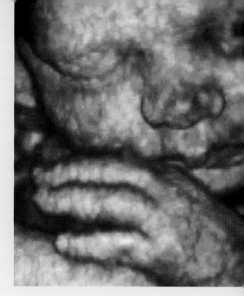

## BABY DATA

Baby is hanging in there, doing his or her part to prepare for the big birth day coming up. This consists principally of growing, developing, and preparing to breathe and regulate body temperature. Your baby is now about four and half pounds (2.25 kilograms), though at this stage of the game there is more room for variance and where diet and genetics play a significant part. Your baby is approaching eighteen inches (46 centimeters) from head to toe.

Babies born at this gestational age often do well with special care nurseries, but it is still considered early. Babies who are born early often have respiratory illnesses and breathing difficulties, which can lead to an increased risk of SIDS and lifelong issues such as asthma and learning disabilities (although the greatest risk is during the first year of life).

**PREGNANCY PARTICULARS**

## Finalize Your Birth Plan

As you are getting down to the last few weeks of pregnancy, it is important to finalize your birth plan. While a birth plan is not a rigid document that plots every movement in labor, it is something to share with the people you are working with on your baby's birth to provide them with a sense of your wishes and preferences.

To that end, your document should be brief. Busy nurses, doctors, and technicians do not have the time to read lengthy documents. They need to find the information that pertains to their jobs quickly so that they can appropriately and adequately help you.

Your birth plan should fit on one piece of paper, single sided. Think about dividing it into sections, such as labor, postpartum, and baby care. Under each heading, you might have a short bulleted list of your main points. Here's an example:

Labor Plan:

- Freedom to move around
- Saline lock or clear liquids
- Intermittent monitoring of the baby
- Pain medicine as requested, but do not offer

Your birth plan should be positive and realistic in tone. Avoid a long list of things you do not want done to you or your baby. Instead offer positive suggestions for how people can help you. Be realistic. For example, do not write that a water birth is your highest priority if you know that the hospital or birth center does not do water births. Knowing the policies of your birth place is the best way to avoid this type of problem.

Once you and your partner have finalized your birth plan, you should show it to your practitioner and your doula. They can help spot any issues with policy or wording that you may have missed. When you are done, ask your practitioner and the baby's pediatrician to sign copies. This tells the nurses and other professionals at your place of birth that this is what your practitioner and pediatrician want for you and your baby as well and that they have approved the plan.

Make extra copies of your signed birth plan to distribute. Be sure to keep some for yourself, but you should also give copies to your practitioner, your place of birth, the baby's pediatrician, and the nursery if you are planning a hospital birth.

## Visit a Breastfeeding Group or New Mothers' Group

Late in your third trimester is an ideal time to visit a breastfeeding and/or new mothers group. They offer you the chance to make new friends with women who also have small babies, and they are places for you to seek out advice.

To find a new mothers' group, check area birth centers, churches or synagogues, libraries, and even maternity shops and toy stores. Most are for new mothers in general, but some have a particular focus such as mothers of young boys, mothers of multiples, etc.

For groups with a set theme or focus, the members might meet to discuss specific topics rather having a simple play group. It is your choice to decide if you would like a time of interactive learning or a time to connect with other moms. Many groups are successful at combining both interests.

You simply cannot get all your learning and tips from a class or book, so being around other

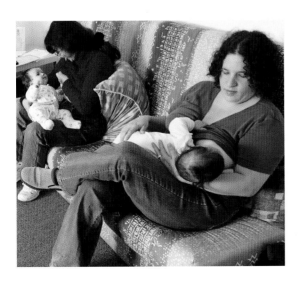

## PREGNANCY AFFIRMATION FOR WEEK 35

+

## I know how to take care of my baby.

parents is ideal. There are so many things to discuss and discoveries to share as new parents. Joining a group now also provides you with a whole new support network that you can rely on before your baby is born and look forward to growing with after baby arrives.

## Learn about Breech Babies

At the end of pregnancy, only about 3 to 4 percent of babies are in a breech position. This means that rather than being head down, your baby is presenting with one of the following body parts:

- Frank breech: bottom first, feet near baby's head
- Footling breech: one or both feet first
- Kneeling breech: knees first

Any of these positions can complicate the birth for you and the baby. Your practitioner might make recommendations to encourage your baby to turn head down. This can range from simple exercises to visits with specialists.

Simple exercises that you can do at home include the following:

- Breech tilt: Lie with your feet higher than your head. (Reclining on a collapsed ironing board that has been propped on a chair or sofa works well.) Your baby will then be able to move out of the pelvis and shift to a head down position.

*Being around other nursing mothers is a great way to learn to breastfeed and to pick up great tips for caring for your new baby.*

- Music or light therapy: Using a handheld device, play music directed at your pubic bone. This is meant to encourage your baby to move toward the music. The same trick can work using a flashlight.

Some mothers and practitioners prefer to use something that encourages the baby to move away from the top of your uterus. An example might be doing light therapy aimed at your public bone while placing a bag of frozen peas toward the top of your uterus.

Among approaches that are more medically driven, a visit to your local chiropractor may be in order. A chiropractor trained in the Webster technique can help your body naturally turn the baby with a chiropractic adjustment. It may take more than one visit and can be used in conjunction with other practices.

Some research indicates that the ancient Chinese art of moxibustion can help with breech babies. This involves a practitioner of Chinese medicine burning a moxi stick near certain pressure points on your body to help rotate the baby into a head-down position.

Another technique, known as an external cephalic version, is typically done in a hospital. Using medication to relax your uterus and an ultrasound that guides the practitioner away from the placenta and monitors the baby, the practitioner moves the baby from the outside by placing his or her hands on your abdomen. This is not a gentle or easy technique, but most mothers agree that this is easier than giving birth to a breech baby or having a Cesarean section.

How likely any of these techniques will work varies from mother to mother and practitioner to practitioner. You should have a lengthy discussion about the benefits and risks or every option before you attempt a procedure. If the procedure you choose to undergo is successful, your pregnancy will continue on as before.

While many practitioners are not comfortable allowing women to give birth vaginally to a breech baby, some practitioners are well trained in vaginal breech birth and will assess each woman individually. A woman who has previously had a vaginal birth and is carrying a baby who is not too large and is in a frank breech position is a good candidate for a vaginal breech birth. You may need to seek out another practitioner if your practitioner is reluctant to perform this procedure.

## Prepare Your Pet for the New Baby

Whether you have a cat or a dog, or even some other exotic pet, you will need to prepare for an adjustment period—for both you and your pet—once the baby is brought home. This does not have to be a huge deal, and for many families it never becomes an issue.

For typical household pets such as dogs or cats, you should consider if there will be changes in schedules and places your pets are no longer welcome. Occasionally pregnancy provides the impetus to take a puppy (or stubborn older dog) for obedience training, just to get the ball rolling.

You hope everything will go smoothly, but introducing a new baby into the family might not be as easy on your pet as you assume it will be. Your pet does not understand what a baby is or why it lives with you, and jealousy can result. Remember to spend time with your pet before and after the baby's arrival. Once the baby is born, bring home a blanket that your baby has slept in at the hospital and let your pet smell it. This can help your pet get used to your baby's scent. Some experts agree that you should greet your pet without the baby in your arms when you arrive home for the first time.

## KEEP THE CAT OFF THE BABY STUFF

Cats seem to be drawn to all things baby, even before your baby is born. Cats are frequently found curled up in car seats, cribs, and bassinets. The small, enclosed spaces make great napping spots for them. The problem is that your cat and the baby cannot share the same space once the baby is born.

Some families use the water bottle method to train cats. This involves spraying the cat with water every time you catch it doing something wrong. Other families drape blankets and other covers over items or areas they don't want the cat to wander into. Do whatever works for you and your pet; just remember that your baby doesn't want a crib mate just yet.

If a new baby keeps you busy around the clock, find someone who's willing to spend some time with your pets. Start by having someone come and feed them while you are away having the baby. Then invite them back to take your dog for walks or go on play dates when possible. Some new parents rely on pet day cares for socialization purposes.

With more exotic pets, you may need expert advice from someone who specializes in that type of animal. Certain pets can be dangerous with babies if you are not careful because of potential diseases. Other animals are perfectly fine to have around a new baby, but you may need to follow some common sense precautions.

**HOT MAMA**

Shaving your legs can get pretty tricky at the end of pregnancy. It may be time to give up trying to shave in the shower or in the bathtub. Instead, sit on the side of a half-filled tub, rinsing the razor in the running tap. You have a bit more balance and you are not quite as slippery as when wet. Some mothers say their husband was more than willing to help shave their legs, which went a long way toward helping them feel pretty and put together.

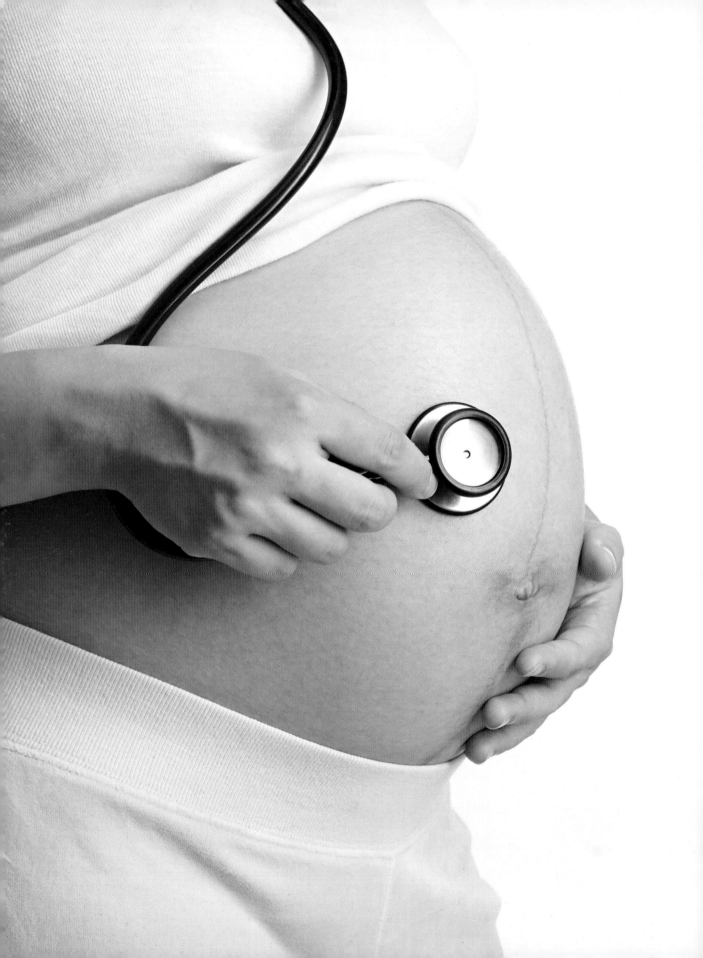

# WEEK 36

## CHECKLIST FOR WEEK 36

[ ]  Celebrate your baby.

[ ]  Practice comfort measures for labor to aid in relaxation and pain relief.

[ ]  Learn about cord blood banking.

[ ]  Schedule weekly prenatal visits.

[ ]  Revisit your birth place.

## WHAT TO WATCH FOR THIS WEEK
*Double Check*

**Decrease in fetal movement:** Your practitioner can help you figure out if any decrease in fetal movement signals a problem with your baby. It's possible that your baby has changed his or her kicking routine or has less space and therefore kicks less, but it's worth discussing the change with your midwife or doctor immediately.

**Swelling:** Keep an eye out for swelling that appears suddenly in the face or hands. These are signs of pregnancy induced hypertension (PIH) or preeclampsia.

**Headaches:** Tell your practitioner if you develop severe headaches, which can be a sign of problems with your blood pressure. Pregnancy hormones can cause mild headaches. But in their more severe form, headaches may be linked to PIH or even preeclampsia, which is a severe illness in pregnancy related to blood pressure, protein in your urine, and other complications.

**Blurred vision:** Report blurred vision immediately to your practitioner. Along with severe headaches, it is associated PIH and preeclampsia.

**Bleeding or spotting:** Unless you've undergone a vaginal exam or vaginal ultrasound or have had sex, you should report any incidents of bleeding or spotting. Your practitioner will examine you to rule out the possibility of infection, premature dilation of the cervix, or issues related to your placenta.

**Back or abdominal pain:** Pain in your back or abdomen can be a sign of contractions or premature dilation of the cervix, a sign of potential preterm labor.

**More than six contractions per hour:** Contractions that happen this often suggest preterm labor and should be brought to your practitioner's attention.

**Gush of fluid from the vagina:** This can be a sign that your water has broken prematurely. Your practitioner can determine if fluid leaking from your vagina is amniotic fluid or normal vaginal discharge.

*Report any strange or troublesome symptoms to your practitioner immediately.*

##  BODY BASICS

As you come to the end of your pregnancy, you will most likely experience more discomfort from the physical changes in your body. Your baby will be nestling downward into your pelvis, which increases pelvic pressure and the urge to urinate frequently. More than one mom has felt certain that her baby was about to fall out because the pressure is so intense. For most women, this is a normal sensation, and without contractions, pain, or bleeding it is nothing to worry about.

Once your baby settles down into your pelvis—which is called lightening, engaging, or dropping—you may feel relieved that you are able to breathe more easily. You may also notice more Braxton-Hicks contractions. These practice contractions are a great opportunity for you to try out what you've learned in your childbirth class about comfort measures for labor, such as breathing, massage, and relaxation. You can also practice timing contractions.

### 🛒 BABY DATA

Your baby weighs about six pounds (2.7 kilograms) at this point. Most of the weight your baby will gain between now and birth will be brown fat, which is a layer of fat that will help your baby regulate his or her temperature after being born—a skill that is needed right from the start. Lengthwise your baby is about 18 inches (46 centimeters) long, and growing.

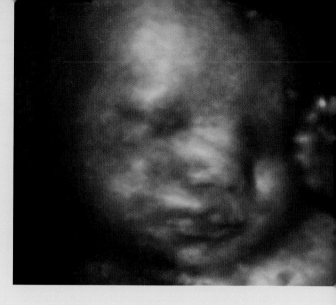

Toward the end of pregnancy, the weight and length differences between babies tend to be more pronounced. This is because humans are all slightly different. Genetics come into play as well as personal health, nutrition, and wellness. Your practitioner may try to guess how large or small your baby is, but even with ultrasound, these guesses are usually off, sometimes by quite a lot. If these guesses make you anxious, say that you'd prefer not to be told.

PREGNANCY PARTICULARS

## Celebrate Your Baby

This is the perfect time to have your baby shower or mother blessing ceremony. No matter which you choose, most moms need a bit of pampering toward the end of their pregnancies. It is also nice to pause amid all the planning for new parenthood to focus on the baby and your future together.

The baby shower is a traditional American ritual where partygoers gather to celebrate a new life. Typically one can expect food, baby gifts, often silly baby shower games and lots of people.

While some families reserve baby showers for first babies only, there are many who are less rigid and welcome the idea of a shower when:

- Second (or more) baby of the opposite sex
- Long period of time between babies
- One parent is a first time parent

Most showers remain women-only, although progressive baby shower goers believe that it is great fun to invite the dad-to-be and other men to these celebrations. And while the rules are changing in terms of who throws baby showers and where they take place, it is most common to see work place baby showers or parties given by close friends and family. Some first time mothers wind up attending three or four showers before all is said and done.

While the traditional baby shower is still the most popular way to celebrate an upcoming birth, some mothers are bypassing tradition and opting instead for a birth blessing, also called a blessing way. A more mother focused event than the conventional baby shower, this can be done for any mother with any number of previous children.

Gifts at a birth blessing tend to be less traditional than baby clothes or stuffed animals. You might find that the guests gather to make a necklace for the mother or offer her prepared meals to have on hand after the baby is born. The guests might share uplifting birth stories or offer practical advice on baby raising. In addition, there could be a ceremony portion that includes prayer, songs, henna tattoos, belly casting or any number of activities that are meaningful to the mother-to-be. At its core, the celebration is meant to honor the mother and her baby by providing love and encouragement through a circle of friends and relatives.

Whether you opt for a traditional baby shower, a co-ed party, a birth blessing or something else entirely, you should remember that each baby is a blessing, and therefore each birth deserves to be celebrated. Figure out what feels best for you and your situation and then follow your heart.

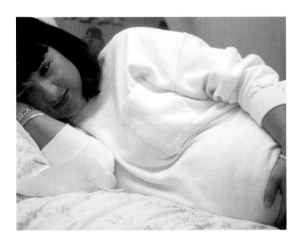

# PREGNANCY AFFIRMATION FOR WEEK 36

## My baby knows when it is safe to be born.

## Practice Comfort Measures for Labor to Aid in Relaxation and Pain Relief

What you learned in childbirth class may seem very far off or abstract at this point, but a little practice could go a long way when the time comes. Even if you are planning to use medication during labor, practicing and applying the skills you learned in childbirth class can make you comfortable prior to getting medical or medicinal help.

It's hard to mimic labor, especially if you've never felt it before, but the aches and pains that come with late-term pregnancy can provide a somewhat realistic setting in which to practice the comfort measures. For example, if you have a backache, try various positions described in class to relieve the pain, such as the hands and knees position. Testing out your comfort measures now will reinforce in your mind which skills go with which symptoms, in a much less urgent situation than labor.

In addition to practicing physical comfort measures, you can practice relaxation and other emotional techniques to help you relax because tension and frustration tend to increase pain levels.

Even if you are not having issues with pain that require your attention at the end of your pregnancy, it is a good idea to practice what you

*Practicing positions and comfort measures for labor will help them feel more natural once your baby's birth is imminent.*

learned in your childbirth classes. Trying to do relaxation or remember positions once labor starts is much harder if you haven't practiced. While many people say that they have trouble practicing, you will rarely hear anyone say that they regret making the time to try.

Many couples find it best to work on relaxation right before going to bed. It tends to be a quiet, calm time and, if you've been battling sleep issues, practicing the techniques you've learned could ease you into a restful night's sleep.

It is also important to practice during your waking hours because you never know when labor will happen. Try to think about it as you go about your daily routine. Ask yourself, "What would I do right now if I were having a contraction?" If you work in an office, look around and scope out places to sit quietly or things you can lean against that are tall and sturdy enough to support you. Think about how you would get home from work if you were in early labor. By visualizing yourself in labor in various places, you will make the actual event more manageable and less frightening.

## Learn about Cord Blood Banking

It's very likely during your pregnancy that you received solicitations from cord blood banks (lots of them). These companies will store your baby's cord blood, for a fee, in case it is ever needed, such as to treat a medical condition. Cord blood contains stem cells, which are young cells that have not yet specialized to become specific cells, such as liver cells or skin cells. These cells are young enough to become whatever you need them for, such as battling certain cancers.

Cord blood banking for stem cells is not a routine procedure at many hospitals or birth centers. The process involves taking blood from the umbilical cord immediately after birth to retrieve the stem cells. Because the cord must be clamped nearly immediately, it does not allow for delayed cord clamping. Delayed cord clamping is when you wait until the cord stops pulsating, usually within a few minutes after birth, before cutting the umbilical cord. This allows the baby to get all of the fetal blood and can help prevent anemia in the baby. If your baby is having a bit of a rough start after birth, the umbilical cord being left intact also serves as a protective measure because your baby is still getting oxygen from the cord.

This blood collection procedure would be done by your doctor or midwife. If you are doing private banking, you will be sent a kit to take to your birth. The kit will include instructions for your practitioner to draw the blood as well as shipping instructions.

Currently the American Academy of Pediatrics does not recommend personal cord blood banking unless you have a specific, known concern. However, they do recommend donating cord blood to a public banking system. These are becoming more popular, but they are still not easy to find. Public banking does not cost anything, unlike the hundreds of dollars spent on private banking and storage.

Even if you plan to bank your baby's cord blood, sometimes it cannot be collected because of how the birth proceeded or simply because the collection was inadvertently forgotten.

## Schedule Weekly Prenatal Visits

Around the 36-week mark, you will begin to see your practitioner every week. Go ahead and schedule appointments for the next six weeks to ensure that you get times and dates that work well for your schedule. These dates can always be canceled or moved, should the need arise or should you have the baby!

These last visits are very important, and they may involve decisions in which you want your husband or partner to participate. This might mean scheduling them at a time when your practitioner is not likely to cancel or show up late. The office staff can help you figure out the best time, which is typically not at the end of the day when delays and emergencies have played havoc with the schedule.

Bring written questions with you and a pen and paper for recording the answers. Some questions you may have at this point include the following:

- Have you reviewed my birth plan?
- Have your partners also seen it?
- When would you like me to call you when I am in labor?
- When would you prefer I head to the place of birth in labor?
- Are there warning signs I need to look for at this point in my pregnancy?
- Can I have access to the call schedule so I know who is on call when?
- Other questions that have been unresolved at previous visits

You may see a variety of practitioners in these last few weeks. This will depend on the philosophy of your prenatal care group. Many larger practices prefer that you spend the last few weeks of your pregnancy rotating through to see different people, because you do not know who will be on call when it's your baby's birth day. While it may be disconcerting to see a different doctor or midwife every week, use it as a chance to double-check that each of them knows your preferences for your labor and birth experience. Always have a copy of your birth plan available for them to see, so they can also ask questions of you.

## Revisit Your Birth Place

You should already have taken a tour of your birth center or hospital, and now is a good time to make a return trip. You've learned so much about pregnancy and birth since your first visit, and you probably have more questions to ask the staff.

This is also a great time to remember some of the tips they give you about preregistration. For example, some hospitals will allow you to preregister online or even during the tour. Others may give you a special form to send in with a copy of your insurance card. They are also likely to

discuss where to come when you are in labor and provide you with a basic overview of the intake process. Be sure to ask about the use of triage and times that you may be separated from your family. Triage is an area where you are asked to wait, sometimes separated from your support people, while the staff determines if you are really in labor. It involves a vaginal exam and monitoring, followed by a second vaginal exam an hour later. If you progress in dilation, you are admitted to a labor room; if not, you are held for continued observation or sent home. If you do not want to be separated, be sure to ask what you can do to avoid this from happening.

If you are planning a home birth, you will usually have a home visit at this point in your pregnancy. Because the 36th week is the earliest you can safely have a home birth, your midwife or doctor will usually wait until now to visit your home. This visit gives you a chance to invite other people who may have questions or will be attending the birth to meet your practitioner. It also gives the practitioner a chance to find your home and offer practical advice for keeping your home ready for the impending birth.

Don't fret if your house isn't spotless. Your practitioner is not there to judge your housekeeping skills, but rather to ensure that he or she knows where you live, that you have your birth kit, and that everything is ready. This might also be the right time to review your birth plan with your midwife and everyone who will be attending your birth. You should also be sure to discuss transport, in case you need to go to the hospital during labor.

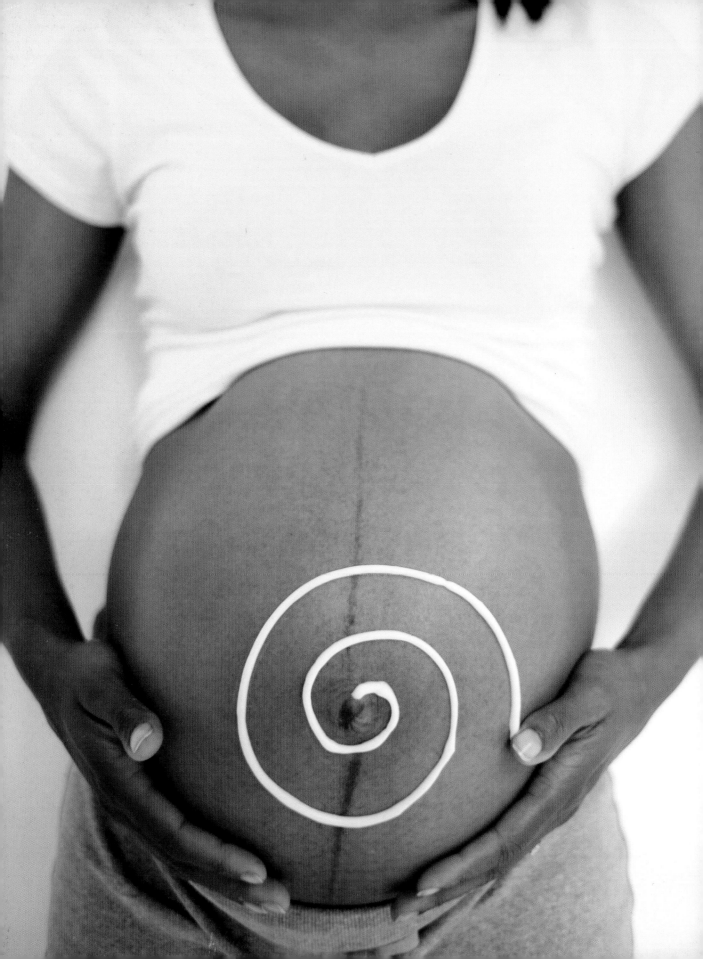

# WEEK 37

## ✏ CHECKLIST FOR WEEK 37

[ ] Install your baby's car seat.
[ ] Know the signs of labor.
[ ] Pack a labor and birth bag for the big day.
[ ] Get a henna tattoo.
[ ] Take pictures of your pregnant belly.

## 🔎 WHAT TO WATCH FOR THIS WEEK

**Signs of labor:** Once you are at the 37th week, your practitioner will not try to interrupt or stop your labor once it starts. You should record the signs and follow the instructions your practitioner has given you for when to call them.

### Double Check

**Decrease in fetal movement:** A reduction in fetal movement can suggest there are problems with your baby. Some people report that they notice a decrease in fetal movement as labor nears, but this is not true. You should still report any decrease in fetal movement to your practitioner immediately.

**Swelling:** If you experience a sudden swelling in your hands or face, tell your doctor or midwife. He or she will evaluate you for pregnancy induced hypertension (PIH) or preeclampsia.

**Headaches:** Headaches that are severe in nature are a sign of possible blood pressure trouble and should be reported to your practitioner. Earlier in pregnancy, headaches can be the common response to pregnancy hormones, but when presented with other symptoms, severe headaches might be a symptom of PIH or even preeclampsia, which is a severe illness in pregnancy related to blood pressure, protein in your urine, and other complications.

**Blurred vision:** Call your practitioner right away if you start to experience blurred vision; it can be another sign of PIH or preeclampsia.

**Bleeding or spotting:** At this point in pregnancy, bleeding can happen after sexual intercourse, a vaginal exam, or vaginal ultrasound. Hopefully you were warned in advance of this possibility to save you from worrying. In the absence of these activities, however, report bleeding or spotting immediately to your practitioner, because it may be a sign of infection, dilation of the cervix or, issues related to your placenta. *Report any strange or troublesome symptoms to your practitioner immediately.*

##  BODY BASICS

You are probably excited at the thought that your baby could be born any day now. While it is always smart to be prepared for that possibility, remember that many women do not have their babies at this juncture.

Remember to take care of yourself during the final weeks. You may feel more tired and strung out. Some mothers-to-be feel teary, as if they could cry at any moment, while others feel angry. These emotions are normal and will pass; they are simply responses to the hormones surging in your body.

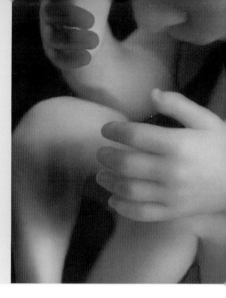

Your baby is nearing his or her final birth weight and getting ready to be born. You may feel like the baby is moving around a lot, though not with large movements. Your baby is looking for the path of least resistance to be born most easily. Your baby is more than eighteen inches (46 centimeters) long.

PREGNANCY PARTICULARS

## Install Your Baby's Car Seat

Although your baby may or may not show up this week, having your baby's car seat installed properly is a huge item to check off your list of things to do. If you haven't purchased a car seat prior to this week, now is the time to do so. No more procrastinating! Here are the types of car seats available.

INFANT CAR SEAT: This car seat is rear facing and is designed to accommodate a newborn until he or she reaches twenty pounds or more. This cannot be used for bigger babies and does not face forward. This type of car seat normally comes with a base that securely attaches to your car. A second base can be purchased for additional vehicles. This car seat can usually be attached to a stroller made by the same manufacturer and can double as an infant carrier.

CONVERTIBLE CAR SEAT: This car seat can accommodate a newborn to a toddler. It is rear facing for younger infants and can face forward for older children. This car seat is not as easy to install and may need to be reinstalled every time you use it for a younger baby. Because these car seats are not designed to be taken out easily, they do not double as infant carriers, nor do they it attach to strollers.

TODDLER CAR SEAT: This car seat is forward facing only. It is usually designed for toddlers who weigh more than twenty pounds, though some car seats are designed for toddlers weighing more than thirty pounds.

SPECIALTY CAR SEATS: If your baby was born very premature or with certain conditions, you may need a specialized car seat. You can usually find these through your pediatrician or the social worker connected with your baby's care facility.

Each of these car seats has distinct advantages and disadvantages. Some car seats take more work to install but are very easy to use on a day-to-day basis. Other car seats can only be used for brief periods of time, determined by a baby's weight and size. Only you can decide which works best for your family. Some two-car families split the difference and purchase one infant car seat and install a convertible car seat in the car they use less frequently.

Your baby's car seat is a critically important safety feature that protects your baby when you are driving. Most problems arise from the user end when parents use car seats incorrectly.

Among the biggest problems related to misuse of car seats is the failure to have it installed correctly. To prevent this from happening, you can have your car seat professionally installed. To find an installer, call your local car dealer or check with your local fire departments. These groups normally have clinics that teach you the proper use of your car seat and include help installing the car seat.

For additional safety tips, read your car seat instruction manual. Keep this manual with you, in the glove box perhaps, to help answer questions you may have at a later time. Some car seats are designed with a special area for storing the manual. Some newer cars also have great sections in their manuals about installation of the car seat. They can explain to you the specific safety features of your car that will help you protect your baby.

## Know the Signs of Labor

Knowing the signs of labor is a very good idea. Even though this is covered in childbirth class, it is handy to have a list close to refresh your memory. (For more on labor, see "Labor and Birth," beginning on page 269.) Here are some of the most common signs of labor.

NESTING: This is often described as an overwhelming urge to prepare for baby's arrival. While this can happen at any point in the third trimester, it is most common in the last days and weeks before your baby's birth. It can prompt you to fold baby clothes over and over, rearrange the baby's room, or simply want to be in the space that you have created for your baby.

MUCOUS PLUG: The cervix has done a beautiful job of protecting your baby during pregnancy. It has been holding a piece of mucous that helps guard your baby against infections and other things. As your cervix prepares for labor by thinning and opening, the mucous becomes dislodged. You may notice the mucous plug as a single chunk of mucous, much like blowing your nose, or you may notice an increase in mucous discharge. Seeing the mucous plug can mean that your labor is coming sometime in the next few days or weeks.

PREGNANCY AFFIRMATION
FOR WEEK 37

✛

# My baby knows its birthday.

BLOODY SHOW: A bit of blood-tinged mucous is normal after a vaginal exam or sexual intercourse. The cervix is very sensitive at this stage of the game, and the tiny capillaries near the surface break very easily. You may notice what's referred to as a bloody show immediately after an exam or sex, or a slightly brownish discharge the following day or so. If you see this when you haven't had a vaginal exam or sex, it could be that your cervix is beginning to dilate.

LOOSE STOOLS: This is nature's way of cleaning out your body for birth. You may have more frequent bowel movements or you may notice what looks like diarrhea. Be sure to stay well hydrated. Labor often follows approximately seventy-two hours after this sign, particularly when it is accompanied by other signs.

BACKACHE: Increase in backache may also be a sign of impending labor. It can be caused by the baby moving down or contractions you may not have noticed.

FLULIKE SYMPTOMS: Some women report feeling "yucky" in the days before their babies were born. They're achy, tired, nauseous, and run down. As long as you're not running a fever, there is no cause for alarm, but remember that dehydration can trigger contractions.

BABY DROPS: This means that the baby can move lower in your pelvis. While this happens more frequently in first-time mothers, it can be a sign that labor is near.

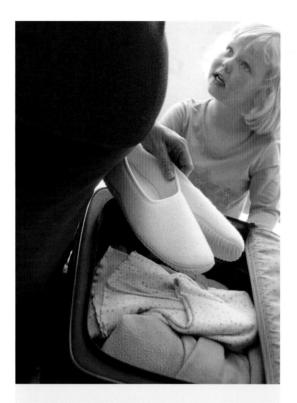

## A QUICK TRICK TO PACKING YOUR BAGS

Certain things can be packed away in your bag for months and never missed. You will need to add other things at the very last minute, which can make you worry you'll forget them.

One idea is to tape a list of what's not included on the bags you plan to bring. Whoever picks up the bags will see the list instructing them to gather what's missing and where to find the items.

You can limit the number of things on this list by purchasing spares. Toss in new toothbrushes for you and your spouse and sample-sized tubes of toothpaste, hair products and other items, which also have the virtue of using up less space in the bag.

CONTRACTIONS: An increase in contractions is a signal that labor is coming. It's possible for the contractions to continue for a few hours and, just when you're ready to declare this the real thing, they stop. Do not despair. Every contraction helps you progress toward birth, even if you don't feel that way at the time.

You may experience all or none of these signs. The more signs you have together, the more likely that labor is on its way. Having signs that seem to come and go can be really confusing and irritating, but it is a part of the process. Try to keep a sense of humor about it all, even when it doesn't seem all that funny.

## Pack a Labor and Birth Bag for the Big Day

Planning ahead is a good thing, particularly when it comes to having a baby. That includes packing a bag for your labor and birth experience. By having a bag packed or mostly packed, you can save yourself the hassle of doing it during early labor or worse, being in labor when you realize that something important did not make it into your bag.

The first thing to do is to make a list of items that you might need. It is easier if you break the list into categories such as the following:

- Mom's needs during labor
- Dad's needs during labor
- Baby's needs after birth/going home
- Mom's postpartum needs
- Dad's postpartum needs

Savvy families pack two bags. Think about it: When you're in the labor and birth area, you aren't going to need your baby's going home outfit and birth announcements. Every hospital and birth center is a bit different, and you may find yourself moving from room to room. The less stuff you have with you, the less lugging there is to do. So pack one bag for the labor room, and leave the rest of the stuff in the car until after your baby is born and you are settled in your postpartum room.

Things to pack might include the following:

- Toothbrushes and toothpaste
- Hair brushes and hair supplies
- Makeup and other essentials, including razors for dad
- Clothes for labor for mom and a change for dad
- Postpartum clothes, such as a robe and slippers
- Going-home clothes for mom (mid-pregnancy size)
- Nursing bra and breastfeeding gear, such as pillow, pads, book, and nipple ointment
- Going-home outfit for baby, including diapers
- Camera, batteries, and film (if needed)
- Labor items, such as birth ball, comfort measures, and music
- Snacks for labor and postpartum

Once you have your list, look for any redundancies. You do not really need two tubes of toothpaste. You can also eliminate anything that might be supplied by the hospital, such as a hair dryer. Ask what is supplied during your hospital or birth center tour. Do not be tempted to pack everything but the kitchen sink. Focus on what you will need for labor because someone can always come back later with items for you postpartum.

## Get a Henna Tattoo

Before you think that a henna tattoo is the worst idea you have heard in a long time, realize what it is: a temporary tattoo created with a plant-based substance that acts as a nontoxic dye. Many pregnant women choose to get henna tattoos on their abdomens.

Most practitioners of henna allow you to select a design from a book of art work or to bring your own design. The tattoo takes anywhere from a few minutes to an hour to do, depending on the complexity of the design. The henna then dries and flakes off, leaving behind an orange/yellow image.

Some women choose to do this at a blessing ceremony, or you may wish to do it in time for belly photos at the end of your pregnancy. If the idea appeals to you, celebrate your pregnancy by choosing art work that is personally meaningful.

## Take Pictures of Your Pregnant Belly

Hopefully you've been taking photos of your growing belly at various stages along the way, but 36 weeks is a great time to do so with a bit more "focus." In addition to the photos you take yourself, consider getting professional photographs done. Consider the following shots for creating memorable photographs:

- You alone
- With your husband (Belly to belly is cute!)
- With your children (Head or hands to belly works well.)
- Decorated belly (pumpkin, basketball, henna tattoo, etc.)
- Nude photos
- Inside or outdoors
- In your nursery

Talk to other mothers and even local artists for ideas on photo shoots for the end of pregnancy. When talking to local photographers, ask about maternity photo shoot specials. Sometimes you can get a package deal that includes photos of the newborn for the birth announcement.

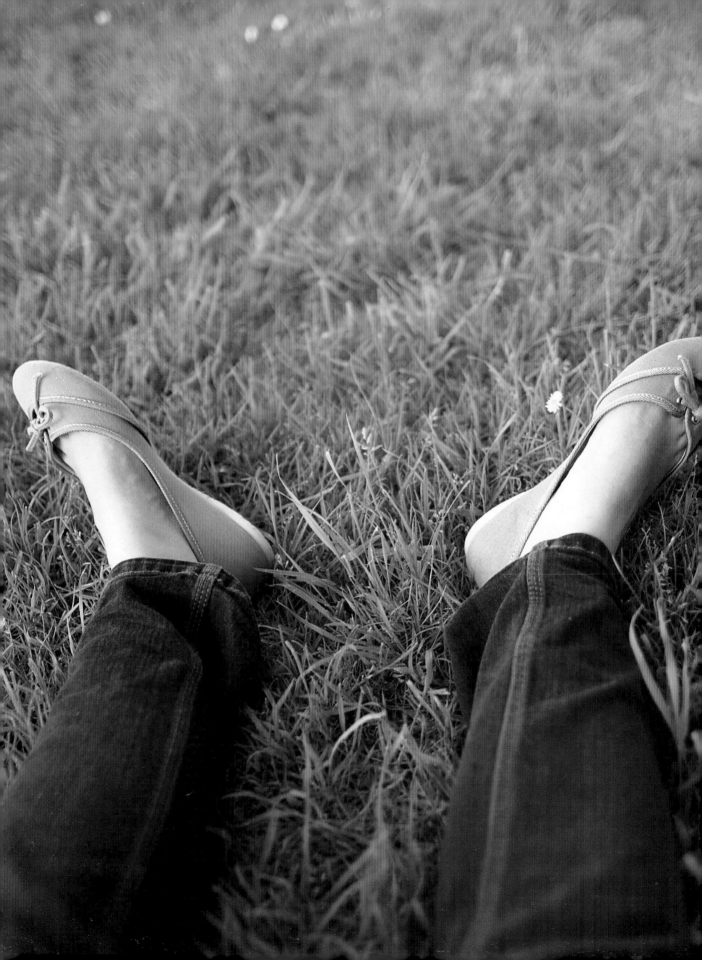

# WEEK 38

## ✏ CHECKLIST FOR WEEK 38

[ ]  Make a trial run to your place of birth.
[ ]  Learn about vaginal exams before labor.
[ ]  Have a neonatal intensive care nursery plan.
[ ]  Deal with comments about pain medication in labor.

## 🔍 WHAT TO WATCH FOR THIS WEEK

### Double Check

**Signs of labor:** Starting at the 37th week, your practitioner will not stop your labor once it begins. Be alert to the signs of labor and follow the instructions your practitioner has given you for when to call him or her.

**Decrease in fetal movement:** A potential sign of trouble, report a lessening of fetal movement—even as labor approaches—to your practitioner immediately.

**Swelling:** Watch for sudden swelling in the face or hands because it is an indicator of pregnancy induced hypertension (PIH) or preeclampsia. Normal swelling in pregnancy is not severe and tends to go away after sufficient rest.

**Headaches:** Severe headaches can be a sign of issues with your blood pressure that can be determined by your practitioner. Sometimes headaches are caused merely from pregnancy hormones, or they may be tied to other symptoms that together can be called PIH or even preeclampsia, which is a severe illness in pregnancy related to blood pressure, protein in your urine, and other complications.

**Blurred vision:** With or without a headache, report blurred vision immediately to your practitioner because it can also be a sign of PIH or preeclampsia.

**Bleeding or spotting:** Report reddish or brownish spotting, unrelated to having sex or vaginal exams, to your practitioner; it could be a sign of infection, dilation of the cervix, or issues related to your placenta.

*Report any strange or troublesome symptoms to your practitioner immediately.*

##  BODY BASICS

You may have noticed an increase in vaginal discharge as you get closer to labor. This is very normal and does not signal a problem. You only need to seek medical advice if you detect a foul odor or odd color, or you experience itching, burning, or a fever. As your baby drops lower into your pelvis, you may have an easier time breathing. The trade-off, however, may be a few more trips to the bathroom.

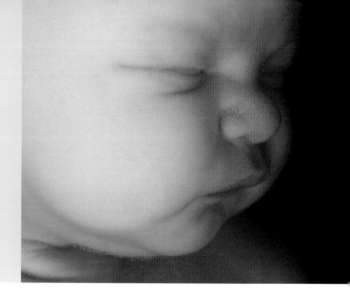

## BABY DATA

Your baby has been gaining quite a bit of weight up until this point. Starting now the baby's weight gain slows dramatically or even stops. Your baby is still moving around, but there is usually a pattern to which times of day your baby becomes active.

# Make a Trial Run to Your Place of Birth

We have all seen the television version of the mad dash to the hospital. The dad usually does something crazy, such as forgetting his wife, or drives like a maniac or some other form of slapstick comedy. It would probably be safe to say that this scenario, while amusing, is not what you have in mind for your trip to give birth.

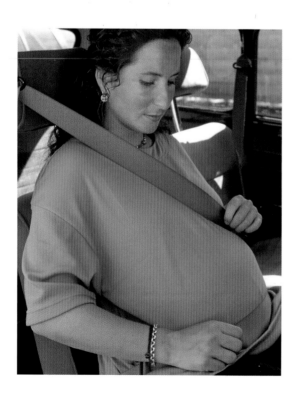

You can plan around this kind of drama. For starters, think about the different times of day that you might travel to your place of birth and then come up with the routes that work best for those particular times. For example, if you are driving to the birth center at 2 A.M., you will probably take a different route than you would at 5:30 P.M. at the height of rush hour. Besides traffic, do a quick study of any construction in the area that might necessitate finding a different route. If you are unsure of the best way to reach your destination, you should take some test drives to find out.

When you are driving to the hospital or birth center for real, make certain that whoever is driving knows the way, obeys the traffic laws, knows where you need to go and where to park. These sound like basic things, but they become hugely important if you are in labor and the driver doesn't know where to go.

You may also want to take note of any major potholes, railroad tracks, and the like. While the old wives' tale says that bumpy roads are good for kicking a woman's labor into gear, they are not much fun when that woman happens to be you. You may also remind the driver that you will not be available to dispense advice and that you may make requests such as, "Drive more slowly!" or "Don't hit that pothole!"

*Your seat belt is not optional, no matter how far along you are—even on your way to give birth.*

A couple of test drives at different times of the day and night should be enough to quell the nerves of any anxious dad or mom. You could tag it on as a side trip after visiting your practitioner or on the way to a child-care class.

## Learn about Vaginal Exams before Labor

A vaginal exam is not anyone's favorite way to spend time, pregnant or not. Late in pregnancy, it is done to assess if your cervix is dilated (open) or effaced (thinned), where it is located, and how ripe (soft) it is. A vaginal exam may give you numbers, but it will not tell you how close you are to labor.

The practice of doing vaginal exams to assess the cervix prior to labor varies from practitioner to practitioner. Some practitioners don't do exams prior to labor, or they wait until the pregnancy has passed the 41 week. Other practitioners prefer to do them weekly starting around 36 weeks.

You can be four centimeters dilated and not in labor. Hearing this can make some women feel discouraged—in the same way that hearing you are not dilated at all can be upsetting news. Other than using vaginal exams for an induction evaluation (how likely it is that an induction will work, what type of induction to do, and whether it's wiser simply to wait), there are very few reasons to do them prior to labor. In fact there are reasons to avoid vaginal exams, such as discomfort, potential infection, and accidental rupture of membranes.

Talk to your practitioner about routine vaginal exams prior to labor. Discuss what information he or she is trying to gather and see if there are other ways to get it. In the end, you have the right to agree or disagree with the decision, and whether or not you have an exam done is between you and your practitioner.

*A premature baby can be overwhelming. Get hooked up with a parent's group for preemies.*

## Have a Neonatal Intensive Care Nursery Plan

No one plans or expects to have a baby who is ill. If you are at a higher risk of having a baby who is sick or may need special care, your doctor or midwife has probably already notified you. If you fall into that category, it is important to familiarize yourself with the resources available before your baby is born. Babies who are likely to need special care include the following:

- Multiples, even born after 37 weeks
- Low-birth weight babies, regardless of gestation
- Babies with congenital anomalies
- Babies born via Cesarean section
- Babies who had meconium present at birth
- Babies born to mothers who had chronic or acute illnesses, such as diabetes and high blood pressure

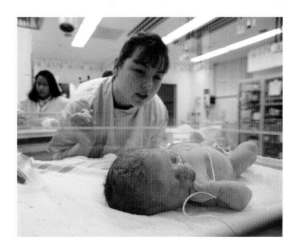

**KNOW YOUR PLACE OF BIRTH'S POLICY ON PAIN MEDICATIONS**

Every place of birth has its own ideas, philosophies, and policies regarding pain medication. It can be a big shock to learn about these policies after you're in labor, particularly if your plans differ from what the place of birth prefers. Examples of different policies might include the following:

- Early epidural use: Epidural anesthesia might not be allowed until you have reached a certain dilation.
- IV medications only: This means intravenous medication is the only form of pain medication used at the facility.
- Pain medication limits: There may be certain restrictions on pain medications given how long you have been in labor. For example, certain IV medication cannot be administered late in labor.
- Use of certain equipment: Some medications preclude the use of certain items such as birth balls and squat bars.

By asking questions while touring your birth center or hospital, you can get clarity around these policies and plan accordingly.

This is by no means a complete list of babies who may require special care at birth, but it gives you a sense of whether or not you should take a tour of your local special care nursery. Find out what they can and can't do and which practitioners they will and won't work with. If you need advice about which facility to contact, start with the pediatrician you have chosen, who may also recommend that you meet with a neonatologist or newborn specialist.

# Deal with Comments about Pain Medication in Labor

The decision whether to use pain medication in labor is entirely up to you. It requires careful thought and will depend on what your labor brings, how you have prepared for labor, and a dash of plain luck.

The problem is that people often want to inject their opinions, just as they have with everything that has to do with pregnancy and birth. You will have women stop you to say, "Get an epidural in the parking lot!" or "Natural birth is the only way to go!" Both approaches have their supporters, and you must decide where you fall in the mix.

Your decision will rest on many factors, including the following:

- How you feel when labor begins
- How your labor progresses
- How prepared you are for labor
- Your support team
- Practices at your place of birth
- Whether you're hungry or tired

You have a degree of control over your preparedness for labor, but other factors are beyond your control. It is wise to talk about this decision with the members of your support system, as opposed to strangers on the street.

Your husband is not immune to this type of talk. Around the water cooler, men get tips on pain medication in labor. Rather than providing constructive advice on how to help a woman through labor, many men just huddle and say things such as, "Call the anesthesiologist as soon as you can."

Try to put labor horror stories out of your mind where they belong. If you can nip a story in the bud, try that as well with a simple, "Oh I think I've heard quite enough about labor. Let's compare stories later ..." This or whatever else works for you is the way to deal with these comments.

## HOT MAMA

Just as you plan what you wear every day, think ahead to labor. Some mothers are fine wearing hospital gowns, while others prefer to wear their own clothing. You may worry that if you wear your own clothes to the hospital, it may have to be cut off in an emergency. There is a happy medium: clothes just for labor! New lines of clothing specifically for labor are cropping up. From fashionable hospital gowns to really cool skirts and tops that allow you to labor with your "buns" covered. If fancy isn't your thing, consider wearing a sports bra and a nightgown or a large T-shirt that you are not attached to during your labor and birth.

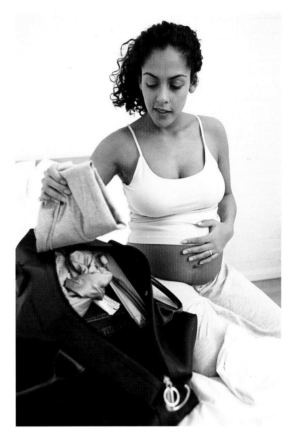

*Choosing each item you pack very carefully will ensure you have what you need but haven't over packed.*

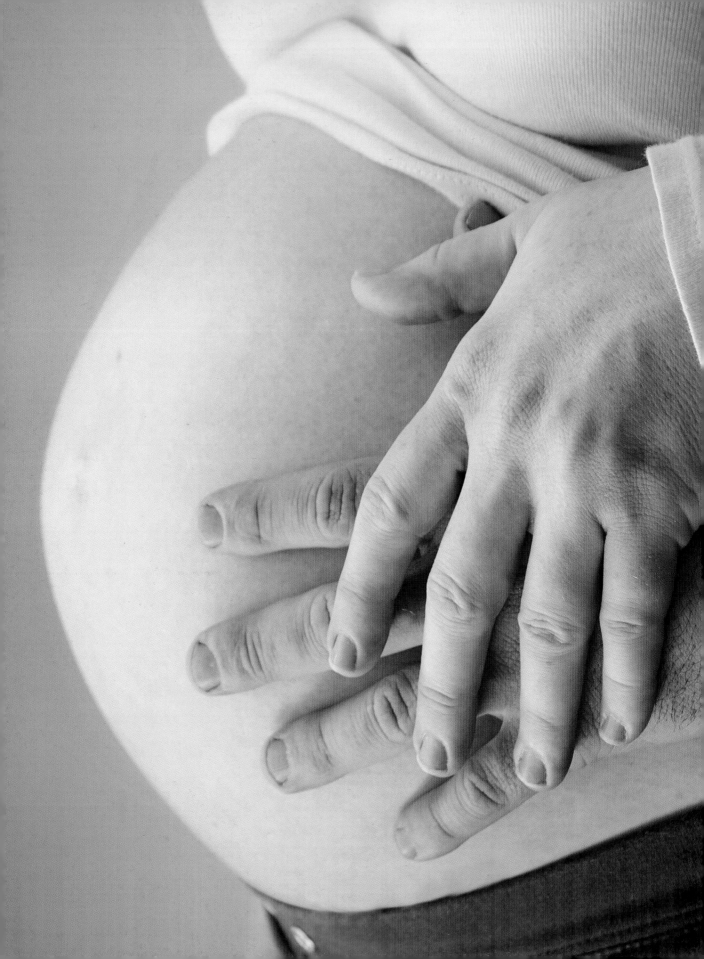

# WEEK 39

## ✎ CHECKLIST FOR WEEK 39

[ ] Verify that everyone has a copy of your birth plan.
[ ] Purchase postpartum meals and supplies.
[ ] Learn about water breaking.
[ ] If necessary, schedule a Cesarean.
[ ] Buy a book on motherhood or the postpartum period in particular.

## ⚲ WHAT TO WATCH FOR THIS WEEK

### Double Check

**Signs of labor:** Beginning at week 37, your practitioner will not try to stop your labor. Simply take account of your labor signals and follow the instructions your practitioner has given you for when to call him or her.

**Decrease in fetal movement:** Some women think they notice a decrease in fetal movement as labor gets closer, but the truth is any decrease may be a sign of problems with your baby. Report it to your practitioner immediately.

**Swelling:** While regular swelling during pregnancy develops slowly, diminishes after resting, and isn't cause for concern, sudden swelling in the face or hands can be a sign of trouble, specifically pregnancy induced hypertension (PIH) or preeclampsia.

**Headaches:** Tell your practitioner if you've been having severe headaches. It is possible that you are suffering from PIH or even preeclampsia, which is a severe illness in pregnancy related to blood pressure, protein in your urine, and other complications.

**Blurred vision:** Report blurred vision immediately to your practitioner because it can also be a sign of PIH or preeclampsia.

**Bleeding or spotting:** Report any bleeding or spotting that cannot be explained by sexual intercourse, a vaginal exam, or vaginal ultrasound to your doctor or midwife. He or she will want to rule out the possibility of an infection, dilation of the cervix, or issues related to your placenta.

*Report any strange or troublesome symptoms to your practitioner immediately.*

##  BODY BASICS

You might be looking closely for signs of labor but not finding many. This is not a problem, and you should not worry. You are probably not gaining weight anymore and may even be losing a small amount as you prepare for labor. This is normal. Staying busy will help keep your mind off labor and being pregnant.

### ![stroller icon] BABY DATA

Baby is settled into your pelvis and preparing for birth. Not every baby is perfectly ready at the 37 week mark, which is why there is a range given for due dates. The last to mature on babies is their lungs.

In other news, your baby's weight gain has slowed considerably. Some babies will gain a few ounces here or there, but the weight gain has pretty much stopped. On average, babies weigh seven and a half pounds (3.4 kilograms) by this point and measures twenty inches (51 centimeters) long.

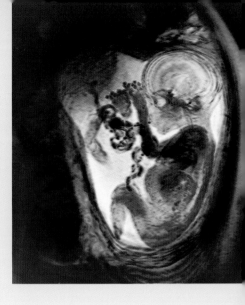

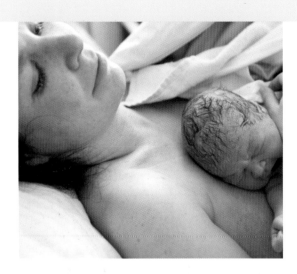

*The moment you are handed your baby is a special one. Remember skin-to-skin contact is exactly what you and your baby need.*

**PREGNANCY PARTICULARS**

## Verify That Everyone Has a Copy of Your Birth Plan

In these last remaining weeks, most everything should be in order for your birth and postpartum, but there are still a few things worth double-checking. One of those things is your birth plan.

Place a quick call to your place of birth to be sure that they have a signed copy in your file.

You should also give your baby's pediatrician, your practitioner, and your doula a call for the same reason.

If anyone does not have a copy, offer to fax it right over. Some places will even accept scanned copies via email. If you are not sure whom to call at the hospital or birth center, ask for the nurse manager at the labor and birth unit. Even if your team has copies of the birth plan, you should still tuck a few extras in your labor bag.

## Purchase Postpartum Meals and Supplies

Before the baby's arrival is an excellent time to plan your postpartum meals. When you're making dinner, simply double the quantity and instantly freeze the second helping. You can also see if there's a "meals for a month" type of store near you where you can quickly assemble seven or eight meals for your freezer. If you have limited freezer space, consider asking a neighbor if you can temporarily store frozen meals at his or her house.

Besides meals, you will need many other items during the postpartum period, and now is the time to plan for them so they are readily available once you give birth.

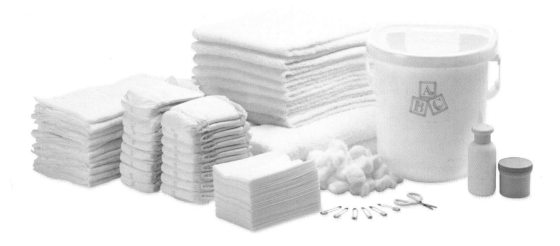

*Having baby supplies around before the baby can be helpful. Ask other parents what they consider the necessities.*

Here's a starter list of items to help care for yourself at home after the baby's born.

MAXI PADS: After you give birth, either vaginally or by Cesarean section, you will bleed vaginally. This is because the section of your uterus where the placenta was located is healing. As it heals and your uterus begins the process of shrinking or involution, you will bleed. Wearing tampons or other items that are inserted into the vagina can promote infection. It may also be less comfortable because you just had a baby. The bleeding can last up to six weeks postpartum.

FIBER-FILLED FOODS: Constipation can be quite common after giving birth, particularly if you were given a lot of pain medication or had a Cesarean section. Constipation, in turn, can make you fearful about having a painful bowel movement after baby. For these reasons (and because fiber-rich foods are good for general health), the sooner you return to normal stools with the help of a nutritious diet with lots of fiber-

## PREGNANCY AFFIRMATION FOR WEEK 39

### My body knows just what to do.

rich foods, such as fruits, vegetables, and whole grains, and stool softeners (if necessary), the better you will feel.

TOILET PAPER: You will need a supply of ultrasoft toilet paper that will be gentle on your sensitive tissues. You can also expect to urinate quite frequently for a few days after birth.

SNACKS: Have plenty of food that you can grab and eat while you are doing something else, probably baby related. Many new mothers skip good nutrition or eating in general when taking care of new babies. By having handy snacks in strategic locations, such as near your bed or chair, you can increase the odds that you will eat a bit here and there. Trail mix, nuts, cereal bars, fruit leather, cheese, and fresh fruit are all great snacks. A bag filled with items such as these also makes a thoughtful gift for new mothers.

WATER BOTTLE: Instead of having to get up every time you are thirsty, a water bottle will make it easier to stay hydrated and can be carried from location to location.

NOTE CARDS: Have note cards and possibly even birth announcements ready for when you are sitting around with the baby and can grab a few minutes to write a thank-you note or address a few announcement cards.

As a general matter, it is wise to stock up on items you and your family tend to go through. This could be anything from laundry detergent to frozen foods. The goal of this sweep of preparation is to prevent you from discovering at 3 A.M. that you are out of paper towels. This is bad enough on a regular day, but it feels much worse when that day is four days postpartum.

## Learn about Water Breaking

One of the biggest fears that pregnant women have toward the end of their pregnancies is that their water will break while they are out in public. Take a deep breath and relax, because only about 13 percent of women have their water break at the start of labor. In fact, when left undisturbed, the water does not break until after the woman is nine centimeters dilated in 75 percent of the cases.

If you are concerned about your water breaking, the following are some handy tricks to minimize any resulting mess:

- Carry a change of clothes with you.
- Sit on towels or plastic-backed pads in the car.
- Cover your bed with a waterproof pad, at least your side of the bed.
- Wear a large sanitary pad at all times.

These will not keep your water from breaking at the beginning of labor, but it can be comforting to have a plan in the event it should happen.

## If Necessary, Schedule a Cesarean

In the rare circumstance that you know ahead of labor that a Cesarean section will be required for your birth, it will most likely be scheduled to take place this week. Some of the reasons that you may need to schedule a Cesarean birth include the following:

- Placenta previa
- Known fetal anomaly
- Uterine anomaly
- Higher order multiples, such as triplets or quadruplets
- Certain fetal positions, such as some breeches and sideways
- Active herpes infection
- Certain maternal illnesses, including heart or lung disease
- Previous invasive uterine surgery

If any of these apply to you, your practitioner will let you know as soon as possible that a vaginal birth is not an option. This will give you adequate time to shift to your Cesarean birth plan as well as a chance to reframe your birth thoughts in your mind. While not everyone will be disappointed to not be able to labor and give birth vaginally, some mothers are. Organizations are available to help you mentally and emotionally come to terms with this decision both before and after your Cesarean birth. (For more information about a scheduled Cesarean birth, see "Labor and Birth" on page 269.)

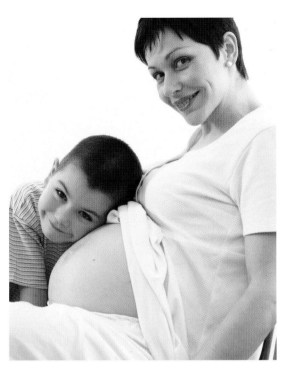

*As you prepare yourself and your home, also remember to include your older children in baby prep 101 at your house.*

## Buy a Book on Motherhood or the Postpartum Period in Particular

Whether you prefer a book with a serious or light-hearted tone, learning about what women go through in the first weeks postpartum can be both useful and a source of relief. It will tell you at 3 A.M. that you are not alone, even if you can't call your friends at that hour. Many books are available in this category, and they range from practical to hysterical. Some books have a specific focus, such as a book on postpartum depression, while most speak to a more universal experience of life with a newborn.

**HOT MAMA**

Maybe you treated yourself to a haircut in anticipation of caring for your new baby, but have you thought about what to do with your hair in labor? Ponytails may be a mommy's go-to hair do, but it's not your only choice. If your hair is long, you will certainly want a style that keeps it off your face and neck when you're hot and sweaty from the effort of labor. Think about how you wear your hair at the gym, playing sports, or doing other strenuous physical activity. This is sure to work well for labor.

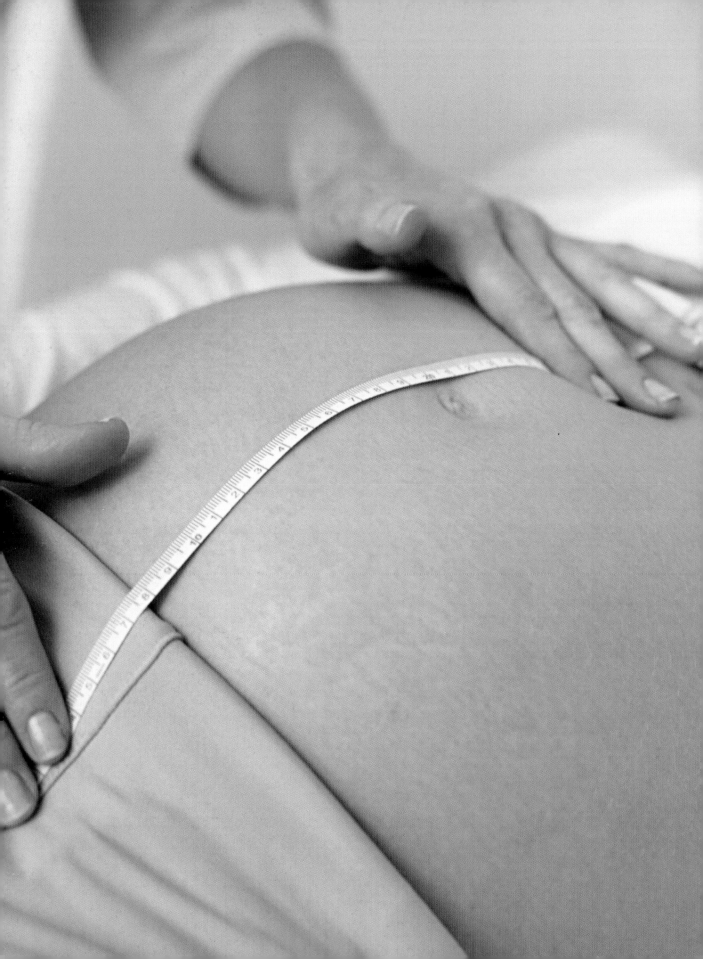

# WEEK 40

## ✏ CHECKLIST FOR WEEK 40

[ ] Have a pedicure.

[ ] Discuss pictures for labor and birth.

[ ] Prepare a list of helpers for after the baby arrives.

[ ] Plan a date night.

## 🔍 WHAT TO WATCH FOR THIS WEEK

*Double Check*

**Signs of labor:** From the 37th week on, your practitioner will not try to stop your labor. Your job is to record your signs of labor and follow the instructions your practitioner has given you for when to call him or her.

**Decrease in fetal movement:** When fetal movement slows, it can be a sign of problems with the baby. Make sure to alert your practitioner immediately.

**Swelling:** Should your face or hands start to swell suddenly, it could be a symptom of pregnancy induced hypertension (PIH) or preeclampsia, and you should tell your practitioner right away.

**Headaches:** Similar to sudden swelling, a severe headache can be a sign of elevated blood pressure and PIH or even preeclampsia, which is a severe illness in pregnancy related to blood pressure, protein in your urine, and other complications.

**Blurred vision:** Tell your doctor or midwife about any problems with your vision because it can be a sign of PIH or preeclampsia.

**Bleeding or spotting:** Unless you can point to intercourse, a vaginal exam, or vaginal ultrasound as its cause, you should report bleeding or spotting to your practitioner; it may be a sign of infection, dilation of the cervix, or issues related to your placenta.

*Report any strange or troublesome symptoms to your practitioner immediately.*

##  BODY BASICS

While your fundus's measurements have been keeping pace with your weeks so far, it now actually measures slightly less for most women. This is because your baby is settling into the pelvis awaiting birth. Occasionally you will find a mom who has a forty or more centimeter fundus, which probably means she is having difficulty breathing deeply. Stretching the upper back and moving should relieve some of the pressure.

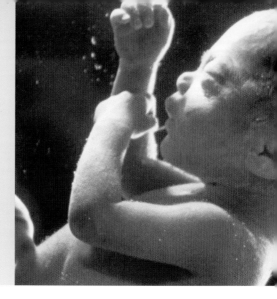

## 🍼 BABY DATA

Your baby has everything he or she needs to be born. Your baby's intestinal tract is lined with meconium, your baby's first stool. About 30 percent of babies will pass this before birth, which means that your baby will need to be deep suctioned at birth to prevent the baby from inhaling the sticky substance.

## Have a Pedicure

A pedicure never fails to soothe the body and soul, particularly when your due date is near. You probably haven't seen your toes in a while, and a pedicure can make them look their best for the big day. A shot of your painted toes, peeking out from under your bare belly, makes for a great photo.

A pedicure is sure to make your toes look great, and the foot and leg massage is heaven-sent for tired and aching feet. In addition, the foot has a plethora of pressure points that can help stimulate labor. So a good rubdown at this juncture may prove beneficial in other ways.

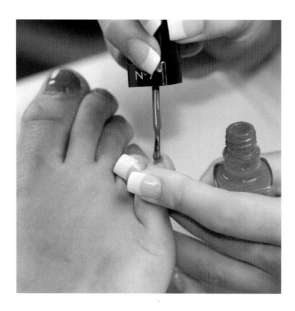

Turn a trip to the spa into a fun outing with your girlfriend or close relative. Treat yourselves to lunch out, have pedicures, and talk about whatever you want, whether that's the baby or a recent movie. Just enjoy yourself!

## Discuss Pictures for Labor and Birth

Pictures during labor can be a contentious issue. Some mothers really want them, and others really do not. By the time you throw in the wishes of family members and the policy of your birth place, it's hard to know what you want.

You can approach this topic in a couple of ways. One side says that giving birth is a special moment—one you can never come back to and take photos of if you change your mind down the road. Some mothers feel that they will be so busy in labor that they will miss the birth of the baby or some other special moment. So they decide to take pictures.

The other side agrees that this is a special moment—one that should never be captured on film but always remembered in your heart for what it was. This group does not take photos.

The thing is, if you take pictures, you never have to look at them. You can lock them away and forget about them. You even have the choice not to

*A pregnancy pedicure can liven your spirits, beautify your toes, and stimulate potential labor vibes.*

## THE ODDS OF YOUR BABY BEING BORN ON YOUR DUE DATE

Everyone circles their due dates in red or otherwise highlights it on a calendar. And even though pregnant women are told, "It's just an educated guess," they get their hearts set on this date, even when they don't mean to.

Some practitioners are beginning to move away from assigning due dates for this very reason. They feel it nearly terrorizes mothers who give birth before or after that date. Instead, they give due weeks or months. So rather than being told "August 22," you would be told you're due toward the end of August or the beginning of September. This means that even if you are among the 4 to 5 percent of women who actually give birth on their due dates, it's within the range you were given.

If it's too late and you already have the red circle on your calendar, don't stress. You probably realize by now that the baby will come when he or she is good and ready, and the date on the calendar is merely the best guess and not an exact target.

develop the film. If you do not take photos, however, you will never have the chance to go back and take them because the moment has passed.

Hospital or birth center policy may play a part in your decision. Some allow still photography only, with or without flash. Others say you can't use flash. They may also dictate when you can take photos; for instance, you can take photos of the labor but not the birth and not of your doctor or midwife.

## PREGNANCY AFFIRMATION FOR WEEK 40

## I am ready to meet my baby.

Similarly, videography may or may not be allowed. Some will allow it for labor and not birth, or only if it is done with the video camera on a tripod.

When you tour your hospital or birth center, ask about the photographing and videotaping policy. If you find that the policy is not in keeping with your desires, try talking to your practitioner or someone at the hospital or birth center to see if there are exceptions to the rule.

## Prepare a List of Helpers for After the Baby Arrives

Postpartum is a time when you will need help. You might not believe it now, or you might not know what others could do to help, but it is best to be ready to ask for help. Part of that is knowing who you can turn to, depending on what the need is. It is always a good idea to make a list ahead of time.

Sit down with a piece of paper and a pen. List every kind of help you might need, such as the following:

- Help with breastfeeding
- Help with meals
- Help with cleaning the house
- Help with yourself (emotionally or physically)
- Help with your other children

Anything you can think of belongs on the list. Then go back and list people you might feel comfortable calling for help. This might include

## THE IMPORTANCE OF SLEEP

Even if the sleep you get is not in the middle of the night, resting whenever possible will help ensure that you are ready when labor comes. Labor is difficult enough when you are well rested, but add exhausted to the mix and it becomes much more difficult.

So wherever you can eke out more time for sleep, go for it! Even if you only find a few minutes to rest and relax, that will help. And the same goes for your partner, particularly if he doesn't function terribly well with inadequate sleep.

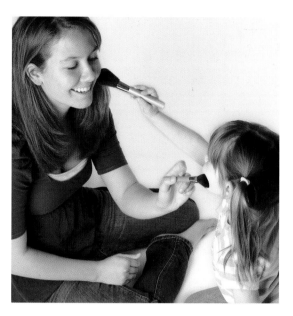

*Before the new baby invades your home, be sure to spend some extra time with your other children. This can go a long way to making them feel better.*

friends and family, and it may include also professional people. For example, under help with breast-feeding, you might list a friend who successfully nursed her baby, a lactation consultant, and La Leche League. Help with the house might include your neighbor, your sister, and a housecleaning service. Having a list makes it easier for you to simply pick it up and get the help you need.

When your baby is born, people will want to help you. This may be good friends or family, or even neighbors or acquaintances from social or religious organizations to which you belong. Sometimes people will offer something specific, such as bringing over meals, or they may set up something in advance, such as play dates for an older sibling. The majority of the time, though, these calls come in spontaneously and can leave a new mother wondering what she needs help with. With your list, you'll be prepared.

In addition to a list of people you can call for help after your baby is born, be sure to have a list of things that people can do to help you. This prevents you from telling someone that you don't

need help, simply because you can't think of anything. Preparing a list ahead of time is not difficult when you write down all the tasks and errands you typically do or need during the day, such as the following:

- Grocery run
- Pick up postage stamps or mail letters
- Bring/prepare a meal
- Play with baby's older sibling
- Do laundry

Now when someone calls, you can say "I have a list, and here are some of the items on it." This allows the person to help in a way that is truly helpful, and it also allows her to choose something that best suits her availability and abilities. Everyone wins.

## Plan a Date Night

Date night! You are probably thinking that's crazy, but it is so important to stay connected as a couple, even at the end of your pregnancy. During these

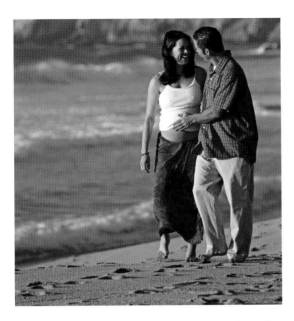

*It's really easy to rush the end of pregnancy. But the truth is that postpartum is a different kind of difficult. Try to enjoy the last days.*

**HOT MAMA**

Have you already thought about what you are going to wear after you have the baby while you are at the hospital or birth center? This is where bed jackets could make a big come back. A soft cardigan also works well to cover ugly hospital gowns, keep you warm, or just add a touch of class to your nightgown. Its design, moreover, is tailor-made for nursing a new baby.

last few weeks, it is very normal for pregnant women to draw inward and focus only on themselves and the baby. Your husband is probably not feeling the same way, and, in fact, some guys report feeling a bit neglected, and the baby has not been born yet!

Making an effort to reconnect with a surprise date night at a favorite restaurant or even an elaborate meal at home can mean the world to your husband. It shows him that you care and helps the two of you come closer together. Let's face it, after baby, it will take at the very least a couple of months to juggle all of the balls in your life, and that means your relationship too.

Your date night can include anything that is fun or special for the two of you. Movies can be nice, but it can also be difficult for you to sit through a movie without a bathroom break, plus it does not allow for much conversation between you and your husband. The time of year will come into play: A picnic might be perfect, but if it's winter, you will want to plan something indoors.

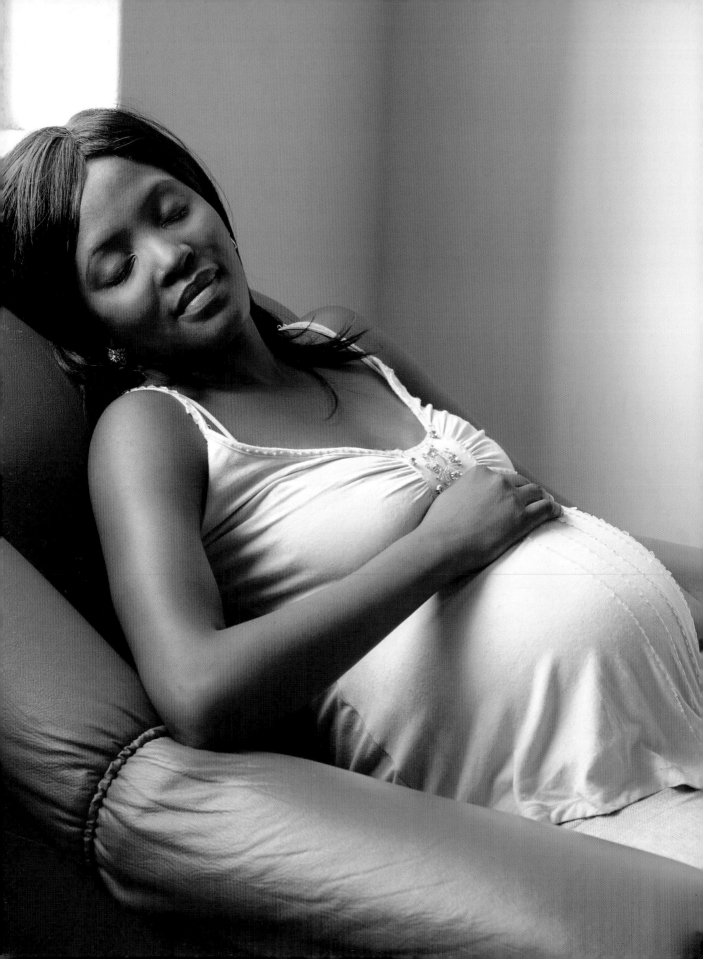

# WEEK 41
## AND BEYOND

### ✎ CHECKLIST FOR WEEK 41 AND BEYOND

[ ] Schedule a nonstress test for fetal surveillance.
[ ] Handle annoying phone calls from well-meaning people.
[ ] Consider induction of labor at forty-two weeks.
[ ] Celebrate your pregnancy.

### ⚲ WHAT TO WATCH FOR THIS WEEK

*Double Check*

**Signs of labor:** Once you reach your 37th week, your practitioner will not try to stop your labor. Be aware of the signs of labor and follow the instructions your practitioner has given you for when to call them.

**Decrease in fetal movement:** If you notice a reduction in fetal movement, tell your practitioner right away because there may be a problem with your baby.

**Swelling:** One of the symptoms of pregnancy induced hypertension (PIH) and preeclampsia is a sudden swelling in the face or hands. You can distinguish this from normal pregnancy swelling because it comes on fast, is severe, and does not go away even after a period of rest.

**Headaches:** Elevated blood pressure can trigger severe headaches, which should be reported to your doctor of midwife. If headaches are tied to other symptoms, you may be suffering from PIH or even preeclampsia, which is a severe illness in pregnancy related to blood pressure, protein in your urine, and other complications.

**Blurred vision:** Another symptom of PIH and preeclampsia, report blurred vision immediately to your practitioner, whether or not it is accompanied by headaches.

**Bleeding or spotting:** Bleeding or spotting may be a sign of infection, dilation of the cervix, or issues related to your placenta, so be sure to contact your practitioner to discuss.

*Report any strange or troublesome symptoms to your practitioner immediately.*

###  BODY BASICS

You might be wondering if your body is paying attention. Yes, your body is paying attention, only not to the calendar. It is listening to your baby and waiting for the sign that your baby is ready for labor. This means that in the last few weeks of pregnancy, you might experience contractions that appear to be labor but do not progress to that point. These contractions are useful for preparing your body and baby for what's to come, but they can be mentally and emotionally tiresome. Be kind to yourself. And remember: Every labor is different. Some pregnancies simply take longer to gestate.

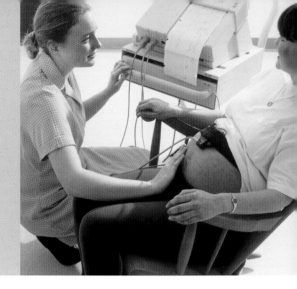

## BABY DATA

Yes, your baby is still in there. Between you monitoring the baby's kick counts and your prenatal care provider monitoring the baby's health, your baby is simply enjoying the last few days of pregnancy. Baby has it good: easy food, no stress, no diapers or clothes. Why give up a deal like that?

## Schedule a Nonstress Test for Fetal Surveillance

Because your pregnancy has gone past the 40-week mark, your practitioner will want to watch your baby more closely to ensure his or her health and safety. This will mean more prenatal visits, usually every few days, until you give birth. You also may be asked to do additional testing, including the nonstress test.

The nonstress test is basically a fetal monitor. You will wear one belt that monitors your baby's movements via ultrasound and another belt that measures any contractions. While you are being monitored, you will also be given a button to push to note when your baby moves. Your doctor or midwife will note how your baby responds to contractions, if you are having any, and how they move and what their heart rate does during the period of movement.

Sometimes babies want to sleep during the nonstress test. You can choose to eat or drink something just prior to your test, which can help wake baby up. Your practitioner may also use a buzzer to rouse a sleeping baby. If your baby is asleep, it is not a sign of a problem, as babies sleep many times throughout the day, oblivious to how you are moving or what you are doing.

Based on the outcome of the nonstress test, you will either be released for another prenatal appointment or you will discuss additional testing. Other tests might include the stress test (oxytocin challenge test) or a bio-physical profile.

## Handle Annoying Phone Calls from Well-Meaning People

Once your due date passes, people will start eyeing you like an expired bottle of milk or a ticking time bomb. You have neither "expired" nor will you explode on contact, but this doesn't shield you from rude or inexplicable comments from people.

Consider changing your outgoing message on your answering machine to something like, "Thanks for calling. I'm resting up for labor right now. When we've had the baby, we'll post an announcement on our machine." You could obviously leave snottier comments, but that's up to you. The message you want to get across, either on the phone or in person, is that you are perfectly well and, yes, still pregnant.

## Consider Induction of Labor at Forty-Two Weeks

The American College of Obstetricians and Gynecologists (ACOG) recommends that labor be induced when you have reached the end of 42 weeks. Induction prior to the completion of 42 weeks can be considered if the mother has an illness that is complicated by pregnancy, or if fetal testing shows that the baby is not doing well in the uterus.

ACOG does not agree with what they call social induction or induction for nonmedical reasons. Their belief is that inducing labor carries sufficient risks and so it should only be done in cases where the medical needs outweigh the risks. They therefore frown on inductions that are arranged to ease family, physician, or midwife scheduling, to pick the baby's birthday or zodiac sign, or simply because the mother is tired of being pregnant.

If your practitioner decides to induce, the method he or she will use will depend on a number of factors, including the following:

- Your cervical dilation
- Your baby's station, which is his or her position in relation to your pelvis
- Your health history
- Your previous birth history
- Your preference

Some methods of induction are more gentle than others, so you should gather information on the different methods that are available. (See "Labor and Birth" on page 269.) This will give you a good idea of the types of labor inductions that can be done, how they are done, and which you prefer. While an induction is likely to change aspects of your birth plan, it does not necessarily mean that you need to scrap your whole plan and start over.

Because induction of labor carries higher risks to your baby and you than births that aren't induced, you will need to ask questions about monitoring in labor. Many practitioners require continuous monitoring with certain types of medicinal inductions, while others have a more lenient policy. Discuss this with your practitioner before arriving at your place of birth.

## PREGNANCY AFFIRMATION FOR WEEK 41 AND BEYOND

✣

# My body knows what to do in labor, and I will let it.

## Celebrate Your Pregnancy

The fact that you are past your due date may seem like a curse, but try to think of it as a blessing. You have had a full pregnancy, and you have grown a healthy baby. Your body is working just as planned.

Look at the extra time as a vacation. Hang out with friends or get another massage before your baby is born. You have bonus days in which to finalize preparations and gather baby supplies. These last few weeks can be a real windfall for the mother-to-be who has procrastinated or who simply needs more time to get everything done.

If your baby planning is complete, try to find a way to celebrate. Have you had a belly cast made? What about a henna tattoo for your belly? Do you have pictures from the last week? Have you taken time to write in your journal? Most of all, enjoy yourself!

## HOME INDUCTIONS

There are lots of recipes for home inductions, and many swear that their method is tried and true. The problem is, similar to medical inductions, nothing is a guarantee. In fact, because many home inductions are done without medical supervision, they can be quite dangerous.

Obviously you can try some induction techniques at home without the approval of your doctor or midwife. These include the following.

**Sexual relations:** Orgasm, with or without intercourse, releases oxytocin, which can cause contractions. If you add deep penetrating intercourse and male orgasm, the sperm contains prostaglandins, which can help to ripen the cervix. This powerful recipe also provides relaxation for mom and dad.

**Relaxation:** Using mental, physical, and emotional relaxation can be a great way to help remove mental or emotional roadblocks to labor. This is especially useful if you harbor fears about birth.

**Old wives' tales:** This is where the bumpy roads and spicy foods come in. There are plenty of variations, and some restaurants even sell their versions of labor soup or salad.

Another category of home induction do not strictly require supervision, but you should run these ideas past your practitioner. This is nipple stimulation with a breast pump, although it can be performed using manual stimulation as well. If you're interested, talk to your practitioner, who will give you a list of things to do or watch for, such as contractions that last too long.

Finally, there are home induction methods that need the approval and supervision of your practitioner. This includes castor oil and herbs.

Home inductions are not inherently bad, but they do carry certain risks, which must be discussed before trying them. Some of the risks are emotional, such as what if you try and it does not work? Other risks are physical, such as dehydration. Being prepared will help you prevent or treat any negative consequences.

### HOT MAMA

If you want a new look, other than not being pregnant, a quick trip to the makeup counter can be a big boon to your self-esteem. Many companies offer free makeovers, and having a professional makeup artist design a new look for you can be a fun boost. Maybe you wash everything off after a day, or maybe you'll pick up beauty tips that last long after you have the baby!

# LABOR AND BIRTH

✏ **CHECKLIST FOR LABOR AND BIRTH**

[ ] Know the terms and definitions for labor and birth.
[ ] Have a vaginal exam.
[ ] Learn the stages of labor.
[ ] Recognize labor.
[ ] Guesstimate how long labor will last.
[ ] Learn how to deal with prodromal labor.
[ ] Check if your water has broken.
[ ] Understand what happens in a home birth.
[ ] Get admitted to the hospital or birth center.
[ ] Prepare for common hospital procedures.
[ ] Know what you can (and can't) eat in labor.
[ ] Find a comfortable position for labor.
[ ] Use a variety of comfort measures in labor.
[ ] Cope with a slow labor.
[ ] Cope with a fast labor.
[ ] Cope with back labor.
[ ] Have an unmedicated birth, if you wish.
[ ] Know the positions for pushing.

[ ] Learn how to push your baby out.
[ ] Prepare Dad to catch the baby.
[ ] Learn about fetal monitoring.
[ ] Learn about amniotomy.
[ ] Learn about pain medication in labor.
[ ] See about an episiotomy.
[ ] Find out what happens to the placenta.
[ ] Decide how to spend the first few minutes with your baby.
[ ] Teach Dad about cord cutting.
[ ] Learn about delayed cord cutting.
[ ] Learn what happens to baby after the initial bonding period.
[ ] Learn about rooming in.
[ ] Prepare for a Cesarean section.
[ ] Learn how a Cesarean section is done.
[ ] Avoid an unnecessary cesarean.
[ ] Have a family-centered Cesarean birth.

🔍 **WHAT TO WATCH FOR**

Warning signs in labor include heavy bleeding, contractions that never stop, and other things that are mostly screened by your midwife or doctor that you're too busy laboring to notice.

**LABOR AND BIRTH PARTICULARS**

# Know the Terms and Definitions for Labor and Birth

Lots of technical terms are bandied about in the birthing arena, and you can feel lost if you don't know what's being discussed. The following list of terms will give you a solid understanding of the labor and birth process and will help you speak the language of your practitioners.

CERVIX: This is the end of your uterus that opens into the birth canal to allow your baby to be born.

LIGHTENING: Sometimes referred to as dropping, this is an indication that the baby appears to be lower in your pelvis and more ready to be born. Your belly, from the outside, will reflect the changes.

DILATION: Measured in centimeters, this refers to the degree to which the cervix is open before and during labor. At ten centimeters, you are completely dilated.

EFFACEMENT: Given in percentages, this is a measurement of how thin the cervix is. Suppose your cervix is normally two inches (5 centimeters) long. For example, if you are told at a vaginal exam that you are 50 percent effaced, then your cervix is only one inch (2.5 centimeters) thick. At the end of labor, you are said to be 100 percent effaced.

RIPE: Your cervix goes through textural changes, or a ripening process, toward the end of pregnancy and during early labor. The cervix starts out very tough and softens as hormones prepare your body for birth. The softer your cervix is, the easier it is to dilate.

STATION: This relates where your baby is in relation to your pelvis. Zero station is considered engaged in the pelvis. If your practitioner uses a negative number, you baby is still high in the pelvis, while positive numbers usually show up when you're pushing and are close to having your baby.

ANTERIOR POSITION: The most common position for birth, this is when your baby's head is down and facing toward your back.

POSTERIOR POSITION: This is when the baby is head down but facing upward toward your belly instead of towards your spine. This can mean that you need to use positioning to help turn the baby to an anterior position for an easier birth. You may also experience more labor pains in your back. (See back labor.)

## Consider a Vaginal Exam

The dilation and effacement of your cervix and your baby's position and station are determined through a vaginal exam during which a nurse or your practitioner places fingers inside your vagina. Vaginal exams are done at various intervals during labor.

Sometimes vaginal exams are done by the clock. For example, you might have one when you get to your place of birth and then another every four hours or more frequently if needed. Because vaginal exams can introduce bacteria into your vagina, many women prefer to have them only when needed.

Signs you might need a vaginal exam include the following:

- You just arrived at your place of birth.
- You want information about your cervix or the baby's position.
- You feel like you have to push.

It's helpful if you have already talked with your practitioner about his or her policy on vaginal exams in labor, before you go into labor.

## Learn the Stages of Labor

Labor breaks down into the following three stages.

FIRST STAGE: The first stage of labor is from the point when your uterus starts to contract regularly until you are ten centimeters, or completely, dilated.

SECOND STAGE: At complete dilation, the baby will begin to descend, and you may feel the urge to push and begin pushing. The second stage ends with the birth of your baby.

THIRD STAGE: The final stage of labor runs from the birth of your baby until the placenta is born.

These three stages are the same for every mother, although the times for each may vary. Within the first stage of labor, there are three phases.

EARLY LABOR: In this first phase, your contractions can be from five to twenty minutes apart. You normally spend a great deal of time wondering if this is really labor or just practice contractions. You should alternate periods of rest and activity and do what you can to ignore labor for as long as possible. If you were to show up at the hospital during this phase, you would most certainly be sent home. This is the longest part of labor; it can last from a few hours to longer than a day.

ACTIVE LABOR: During active labor, your contractions become more intense and appear closer together, giving you a shorter break in between each one. You are more engaged in your labor now, working hard with your contractions. You should use comfort measures and rely on your support team, including your doula. You may go to your place of birth toward the end of this phase or in the early part of the third phase.

TRANSITION: This is the toughest but fastest part of labor. Generally, transition lasts from thirty to ninety minutes. Your contractions are lasting longer now, about ninety seconds each, and they come every three minutes. You may feel shaky, nauseated, and scared. Relaxation, comfort measures, support, and possibly medication can be helpful. Your partner and doula will assist you in staying as comfortable as possible.

You should learn all about the stages of labor, what each one entails, and how you and your partner can deal with them in your childbirth class.

# PREGNANCY AFFIRMATION FOR LABOR AND BIRTH

— My body knows how to labor.
— Labor prepares my baby for birth.
— I am making wise decisions for my baby and me.
— Contractions bring me closer to my baby.
— I am excited to hold my baby.

## Recognize Labor

One of the biggest questions on the minds of moms-to-be is how to tell when labor starts. They've heard stories of women who rushed to the hospital thinking labor was underway only to be sent home. The following signs indicate that your labor is the real deal:

- Contractions get stronger, longer, and closer together.
- Movement does not alter the contractions.
- Taking a bath does not alter the contraction pattern, even if it is soothing.
- You have been having contractions for quite some time.
- Rest does not make the contractions go away.
- You are having other signs of labor, such as bloody show.

Having talked to your practitioner about when to go to the hospital or birth center, you will have a good idea of what to look for as far as labor goes. Some practitioners recommend using the 4-1-1 method: You have contractions 4 minutes apart, each one lasts at least 1 minute, and this rhythm continues for at least 1 hour. If you have special concerns, for example if you're carrying twins or you will require antibiotics during labor for group B strep, your practitioner might have you come in sooner. He or she can also give you alternate suggestions to help you stay home longer if you are comfortable and would prefer to avoid medical interventions that aren't necessary.

If you arrive at the hospital and it is determined that you are not in labor or that you are not far enough along to stay there, do not feel badly. Many women, even women who have had children before, have been sent home from hospitals. Consider it a trial run for the real thing.

## Guesstimate How Long Labor Will Last

Labor is different for every woman, and how long it lasts varies greatly. On average, though, first-time mothers have labors that range from twelve to eighteen hours. Remember, this is an average only, and many moms have significantly longer or shorter labors.

If you have had a baby before, conventional wisdom says that your next labor will be half as long as your first labor. If, however, your first labor was very short, you are probably not going to cut that in half, though you may push for less time.

Other factors influence how fast labor progresses, including the following:

- What's the baby's position?
- What number baby is this for you?
- Are you up and moving around during labor?
- Are you being induced?
- Are you using pain medication?
- Are you worried in labor?
- How much sleep have you had?
- Are you hungry?
- Are the people around you being annoying?
- Are you scared of becoming a mom?

This list is just the beginning. Many things—tangible and intangible—will influence your labor. Mastering the art of minimizing as many of these influences as you can is very helpful. You will find yourself more relaxed and better able to focus on labor and the work that needs to be done.

## Learn How to Deal with Prodromal Labor

Prodromal labor is a piddling kind of labor that keeps you guessing as to whether or not it is the real thing. You have real contractions, and just when you're ready to go to your place of birth, they stop. Sometimes this goes on for weeks.

This emotionally and mentally draining, and the strength of the contractions is enough to make you work with them. The contractions may make you lose sleep, but they are also doing things for your body and your labor. Try to see if they follow a pattern. Some women find that when they pay attention, they have contractions at the same time of day or when all the circumstances are similar. An example might be the mother who contracts at night when it is quiet, only to stop contracting as her husband and neighbors wake up and start the day.

Prodromal labor is not dangerous for either mother or baby, but it can be emotionally and physically exhausting. Do what you can to take care of yourself. Nap when you can. Talk to your midwife or doctor about what you can try to alleviate the discomfort from contractions. Labor will kick into gear when your baby is truly ready. Hang in there!

## Check If Your Water Has Broken

Sometimes in late pregnancy, you may think your water has broken, and instead of hauling yourself to the practitioner or the hospital to find out, you wish there was something you could try at home to confirm your suspicions.

You may imagine that water breaking involves a sudden, huge gush, or some other unmistakable sign. Sometimes that is exactly how it plays out, but more often than not, there is a lingering doubt.

One of the easiest ways to tell if your water broke is to put on a clean maxi pad and lay down for about a half hour. When you sit up, if you have a small gush, your water is most likely broken. While you were lying down, even a small trickle will form a small pool of amniotic fluid in the vagina. When you sit up, this pool flows out onto the pad.

Keep in mind that water breaking as a first sign of labor is relatively uncommon and occurs in approximately 13 percent of pregnancies. In fact, about 75 percent of the time, your water will not break until you are past nine centimeters, well into labor.

## Understand What Happens in a Home Birth

The most obvious difference with a home birth is that you do not have to go anywhere once you begin your labor. (Unless you're not at home already, that is!) The big question is usually when to call the practitioner to come to your home.

This is a question you should ask in advance and discuss at great length with your practitioner. The answer will partially be based on your preferences and partially on your labor. For example, you may want to wait until later in labor to have the practitioner come to your home, but your labor may dictate having them there sooner. You should also take into account how your support team feels about going it alone, how far the practitioner has to travel to reach you, and how your labor typically progresses if this is not your first baby.

When your practitioner arrives, he or she will assess you and the baby. If you are doing well, the practitioner may hang out and help as needed or rest in another room. If you are having difficulty concentrating or coping, he or she will be available for advice and support.

When it is time for your baby to be born, your practitioner will set up the necessary items. You, the laboring mother, have already decided where the birth will take place and how. Your practitioner will offer guidance and help you figure out what feels best for you.

After the birth, you will most likely have unlimited time with your newborn. In a normal birth where there are no complications and no one needs anything, baby is not moved until Mom is ready. Your practitioner will then perform a newborn exam and also examine your perineum to determine if sutures are needed. You and your baby will be monitored for the period that your practitioner stays with you. Your practitioner will usually return the next day and a few days after that, followed by additional visits as needed until your six-week postpartum visit.

## Get Admitted to the Hospital or Birth Center

"Getting admitted" means different things at different facilities. While many places offer preregistration, the majority of laboring women would agree that it didn't seem to help, and registration was still a lengthy process.

Be prepared to show your insurance card and to answer questions about your prenatal care, your practitioner, and your labor. You may also be asked basic medical questions and legal questions, such as whether you have an advanced directive or living will.

You will then be escorted to your labor room or to a triage area, depending on the setup of your birth facility. Many places have a policy requiring that you be transported in a wheelchair. Some women say it was great to be wheeled, but others felt like it was too painful to sit down.

If you go to a triage area, you will either be in a very small room with a bed, a chair, and a monitor, or you will be in a large room with a number of beds separated by curtains. During this period, you will have your vital signs taken, your baby will be monitored, and your cervix will be checked. Unless you are already far along in labor, you will usually be asked to stay in this area for an hour. You are then reassessed to see if your cervix has dilated further. The decision will be made at that point to send you home to continue early labor or to admit you for labor.

Some birth centers and hospitals use the early labor "garden and lounge" concept. Instead of sending you home until your labor has progressed, you are welcome to stay at the birth center or hospital and spend early labor wandering around, eating lightly, watching television, walking in a garden (if there is one), playing games, or whatever you want to do to pass the time. You'll have minimal contact with the staff unless you need it, but you are welcome to stay until you are ready to check in, which saves you from the bumpy ride back to the birth center or hospital while in active labor.

Once you are assigned a labor room, you can move your belongs with you and get settled in. Your nurse or OB tech will ask you another series of questions and give you a quick rundown of what is available for your use from ice machines and birth balls to medications.

You may have an IV started at this point. If, having discussed your birth plan with your practitioner, you have prearranged to have only the basic version put in, such as a saline lock, it would be done at this juncture. You may also have blood drawn from the same site or from a different site. If you are group B strep positive, you may also receive your first dose of antibiotics at this time.

Once the admission process is complete, you are usually left to labor on your own for a while. The process time varies depending on staff availability and the speed at which you answer questions. You may notice that your labor has slowed during this process. This is completely normal as you adjust to your new surrounding. Do not panic. Your labor is not stopping. Once you are left alone, you can do relaxation techniques, and your labor should pick up again.

# Prepare for Common Hospital Procedures

You may have heard one too many horror stories about what happens inside the walls of hospitals and birth centers. These stories, along with what's shown on television, can be truly frightening, especially when you don't know what a particular procedure is for or why it is being done. Here's the lowdown on some of the most common procedures performed during the birthing process.

IV LINE: A small catheter is inserted into your vein to facilitate the delivery of medications or fluids as needed, including an epidural or for emergencies. If you choose to have the tubing removed, you would call this a saline lock. This provides vein access, while not restricting your movements.

CATHETER: A urinary catheter, which is a tube inserted into your bladder to drain urine. It is usually left in place until several hours after you have had the baby and, it is most commonly used with epidural anesthesia and Cesarean birth. This is because when you are completely or even slightly numbed, you can't tell when your bladder is full. Because a full bladder can prevent your baby from descending in the pelvis, it is important to keep your bladder empty. A catheter is inserted for the duration of labor, and you do not need to worry about urinating.

An alternative for later in labor is called an in/out catheter. This is a catheter that is inserted long enough to drain the bladder and then removed. This can be done when you are pushing and don't feel like getting up to the restroom.

FETAL MONITOR: Your baby will be monitored to ensure that he or she is tolerating labor well. How your baby is monitored depends on many factors. (See "Labor and Birth" on page 269.)

SHAVING: Shaving the perineum for birth is no longer a routine procedure. It was once thought to be hygienic, but then studies showed that shaving actually increased infection rates, so it has mostly been abandoned. If you normally shave the pubic region, you can trim your pubic hair before labor if that makes you feel more comfortable.

ENEMA: The routine cleansing of the bowels is generally not done any more. If you have been having issues with constipation and are concerned, you and your practitioner may decide that an enema would be beneficial. It is typically recommend that you do this at home where you are more comfortable.

LAB WORK: It is common to draw blood when you arrive in labor to check your platelet levels, iron levels, and blood type among other things. The findings may determine what medications you are able to use during your labor and provide a baseline for comparison with post-birth lab work. You may also have blood work done after you have the baby.

Every hospital and birth center has policies pertaining to birth procedures. Ideally, you've already inquired into these policies upfront during your tour, so you'll be prepared for what labor will bring.

## Know What You Can (and Can't) Eat in Labor

Most laboring women do not want to eat a lot or eat heavy foods. Whether and what you can eat during labor will depend on your practitioner and place of birth. Most home births and birth centers allow a light labor diet. This usually consists of broths, clear liquids, and light food such as toast. Sometimes, depending on your labor and practitioner, you may eat other things or eat as you please.

In a hospital, you are usually restricted to clear liquids or ice chips. This is because if you have anesthesia, may want anesthesia, or require a Cesarean birth, they prefer you to have an empty stomach. If you have food in your stomach, you run the risk of vomiting and aspirating the contents.

If you are low risk and are not planning to use medications, talk to your practitioner about a compromise. He or she may agree that you can bring beverages such as sports drinks or other snack items for labor. If you reach an agreement, make sure to include it in your birth plan. This lets everyone around you know that your practitioner has given his or her approval.

## Find a Comfortable Position in Labor

There are many positions in which to labor and each has a set of advantages and disadvantages. Hopefully, during your pregnancy, particularly in childbirth class, you tried out as many as you could to familiarize you with the positions in case you decide to use them in labor.

Moving through different positions during labor can really help with pain relief. In addition to making you feel better, moving around can help the baby find the best position to be born, because babies continue to shift around even in labor. The upshot is that it might make your labor shorter.

SITTING POSITIONS: This can include sitting in bed, on a rocker or other chair, on the toilet, or on a birth ball. The key to this position is that it uses gravity without causing stress or strain on your legs. The more upright you are, the more gravity can help pull the baby down into the pelvis, closer to birth. On a birth ball, you also engage the hips that keep you balanced. Here you are able to rest and move at the same time, which allows you the benefits of both! A benefit to a rocking chair is that it can also be calming.

STANDING POSITIONS: Standing upright involves gravity in the process while helping to stretch your legs. Try standing, walking, leaning, dancing with your partner, or leaning over a taller object or a birth ball placed on a bed or chair.

SQUATTING POSITIONS: Squatting can help open up the pelvic outlet by as much as 10 percent. This can be very beneficial, particularly when you're pushing. This position should be used when you are certain that the baby is well engaged in the pelvis. (If you are unsure, ask your practitioner or nurse.) You can do this alone on the bed, on the floor, leaning back against someone, or even using a squat bar across your hospital bed. It is suggested that you squat only during contractions and stand or stretch your legs between contractions to prevent cramping and pain.

LYING DOWN: Lying down to relax or to slow the birth is an option when labor is progressing very quickly. It reduces gravity's pull on the baby and slows labor for many women.

HANDS AND KNEES: This position is great to give others access to your back for a massage or to treat back labor. It also can help a baby who is in the posterior position to rotate. You can get down on all fours on the floor, on the bed, or in a bathtub.

Choosing the position that works for you may come instinctually, or you may need help deciding. Select positions that feel good, that give you the sense that the baby is moving down, and that labor is progressing. You will probably want to change positions at least every thirty minutes. You should also remember to try to go to the bathroom every hour or so to avoid a full bladder from preventing the baby from descending into your pelvis.

You should be able to assume these positions easily on your own or with support from others. If you are dealing with monitoring equipment or IV lines, ask for help. You can also ask to be taken off the monitors for a while or ask for telemetry, or wireless, monitoring. Don't worry about being a pest: Maintaining your mobility is absolutely key to managing pain relief.

## What to Do If You Need to Labor in Bed

Sometimes laboring in or near a bed may be the most beneficial approach for you and your baby. This happens in the following circumstances:

- You need a rest.
- Monitors prevent you from moving very far.

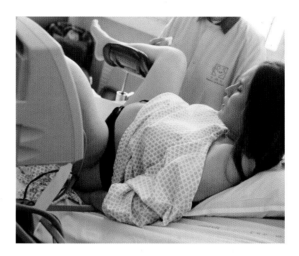

*Laboring in bed doesn't mean that you need to give birth on your back, even with monitors, ask for helping in choosing an upright position for birth.*

- You have an epidural or other medication.
- Your blood pressure is high.
- Your baby tolerates labor better in a side lying position.

If you have the need or desire to stay near the bed, you can sit on a rocking chair or birth ball, or you can stand next to the bed to assume a variety of positions, such as leaning over a taller object or a birth ball placed on a bed or chair. This accommodates monitoring wires that do not reach very far. If you are in bed, you can still do some of the more upright positions, such as leaning over the back of the bed or using a squat bar on the bed.

If you need to lie down, you can still move from side to side, supported by pillows. This works when your movements are restricted but still provides you with some of the benefits of moving in labor. It can also help your baby progress.

## Use a Variety of Comfort Measures in Labor

You can use a range of comfort measures in labor, and it is important to learn as many as you can because you do not know which will be effective once your labor begins in earnest. Whether you're aware of it or not, you already know certain comfort measures because you use them to comfort yourself when you are sick or in pain. These can work well in labor too. Your childbirth class, doula, practitioner, and pregnancy and birth books will give you other suggestions. Here are some to consider.

WATER: Water has been shown to be a very effective tool against pain in labor, second only to the most powerful medications. You can use your tub or shower at home once you hit active labor. You can assume different positions in the tub or shower as well, as opposed to just sitting or standing.

Once at the hospital or birth center, your options may be limited to a shower or possibly a two-person tub. Be creative with how you use water. Don't hesitate to move around and even use the birth ball in the tub or shower; just be sure not to block the shower drain!

MASSAGE: During labor, you could enjoy a full-blown body massage. Something as simple as a foot or hand massage or having someone rub your back can work wonders. There are also special massages for the perineum that practitioners do when the baby is crowning.

TOUCH: Touch relaxation (where you tense a muscle and then release it when a doula or other person touches it) or simply touching an area that is experiencing pain is beneficial for many women in labor. (If you prefer not to be touched, speak up.) Long strokes in one direction, such as from the shoulder to the hand, can also feel great. You can combine the stroking with soothing words such as, "Feel the tension leaving through your fingers…"

HOT AND COLD COMPRESSES: Heat and cold are commonly used for pain relief, and labor is no different. The key is knowing how and when to use each one. Heat is used for mild to moderate pain, and it is perfect for the lower back, the pubic bone, or stiff, aching joints in labor. Cold is more appropriate for moderate to severe pain. Rice socks make great hot compresses and use moist heat, which is penetrating. For cold compresses you can use frozen washcloths or gloves filled with ice. Be sure to test the temperature of any compress and do not apply compresses to numbed skin, such as from an epidural.

RELAXATION: Relaxing your muscles can be wonderfully soothing during labor. With progressive relaxation, you start with your toes or the top of your head, tense each muscle and release, slowly working through the length of your entire body. Alternatively, you can use mental techniques such as visual imagery or imagining and retelling stories about favorite places or happy events to help you relax.

Combining any or all of these techniques with the various positions should help reduce the pain and anxiety you may feel in labor. Practicing prior to labor is recommended so the techniques and positions become familiar.

## Cope with a Slow Labor

For many laboring mothers, a slow labor can be frustrating. It is not so much the pain of labor, but the emotional tug of war that ensues. Because a longer labor usually means more time in early labor, you can get tired from losing sleep to contractions and anxious to get on with labor and meet your baby.

To help stimulate a slow labor, consider the following suggestions:

- Rest when you can, even if only for a few minutes at a time.
- Alternate periods of rest with appropriate activity, such as walking.
- Eat and drink to comfort.
- Try a bath or shower; it can be refreshing.
- Use different positions and comfort measures to help you deal with contractions.
- Call for reinforcements. New faces can renew your spirit and energy.
- Make sure your support team is eating and resting.

- Consider nipple stimulation or acupressure to stimulate labor.
- Talk to your practitioner about medicinal augmentation of your labor.

The key to successfully managing a slower labor is to rest and relax as much as possible. You need to pace yourself so you don't get worn down early on. Slower labors happen for a reason. Perhaps your baby needs more stimulation before birth, or your body needs the labor to progress slowly.

## Cope with a Fast Labor

During pregnancy, you may have secretly, or not so secretly, been hoping for a speedy labor, but it is a difficult labor to manage. That's because there isn't a gradual build up that tells you: "Here comes labor." If you are lucky, you have a manageable contraction or two before it becomes serious labor.

A fast labor can really throw you off your stride. If you think your labor might be fast, as soon as you realize you are in labor, gather your support team, even if you are not planning to go to your place of birth yet. You will need support sooner than you would with a labor of a regular duration.

You may want to assume positions that are easier on you for contractions, such as side lying or even getting on hands and knees. This can lessen the sensation of contractions and actually slow labor slightly, both of which can be beneficial for your labor and your sanity.

If you are going to the hospital or birth center, you may want to go and get settled in. This means you won't have to travel when you are in transition or trying not to push your baby out. It may also bring you peace of mind.

You should have your partner, your doula, and others there to support you and working intensely to help you. It may take just a short while, but a lot can be packed into a few hours. After the baby is born, you may sit up and think, "What was the name of the truck that hit me?"

## Cope with Back Labor

About one-third of laboring women report that their backs hurt during labor, more so than their abdomens. Sometimes the pain of back labor does not go away during the break in contractions. This was once solely blamed on the baby being in a posterior position, turned to face the mother's front. Now we know that this only makes up a fraction of back labors.

The good news is that there are some tricks to help deal with back labor. Many of the strategies for alleviating the pain associated with back labor also help move a baby out of a posterior position. If your back is hurting more than your belly in labor, try the following.

HANDS AND KNEES POSITION: Getting on your hands and knees reduces the strain on your back. This position is also helpful at making the contractions less painful and will encourage a baby to rotate if he or she is facing forward.

COUNTER PRESSURE: This is a steady, firm pressure on the lower back, per mom's orders. If your support people are pushing too hard, give feedback and tell them how hard they need to push. By pressing against the sacrum, the hard bone at the base of your spine, they are counteracting the pressure from the baby's head on your sacrum, which is where the pain is coming from. It may be necessary to apply this pressure for hours, and it is most easily accomplished with Mom in the hands and knees position.

ICE PACKS: Using an ice pack or cold compress on the area of the back that hurts can help alleviate pain.

WATER: Laboring in a tub or shower has been shown to provide enormous relief for many moms. Feel free to use a variety of positions in the water, including hands and knees.

STERILE WATER INJECTIONS: Not offered everywhere, this treatment involves four carefully placed injections of water, just under the skin around the sacrum. It can provide amazing relief from back pain without medication.

TRANS ELECTRICAL NERVE STIMULA-TION (TENS): This is a small pack that carries a small electrical current delivered wherever you place the pads. A very common device in physical therapy units, TENS has been used widely in labor and birth wards in many countries with great success. The results are best when applied early in labor before the pain becomes too great.

PAIN MEDICATIONS: Sometimes pain medication is the best approach. Choosing an epidural can blunt the pain, but be aware that if your baby is in the posterior position, you should still try to have assistance moving, even if just from side to side to encourage your baby to change positions.

## Have an Unmedicated Birth, If You Wish

Going through labor and birth without pain-relieving medication is called natural childbirth or having an unmedicated birth. Women choose unmedicated births for a variety of reasons, such as it is better for the baby and mom, it is a personal challenge, or they have adverse reactions to medication.

To have a natural childbirth, however, one must be prepared. Here are some things you can do to increase your chances of giving birth without medication.

Get educated. This should include a combination of reading books on the subject, talking to other mothers who have experienced natural birth, reading birth stories, and more.

Hire a doula. Using a doula can drastically decrease your chances of getting medication. Many women who are planning to use medication also use doulas, but the knowledge and skill a doula brings to the process has been shown to greatly reduce requests for pain medication.

Take a natural childbirth class. Not all childbirth classes are created equal. While it is important for you to learn about medications and interventions, it is also important that the class teaches real skills to be used in labor to help with pain management. Ask the teacher how many of her students go without medication; consider asking to speak to some of them.

Talk to your practitioner. Your doctor or midwife should know your plans with respect to medications. If you'd prefer to have natural childbirth, he or she should have concrete suggestions for helping you achieve your goal. There is a huge difference between being supportive of your plans and merely tolerating them.

Talk to your partner. Your partner needs to be on the same page as you throughout the process. If you've chosen to go the unmedicated route, he needs to understand what his role will be and stay committed to helping you with the kind of birth you've planned for.

## Know the Positions for Pushing

Many of the positions that you used for labor are also beneficial for pushing. This is particularly true of the upright positions that employ gravity. While the average pushing stage for first-time mothers is about two hours, it is a very active period compared with labor. But because you only push during the contractions, which have spaced out a bit, you and baby get built-in breaks. .

You should change your position every fifteen minutes or so during the pushing phase of labor, unless you are making substantial progress. If baby is moving down nicely and you and baby are not having any problems, there is no need to move just to move, unless you wanted to give birth in a specific position.

Your practitioner can help you determine if this works for you. Consider the following positions for pushing:

- Standing
- Squatting, with or without a squat bar
- Sitting upright
- Sitting on a birth ball

- Hands and knees
- Side lying (for fast labors)

## Learn How to Push Your Baby Out

The pushing phase of labor comes after your body is completely dilated. As your baby moves further down into the pelvis, you will experience an urge to push. Some women feel this urge almost immediately, while others take a while to feel the sensation. There are two basic variations on this urge to push.

THE SO-SO URGE: You may only feel this urge to push at the peak of contractions, which is usually when your baby is further down into the pelvis, stimulating the nerves that encourage you to push. Even if you only push slightly when you feel the urge, the baby will move down. As the baby moves, the urge becomes more urgent.

THE UNCONTROLLABLE URGE: This urge is very difficult to resist or stop, because your body is acting for you, whether you are trying to or not. The further down the pelvis the baby is, the more likely you are to feel this urge.

If you are completely dilated but don't feel an urge to push, do not worry. The concept of "laboring down" means that you will continue to deal with the contractions as your baby slowly descends. You do not push until the baby is much further down, meaning an easier pushing phase for you and baby.

There are two different ways to push and each has its own style and reasons for use. One is used more frequently for mothers who are medicated because of the decreased sensations for pushing. It is called purple pushing (because the mother's face turns purple from holding her breath) or directed bearing down. As a contraction starts, the mother takes a deep breath in, blows it out, and repeats—but holding her breath in this time. She holds her breath for a count of ten, quickly exchanges her breath and repeats for a total of three breaths. While holding her breath, the goal is to "push" with her uterus to allow the baby to descend. The breath holding supposedly adds force to the expulsive effort. A midwife or doctor provides feedback and advice on whether the efforts are helping to move the baby. Mothers using this method tend to get very exhausted and can even break facial blood vessels because of the strain.

The other way to push is known as spontaneous bearing down, in which your body tells you when to push. It's called an overwhelming urge to push because your body is already doing it; you just help by aiding it. Mothers hold their breath according to their own comfort levels, but rarely more than about six seconds, and each contraction tends to involve more pushes than with purple pushing. With this method, you push when you feel the urge, usually at the peak of each contraction.

If you are having trouble feeling the urge to push, try a different position. You could also switch pushing methods, even if only for a couple of contractions. Remember that your body will push the baby out, without your help. Your help merely speeds things up. Being patient is sometimes the key to having an easier second stage in your labor. Your practitioner will help guide you as well.

## Prepare Dad to Catch the Baby

Some practitioners are open to having the baby's father or some other nonbirth professional assist in the birth. This usually happens at the very end, after the head and shoulders of the baby are outside the mother's body. The practitioner then gently hands off the baby to the other person, allowing him or her to hold the baby as it slips out of the womb.

If your practitioner has experience and is comfortable with this practice, often called a four-handed catch, it should be no problem to arrange. If, however, your practitioner has not participated in many four-handed catches or is otherwise reluctant, you may have some work to do in convincing him or her. Get a head start by including it in your birth plan and discussing it ahead of time.

## Learn about Fetal Monitoring

The goal of fetal monitoring is to assess how your baby is handling labor. How and when fetal monitoring is done will depend on your practitioner and where you are giving birth. Here are the most common forms of fetal monitoring.

DOPPLER OR FETOSCOPE: A handheld device used at various intervals to check on your baby, which is a very low key form of monitoring for low-risk women in hospitals, home births, or birth centers. The benefits: You can move freely, unrestricted by cords, and you have a live person on the other end interpreting the data.

EXTERNAL FETAL MONITORING: Belts are strapped to your abdomen that use ultrasound to transmit the sound of your baby's heartbeat. This can restrict your movement during periods of monitoring.

INTERNAL FETAL MONITORING: Internal monitoring requires that your bag of waters be broken to access the baby. This is a very accurate form of monitoring used for high-risk patients or babies who may be having trouble handling labor. It is also done to get a better read of the pressure, or strength, of the contractions inside the uterus.

Baby monitoring can be done continuously or intermittently. The American College of Obstetricians and Gynecologists recommends that low-risk women have intermittent monitoring in labor: approximately fifteen minutes out of every hour in the first part of labor and five minutes out of every fifteen minutes during the pushing phase. This enables a mother to have more freedom to move around and be comfortable. If your baby appears to be having a rough time or if you are using medications or being induced, additional monitoring of your baby or labor may be required.

Some controversy surrounds the use of fetal monitoring. While its goal is noble—to reduce injuries and stillbirths—it has not been shown to improve the rates of either injuries or stillbirths in the past thirty years. In fact, the only real difference in fetal outcomes has been the marked increase in the Cesarean rate since the invention of fetal monitoring. The least amount of monitoring that you can use is the best idea for you and your baby. Electronic monitoring inhibits mothers

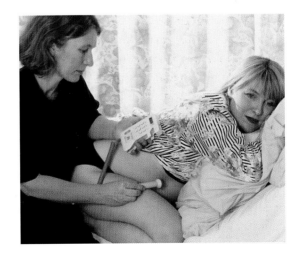

*Many forms of monitoring allow you to stay in a comfortable position while your baby is monitored.*

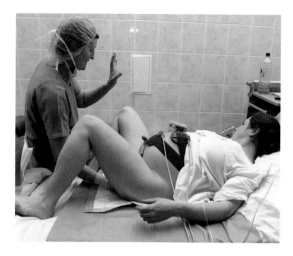

*Breaking your water is done during a vaginal exam while you lay back. It should feel like a vaginal exam with a bit more pressure.*

from moving freely and using all available pain management techniques. As a result, fetal monitoring equipment leads to a greater reliance on medical interventions such as epidurals, catheters, and more.

## Learn about Amniotomy

Amniotomy is the surgical rupture of your membranes, also known as breaking your water. Sometimes this is done as a method of induction while other times it is used to supposedly speed up your labor.

During a vaginal exam, a small crochet-like hook is used to snag the membranes and leave a small hole. This is a painless procedure (the membrane has no nerves), and it does not hurt your baby. It is no more uncomfortable than a vaginal exam for most women, but it does carry the following possible complications:

- The cord can come down, necessitating an emergency Cesarean.
- Your practitioner may implement a deadline for you to have your baby for fear of infection setting in.
- You or your baby may get an infection.

- You and your baby no longer have the cushion of the amniotic fluid.
- Your contractions may feel more severe, causing pain for mom and fetal distress for baby.
- Your labor may not start, and you would require additional interventions.

A recent review of the medical literature showed that there is very little evidence to indicate that breaking the water speeds up labor. And because it can lead to complications, it should be done sparingly. Talk to your practitioner about how often he or she uses this tool in labor.

## Learn about Pain Medication in Labor

Pain medication in labor has undergone a transformation in the past century. The medications that we use in labor and birth today leave mothers much more alert and able to participate in the birth experience.

Pain medication is part science and part art. How medication works is scientific, but how it will work on a particular body cannot be known with the same level of precision.

Of the many medications available in labor, some can be used early in the process, and others should be used later. Some medications are appropriate for the pain of a Cesarean birth while others are not. Here are the major classes of medications.

SYSTEMIC MEDICATIONS: These medications are given orally, via an IV line or as an injection. This can be a narcotic such as Demerol or Stadol, but it can also involve other medications to promote relaxation in very early labor. These medications do not eliminate pain, but they increase your ability to relax and cope with labor. Benefits: These are easy to administer and start taking effect very quickly. It should also be noted that if at a later point you opt for another classification of medication, such as an epidural, these medications can be combined.

REGIONAL ANESTHESIA: This is most commonly the epidural, although it can also include a spinal and other block that numbs an area of the body. Regional anesthesia is given as a continuous line of medication through a catheter placed with a needle through your spine but not inside the spinal cord. The cocktail of medications used in an epidural can vary. You can talk to the anesthesiologist or nurse anesthetist to discuss what you'd like to feel: pressure, the contractions without the pain, or nothing at all. There are no guarantees that you will get precisely what you requested, but it's worth a discussion. Regional anesthesia is usually used from mid to late labor and can also be used for a Cesarean birth.

GENERAL ANESTHESIA: General anesthesia is medication that causes your whole body to be completely "asleep" and unaware of what is going on. It is used only in extreme cases, such as an emergency Cesarean birth.

Each medication carries its own risks and benefits. While the primary benefit of pain relief is obvious, the risks may not be so easily grasped. Risks associated with most medications include the following:

- Fetal distress
- Stalled labor
- Malpositioning of the baby
- Fluctuations in mother's blood pressure
- Vomiting and nausea

If any of these result, you may be subject to additional monitoring or interventions, including the following:

- Continuous fetal monitoring
- More frequent blood pressure checks
- Maternal EKG to study the mother's heart rate and pattern
- Bladder catheter

- Medications to speed labor
- Medications to ease nausea and vomiting
- Oxygen administered via face mask or nasal tubes

If you think you might want to use medications in labor, learn what you can about your choices. Some options are not available at every hospital or birth center. You may also have a condition or disorder that makes certain medication choices unavailable to you. Before you go into labor, have a discussion with your doctor or midwife to clarify your wishes and options.

A good childbirth class will teach you about the various interventions and medications. You can then use what you've learned to ask questions of your practitioner. You will also learn coping skills to assist you in the period before you receive medication. With few exceptions, every woman goes through some part of labor without medication. Relying on skills you picked up from a childbirth class or from your doula, you can make yourself more comfortable until the time arrives to use medications.

## See about an Episiotomy

An episiotomy is a surgical incision made in your perineum to enlarge the birth canal. As a result of medical studies showing that it is rarely needed for mothers or babies, there has been a dramatic reduction in the number of episiotomies in recent years.

You should talk to your practitioner about when he or she performs an episiotomy. Ask what can be done to prevent it, such as positioning the mother and perineal massage. With the help of their practitioners, many women are able to give birth with no episiotomy and no tearing.

Avoiding an episiotomy means an easier recovery and fewer risks, such as infection and urinary or fecal incontinence. Ask your practitioner if prenatal perineal massage might be beneficial in your case. Learn which positions equalize the pressure on the perineum during pushing, such as standing, squatting and sitting completely upright. This allows your baby to exert equal force and prevents a weak spot from getting more pressure. You should also follow your practitioner's instructions in the final few pushes to permit your perineum to stretch.

## Learn about Forceps and Vacuum-Extraction Births

Sometimes mom or baby needs a bit of assistance in the final stages of pushing. This can be accomplished by using a set of forceps or the vacuum extractor.

Forceps have long been used in birth. There was a time, in fact, when nearly 40 percent of births involved the use of forceps because mothers were given general anesthesia, fell asleep, and were unable to push. Forceps are used much less frequently today, although they are more common when medications such as epidurals are used in labor.

Forceps consist of two separate instruments, and each is inserted to slip around the baby's head. When both have been properly placed, the practitioner will pull as you push. In some cases, forceps are used to help a baby adjust its head to a better position.

A vacuum can be used a bit higher in the mother's pelvis than forceps but is not as good at turning babies. It uses high-powered suction that attaches to the baby's head, and as you push, the doctor or midwife pulls.

You should talk to your doctor or midwife about their use of forceps and vacuum extraction. And if he or she suggests using either one, you might ask if changing your position might be helpful before resorting to an assisted delivery.

## Find Out What Happens to the Placenta

The placenta is the only disposable organ in the world. If you become pregnant again, you will grow a whole new placenta. Once your baby has arrived safely in your arms, the placenta is no longer needed.

About thirty minutes after you have given birth, your placenta will detach itself from the uterine wall. You may see a small amount of blood, letting you know that the placenta is ready. Your practitioner will ask you to push once or twice to help expel the placenta.

Pushing out the placenta does not hurt; it has no bones and it is smaller than your baby. Your practitioner will inspect the placenta to make sure it is all out.

You may want to see the placenta. You may even wish to take it home and plant it. It contains nutrients that enrich the soil, and certain cultures believe in honoring the organ that nurtures babies. The decision is yours but be sure to mention your wishes to your practitioner before your placenta ends up in the medical incinerator.

## Decide How to Spend the First Few Minutes with Your Baby

You have probably been imagining the first few minutes with your baby for a long time, that magical moment after birth when you gaze into your newborn's eyes. Your baby is handed to you or placed on your abdomen. You touch your warm, wet baby, pulling him or her to your breast.

You can't believe labor is over. You're not pregnant anymore. You're a mother! All of these thoughts race through your mind. And here is your baby. Whether you are thinking more about the labor you just lived through or falling head over heels in love with your baby, both are normal responses.

Being skin-to-skin with your baby will help keep him or her warm. Blankets may be placed on top of the baby to keep the cold room air away, and a hat may be placed on your baby's head.

If you place your baby at the breast, he or she may start to nurse. He or she may also just stare at the breast or try to latch on slowly. This is good for you and the baby. The American Academy of Pediatrics recommends that you nurse your baby in the first thirty minutes of life.

Your baby will have an alert period for about an hour after birth. Shortly after that, your baby will get tired and fall asleep. This is typically a deep sleep that lasts several hours. Nursing before this period is very beneficial in helping baby get off to a good start with breastfeeding. If for some reason your baby cannot or will not nurse during this time frame, do not be concerned. It is worth trying, but you will have plenty of time to try again once baby wakes up.

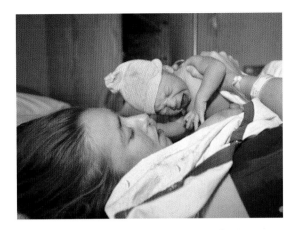

*If you feel like you're a bit tied down with monitors and cords, ask for help in positioning the baby skin to skin.*

## Teach Dad about Cord Cutting

Most practitioners are more than willing to accommodate a request by dad or mom to cut the umbilical cord. It is very simple: First the midwife or doctor places an umbilical cord clamp near the baby and another clamp further up the cord. Then you or your husband is given a pair of scissors and told to cut between the two clamps.

The cord does not have any nerves so it does not hurt mom or baby when it is cut. Sometimes there may be a tiny bit of blood when it is cut, depending on how long ago the cord stopped pulsing. You may be surprised at how thick the cord is. Remember, it had to withstand gymnastic tricks and a baby sitting on it for nine months.

Occasionally the cord will need to be cut before the baby's body is completely born. This happens when the cord is wrapped too tightly around the baby's neck to allow the practitioner to slip it off. About one-third of babies are born with the cords around their necks, but this is generally not a major complication. It might also be that the practitioner needs to cut it quickly. This may be disappointing, but you might be able to help trim the cord if it's too long. If not, you still get to keep the baby.

## Learn about Delayed Cord Cutting

There has been some discussion of late about the benefits of not cutting the cord right away. Proponents of delayed cord clamping point to the benefits to the baby from the blood in the cord. In fact, as long as the cord is still pulsing, even after birth, the baby is getting oxygenated blood.

You may wish to delay cord clamping and cutting for your baby. If this is something you are interested in, talk to your midwife or doctor. This may already be a part of their routine or you may need to put it in your birth plan. Even if it's in your birth plan and your practitioner has agreed to it, be sure to remind them at the birth before his auto-pilot takes over.

## Learn What Happens to Baby after the Initial Bonding Period

After you have spent time with your baby right after birth, the staff at the hospital or birth center will need to have their turn. They have a list of procedures that must be performed according to the state and where the birth takes place (hospital, birth center, at home). This may include the following:

- Weighing
- Measuring
- Conducting a general newborn exam
- Administering eye medication
- Administering vitamin K and/or vaccinations
- Trimming the umbilical cord
- Making footprints
- Banding with identification
- Bathing

Some of these may be optional or can be delayed. Your preferences should be reflected in your birth plan. If you are in a hospital, there may be other procedures that are done later or procedures that are repeated, such as weighing, a hearing test, and completion of birth certificate forms. While touring your hospital or birth center, inquire about their policy and protocol.

## Learn about Rooming In

Rooming in means that the baby stays with the mother for most of the time that they are in the hospital or birth center. Many hospitals have adopted rooming in as the norm, with some closing the newborn nurseries except for the sickest of newborns. They recognize that babies need their mothers.

That said, many hospitals have various policies on rooming in. Some place restrictions on having the baby in your room if you are alone, if you have had a surgical birth, or for other reasons. You may also find that the hospital has a mandatory nursery stay for newborns immediately after birth. This contradicts what much of the medical literature says about the optimal placement of newborns. If this is not something you want to happen, be sure to get an approval prior to labor to keep your baby with you.

## Find Out Why Labor May Be Induced

Ideally, labor should begin on its own. This is the safest way for your baby to be born. Occasionally there are times when the baby needs to be born before nature is ready for it to happen. In these cases labor is induced or forced to start. Reasons for an induction include:

- Your pregnancy has reached forty-two weeks.
- You are too ill to continue the pregnancy, such as pregnancy induced hypertension.
- The baby is no longer growing appropriately.
- There is an improper amount of amniotic fluid.

While an induced labor carries additional risks, including a higher Cesarean rate and an increase in other interventions, it can be a very uncomplicated procedure. Talk to your practitioner about the pros and cons of inducing your labor, what happens if you decide to wait, and what your options are for birth. Be sure to ask how the induction will be done, as there are several ways, and how it will alter your birth plan.

Currently more than a third of women have their labors induced. The majority of these are for nonmedical reasons. The World Health Organization says that the induction rate should be about 10 percent and no higher. If your doctor or midwife suggests induction for social reasons, you may want to wait for spontaneous labor because it is safer for you and your baby. Nonmedical reasons can include the following:

- You are tired of being pregnant
- Your doctor or midwife is on call the day of the proposed induction.
- You want a specific birth date for your baby
- You have family coming to town
- Your practitioner is going on vacation

# Find Out How Labor Is Induced

Labor can be induced in various ways, and the choice is up to you and your practitioner. Some of the more common forms of inductions are the following:

CERVICAL RIPENING: This is used when the cervix is not very soft, dilated, or effaced. It can be done with a gel, suppository, or other substance that is placed directly onto the cervix, taken orally, or administered via IV. If necessary, the dose may be repeated a few hours apart. This method can be used alone, if it works, but many times it is used in conjunction with other labor induction methods.

AMNIOTOMY: Breaking the bag of waters artificially when the cervix is already ripe can be an easy and drug-free way to induce labor. It may also require additional induction agents depending on the mother.

PITOCIN: Given through an IV line, this medication is strictly controlled to bring on contractions. The dosage is increased at various intervals depending on your body, how your baby is tolerating the induction, and your practitioner's orders.

FOLEY CATHETER: A nonmedicinal way to dilate the cervix, a Foley catheter is inserted in the cervix and filled with saline. The weight of the catheter pulls down on and opens up the cervix.

Induction of labor can increase the risks to mother and baby. These can include the following:

- Fetal distress
- Prematurity
- Cesarean section
- Necessity for additional interventions
- Rare complications such as amniotic fluid embolism, which is when amniotic fluid enters the mother's bloodstream, which can pose a severe threat to the mother, including death

## LABOR AUGMENTATION

Labor may start on its own but progress very slowly. Speeding up the process is an option and is called augmentation of labor.

The following are various ways to accelerate your labor. Some are natural and others involve medications or procedures.

- Frequent position changes
- Nipple stimulation (manually or via breast pump)
- Acupressure
- Change of scenery–leave your room!
- Walking
- Relaxation and visualizations
- Discussion of fears that may be holding you back
- Breaking your water
- Medications such as Pitocin

All of these things can work with varied amounts of success. What works well for one laboring mother may not work as well for another. Be sure to talk about the risks and benefits of each approach before you accept the intervention. It is always advisable to try the smallest steps first.

The decision to induce your labor before natural labor starts can be difficult as you weigh the risks and benefits. It will help to discuss what type of induction will be used, what happens if it doesn't work, and what other options are available. Having an open and trusting relationship with your practitioner is very comforting at junctures like this.

## Prepare for a Cesarean Section

A cesarean section may be done in the following circumstances:

- You are too ill to give birth.
- Your baby is in an odd position (some breeches, transverse lie, etc.).
- The placenta is covering your cervix.
- Your baby is not tolerating labor well.
- Labor is not progressing.
- You are having higher order multiples.
- You are having twins, and one is not head down.
- Your placenta is pulling away from the uterus.
- You have an active herpes infection.
- Occasionally if your first birth was by Cesarean.

You and your doctor or midwife will make the decision jointly about how your baby should be born. A cesarean section is usually done after labor is well established, known as an unplanned Cesarean, but occasionally you will know about your scheduled Cesarean before you go into labor. Even more rarely, an emergency may arise during labor necessitating an emergency Cesarean.

If you and your practitioner have determined that the best decision for you and your baby is a surgical birth, the next step will be to pick a date. It is generally recommended that scheduled births that are not urgent be held off until 39 weeks. This is an attempt to minimize the problems that can occur when babies are born even slightly premature.

Your practitioner will help you set the date at the hospital where your baby will be born. If this change in birth plans means a different hospital or place of birth, you may also want to take a tour of the hospital and nursery beforehand to familiarize yourself with it. You may also see if a Cesarean birth class is available for you to take.

If you go into labor prior to the scheduled surgery date, call your practitioner. Many practitioners will have you come in to the hospital for

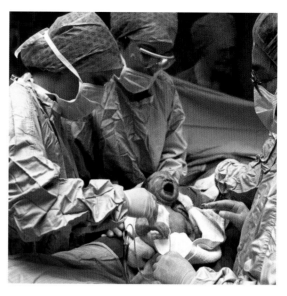

*Consider watching your baby's Cesarean birth with a mirror. The staff at the hospital can help you do this and if you change your mind, simply look elsewhere.*

monitoring. If you are in labor, the Cesarean birth will be performed right away instead of waiting for the scheduled date.

## Learn How a Cesarean Section Is Done

A Cesarean section is a way to surgically remove the baby via incisions in the abdomen and uterus. If it is time for you to have a Cesarean birth, you can expect the following to happen:

- You will be admitted to the hospital.
- You will have blood drawn
- You will be given a gown to change into.
- You will have your vital signs taken.
- Your baby will be monitored.
- You will take medicine to decrease your stomach acids.
- You will have your stomach and lower abdomen shaved.
- You will be given an IV.
- You will have a spinal or epidural administered for pain relief during and after surgery.

- You will be taken to the operating room and given oxygen to breathe.
- Your partner and doula will be invited into the operating room.
- The initial incisions will begin.
- It takes about five minutes for the birth.
- The placenta will be removed.
- The external layers of your uterus and abdomen will be repaired with sutures and staples.
- You will return to the recovery room.
- You will stay in the hospital three to four days to complete your recovery.

These procedures may vary slightly, depending on the hospital. Your practitioner can give you a crash course in Cesarean birth prior to your surgery and answer any questions you have.

After the procedure, you will have the same postpartum care needs as a mother who had a vaginal birth, plus the needs resulting from major surgery. (See "Postpartum" starting on page 291 for more information on Cesarean recovery.)

## Avoid an Unnecessary Cesarean

Cesarean births certainly save lives, but adding surgery to your birth experience can be hard on you, your baby, and your future pregnancies. Most people would agree that the current rate of Cesareans is alarming. The problem is, how do you sort out the necessary from the unnecessary Cesareans?

Studies show that selecting a practitioner and a place of birth that believe in the natural process of birth, while being ready to intervene in a true emergency, will lower your chances of having an unnecessary Cesarean. You can ask questions about beliefs, but the statistics of the practice will speak for themselves. The national Cesarean rate is more than 31 percent. If your doctor or midwife has a lower rate, you can rest assured that you are well positioned to reduce your risk.

A rate that is higher than the national, however, does not automatically mean your practitioner

### MATERNAL CHOICE CESAREAN

This refers to a mother's ability to choose to have a Cesarean section when no medical indications are present. This is a very controversial subject. While practitioners claim they are asked about this repeatedly, numerous studies indicate that the numbers of mothers who actually choose Cesarean births are very low, around 1 percent.

Whether this request is granted or not varies from practitioner to practitioner. It also raises the question of insurance coverage because Cesareans without medical indication are generally not covered. Moreover, Cesareans can be riskier for babies and mothers, as well as more expensive due to a longer and more intensive hospital stay.

doesn't support natural, nonsurgical birth. Some practices have higher overall rates, either because of the clientele or because certain practitioners in the practice perform more Cesareans. It is therefore important to know your practitioner's individual number, in addition to the number for the practice and the place of birth.

You should also look into the following as ways to reduce the risks of an unnecessary Cesarean:

- Hire a doula.
- Avoid an induction of labor.
- Eat well and exercise in pregnancy.
- Stay home in early labor.
- Know your options for labor and birth.
- Discuss your choices with your birth team.
- Move around during labor to help the baby descend.

All of these have been found to be helpful, but they cannot eliminate your risk of Cesarean birth. Doing them, however, will allow you to say that you did everything within your power to have the safest birth possible for your baby.

## Have a Family-Centered Cesarean Birth

Once it has been determined that a Cesarean birth is the safest way for your baby to be born, you may be wondering how to maximize the parts of your birth plan that you spent so much time working on.

For example, what aspects of the plan can still be honored? Was your goal to have a quiet birth? Did you plan to hold the baby immediately? These are the types of items that can be incorporated into your new birth plan.

Talk to your practitioner about how to preserve some of these simple preferences. Many women say that having some of the smaller but important points included in their birth really helped emphasize the birth rather than the surgery. Here are some examples.

HAVE A MIRROR TO WATCH THE BIRTH. Using a mirror for the moment when your baby is born allows you to witness the birth without seeing much of the surgery. Once the baby is out, the mirror can be moved unless you would like to watch the rest of the surgery.

HAVE A HAND FREE TO TOUCH THE BABY. When you are taken in for the surgery, your arms will be extended out to your sides and possibly strapped down to thin boards. Ask the anesthesiologist to leave one of your arms unstrapped so you can touch the baby after birth.

HAVE DAD CALL OUT THE SEX OF THE BABY. Remind the doctor that your husband would like to be the one to tell you if your baby is a boy or a girl. Once the baby is born, have the doctor hold the baby up so you can see the face, and so your husband can announce whether you have a new son or daughter.

BRING THE BABY TO YOU AS SOON AS POSSIBLE. Have your husband or doula bring you the baby as soon as the baby is ready. With support you can even nurse while the surgery is finishing.

HAVE THE BABY COME TO THE RECOVERY ROOM WITH YOU. You may be tired, shaky, or any number of feelings after the surgery and giving birth. But you should still spend time with your baby. Make skin-to-skin contact, requesting help to do so if you need it.

One of the hardest things to deal with after a Cesarean birth is the fact that most people think of it as just another way to have a baby. How would they feel after having their appendix removed or some other abdominal surgery? Having a baby via surgery is extremely strenuous and difficult, and you are entitled to ask for the help you need.

**HOT MAMA**

With the hard work of labor and giving birth, sometimes your hair pays the price. Consider carrying an emergency scrunchie for a quick ponytail. You might even experiment with some fancy buns with your scrunchie beforehand. If you have short hair, a small bottle a liquid gel or curl enhancer can help you spruce up your hairdo in labor. If it's comforting smell, all the better!

# POST-PARTUM

## CHECKLIST FOR POSTPARTUM

[ ] Experience the first few hours after birth.
[ ] Stand up for the first time after you give birth.
[ ] Cope with bleeding after birth.
[ ] Relieve your postpartum pain.
[ ] Deal with after pains.
[ ] Take care of your perineum.
[ ] Take a sitz bath.
[ ] Deal with staples.
[ ] Make the most of your postpartum stay.
[ ] Go home!
[ ] Check out your postpartum body.
[ ] Watch for weird postpartum symptoms.
[ ] Swaddle your baby.
[ ] Understand why babies cry.
[ ] Return to your normal bowel movements.
[ ] Head out for the first time.
[ ] Manage the baby blues.
[ ] Get help for postpartum depression.
[ ] Go to your six-week postpartum visit.

[ ] Select postpartum birth control.
[ ] Have your first period.
[ ] Reconnect with your partner.
[ ] Adjust your diet for breastfeeding.
[ ] Figure out when and how to sleep after birth.
[ ] Get everyone fed.
[ ] Set realistic expectations for yourself.
[ ] Get back to exercise.
[ ] Experiment with positions for breastfeeding.
[ ] Set up a breastfeeding station.
[ ] Ensure that your baby is getting enough to eat.
[ ] Know when to call a lactation consultant.
[ ] Deal with engorgement.
[ ] Use a breast pump.
[ ] Return to work after maternity leave.

**POSTPARTUM PARTICULARS**

# Experience the First Few Hours after Birth

The first hours after having a baby are magical and difficult all at the same time. Toward the end of labor, women say things like they want to be done so they can eat or take a nap, but when that baby is born, everything changes and all you want to do is spend hours just staring at this little person.

That is generally what you get to do, depending on the policy at your place of birth. However, while you are nursing and getting to know your new baby, there is a lot going on. You will be asked a bunch of questions while things keep happening with your body.

Once the placenta is out, you will be cleaned up and examined, a repair will be done if needed, and you can put underwear on. Many times a special type of mesh panty is used to allow air flow to the area, and the biggest maxi pad you have ever seen is placed inside. Sometimes the pad doubles as a cold pack, which feels really good on swollen tissues.

Every fifteen minutes, then stretching to every half hour and then every hour, someone will come in and check your uterus via your abdomen, much like abdominal exams in pregnancy. They are making sure that your uterus has clamped down so that you will not bleed too much. You will also be reminded to empty your bladder because a full bladder can cause your uterus to relax more than you want it to.

You may notice contractions as you nurse. This is normal. Your uterus is beginning the process of involution or shrinking back to (almost) its pre-pregnancy size. The process takes about six weeks.

During this period, you may also be asked if you want to take a shower, which is completely up to you. It may depend on whether your baby is actively engaging you or if you are ready to let Dad or someone else hold the baby while you shower.

After about an hour and a half, most hospitals will move you to a postpartum room for the rest of your stay. If your hospital has labor/birth/recovery/ postpartum rooms or single-room maternity care, you will be in one room for the duration of your stay.

# Stand Up for the First Time after You Give Birth

The first time you stand up after giving birth, no matter how you gave birth, can be interesting. Start slowly by sitting up in bed to see if you're feeling dizzy or anything else. If not, swing your legs over the edge of the bed and stop again for a minute.

Using support, stand up and stop once again, checking how you feel. If you feel dizzy or light headed, sit back down. If you feel okay, you can continue. Don't be surprised if you notice a trickle of blood that pooled in the vagina or if you feeling shaky. Both are perfectly normal, which is why you should have someone nearby to help if necessary.

Following a vaginal birth, you will probably get up within a few minutes of giving birth. If you had an epidural, you will need to wait until you can feel your muscles and move your legs. If you had a Cesarean birth it may take a bit longer, though getting up is important to your recovery, so you may get up within the first six to twelve hours, depending on how you are doing.

The first time you get out of bed after having a Cesarean, you may have a lot of strange feelings. Many women report that the first time they stand, they felt sure their internal organs were about to fall out. It's only a sensation and with time, patience, and practice, you will get used to it and then it will pass.

## Cope with Bleeding after Birth

Everyone bleeds after giving birth. The blood comes from the site of the placenta. You will bleed vaginally and even if you had a Cesarean section, and it will resemble a very heavy period.

While you are bleeding, you should wear absorbent pads, not tampons. This is to prevent infection and allow your vagina to heal. When you get up after sitting or sleeping for a while, you will notice blood leaking a bit. You may also notice that you are passing small clots. Again, this is completely normal.

Your bleeding will gradually lessen, although if you are physically active, you may notice an uptick in the amount of bleeding. The color of the discharge will change from bright red to brownish to pink to clear. Call your practitioner if the following occur:

- You soak a pad or more every hour.
- You run a fever higher than 101 degrees Fahrenheit.
- You have clots bigger than a quarter.
- You notice a foul smell.

## Relieve Your Postpartum Pain

Whether or not you used pain medication during labor or birth, it is available to you after the birth. This pain medication ranges from heavy-duty narcotics that make you sleepy to over-the-counter pain relievers that take the edge off your aches and pains.

If you have had a surgical birth, the heavy-duty medications may be exactly what you need as you recover from major surgery. Sometimes, for the first day or so after birth, you will be given a pain medication pump, which allows you to control the delivery of pain medication, with safeties built in to prevent overdoses. Or you may have been given special medication as part of the epidural to help

# PREGNANCY AFFIRMATION FOR POSTPARTUM

— I am a good mother to my baby.

— I know what my baby needs.

— My baby senses my love.

— I love my baby.

— My postpartum body is temporary.

control pain for several hours after birth. After the first few days, you can switch to over-the-counter medications, which should help manage the pain.

You may want to be stoic and wait until you are in pain to take medication, but that approach will delay how you heal. Women who feel better move sooner and more often, allowing the healing process to take place.

After a vaginal birth, you also have options when it comes to pain medication. Which one you choose will depend on your pain level and how your body feels, which can vary from day to day. Most women find that a steady dose of an over-the-counter pain reliever works wonders for their sore, aching bodies.

Pain medication after birth is geared for new mothers, meaning that it is compatible with breastfeeding. It also means that the types of medication and dosages are safe for your baby. If you are concerned for any reason, be sure to ask.

## Deal with After Pains

After pains refer to the contractions that you may experience after giving birth. For most women these pains are not very noticeable, particularly after their first baby. More of these pains tend to show up during subsequent postpartum experiences. The explanation is that it takes the body more work to return to its prepregnancy shape.

Many women feel these contractions when they are nursing. This is because breastfeeding stimulates the production of oxytocin, which causes the contractions that help the uterus heal. Medication can control these pains, and some women try to time their dosages for about a half an hour before they expect to nurse.

These after pains do not last long; in fact, most women report that after a few days they barely notice them. This comes as a relief to know it is not going to continue for weeks on end.

## Take Care of Your Perineum

Taking care of your perineum after giving birth is very important. Even if you had a vaginal birth without an episiotomy or any stitches, the area will most likely be bruised and swollen. This means keeping your perineum clean and comfortable.

When you urinate after birth, the urine may sting for the first few days. To help alleviate this, fill a peri-care or small squirt bottle with warm water. When you begin to feel the flow of urine, squeeze the warm water towards your perineum. Hopefully it will reduce any stinging sensation.

When you are done urinating, fill the bottle again and rinse your perineum off with warm water. Then pat the area with toilet paper to keep it clean and dry.

For pain relief, besides over-the-counter drugs, there are topical medications in cream or spray form that help numb or dull the pain. Your doctor or midwife can give you a prescription or recommend something over the counter for this purpose.

Ice is always useful to reduce swelling. There are sanitary pads that have cold packs built in, and they can provide significant relief in the first few days postpartum. After that your perineum should feel much better and the swelling should be drastically reduced.

If you have stitches in your perineum, you may wonder when they'll be removed. Most often, the stitches dissolve naturally, and your doctor or midwife can tell you how long it should take, depending on your body and the type of materials used.

When the stitches start to dissolve, you may notice them on the toilet paper. Do not panic; simply continue your perineal care. Call your practitioner if you have questions about your stitches, especially if you notice an increase in pain, redness, or swelling.

## Take a Sitz Bath

A sitz bath is a specially designed to help heal your perineum after birth. Some hospitals or birth centers have shallow tubs meant for this purpose, and you may even be given a portable sitz bath to bring home.

A portable sitz bath requires a toilet and warm water. You place the sitz bath on the toilet seat for stabilization and draining. Fill a bag with warm water, sit on the sitz bath, and allow the water to flow over your perineum.

Some practitioners also say that you can do the same thing in a clean tub in your home. You simply fill a tub with a few inches of warm water and soak for a few minutes. A sitz bath helps most during the first few days to a week postpartum and can be done two to three times a day.

## Deal with Staples

Staples, stitches, and special band-aids can all be used to close the skin following a Cesarean section. What type you come home with will depend on your body type, your practitioner's preference, and how your skin is doing. If you have staples, you may want to wear underwear that doesn't come near your incision. This means going really low or really high with your underwear. Grandma panties may not be on your top ten list of fashionable items, but right after abdominal surgery, it might not feel good to have the slight pressure on your incision. Your practitioner will provide you with specific instructions on how to treat your incision after you give birth.

Steri-strips or special band-aids usually stay on until they fall off. Stitches may be left in until they dissolve or they may need to be removed. If you have some that need to be removed, your doctor will give you a time frame for this removal. It may happen on your last day in the hospital or you may need to come back to your doctor's office for a check up and to remove the stitches.

Staples will be removed within the same time frame as stitches. Neither hurt when they get removed, but it can be disconcerting to watch.

## Make the Most of Your Postpartum Stay

If you had a vaginal birth in a hospital you will stay for a day or two; with a Cesarean or complicated birth you may stay for three or four days. Talk to your practitioner about your preference. Some people rest well in the hospital while others do not.

During your hospital stay, you will have to learn the routine. Meals are brought at specific times, and you may or may not get a say in what is on your tray. You will receive periodic checks from nurses, aides, and lab workers. They have their reasons, but in the middle of the night, having your blood pressure taken can be annoying.

If you have given birth in a birth center, the rules may be completely different. Some birth centers allow you to stay up to twenty-four hours, depending on your preference. Other women prefer to go home much sooner, after just six or eight hours.

## Go Home!

Once you have been given the all-clear to leave, be it six hours or four days later, you may be a bundle of emotions. You probably feel a mix of excitement, nerves, and fear. This is completely normal!

If you are leaving a hospital, you may find that your release is more like an order to "Hurry up and wait." You must be released by your practitioner and your baby must be released by the pediatrician. Then you usually wait for a nurse to draw up your discharge paperwork.

You will then be given prescriptions to fill for home. You gather everything up and wait some more. This time you are waiting for a wheel chair to transport you and your baby. Ask for a rolling cart to help you carry anything that you may have accumulated during your stay, from personal belongings to gifts and flowers. It may help to have your husband or others take as much as possible beforehand.

If your discharge time is close to when you would need your medications, ask for them before you leave. It may take you awhile to get home, and more time to get the prescriptions filled. Taking your medication beforehand ensures that you are as comfortable as possible.

Some states or hospitals require a nurse check the installation of your baby's car seat before allowing you to leave. You may therefore be asked to pull the car around for inspection.

Once you have made it to the car, you are home free. On the way home, you might want to drop off your prescriptions at a drive through pharmacy. Then once you and baby are settled at home, someone can go back and pick up the medications.

## Check Out Your Postpartum Body

After you have given birth, you might be anxious to check out your postpartum body. You've been waiting to see it for nine months, right? Go ahead, but don't be shocked.

You will probably, initially, feel that your belly is small and flat compared to how it looked before giving birth. Then it occurs to you that you still look about six months pregnant and your belly is no longer hard. It has become large and soft. This can feel really rotten, but you shouldn't worry.

Make a point to avoid the scales for at least a few days, if not weeks after giving birth. Many women do not lose as much weight as they think they will from the birth itself. This is partly explained by the fluids you were either given or retained after the birth process, which plays with your weight loss.

The good news is that as your uterus continues to shrink, it will feel and look better—and more quickly than you would think. Most women will lose their pregnancy weight or be within ten pounds of it by the time they return for their six week postpartum visit. Your belly will continue to deflate and firm up.

With exercise, the right clothes, and smart nutrition, you will be back in shape before you know it. Just remember that the time to be concerned about your figure is not moments or even days after giving birth.

## Watch for Weird Postpartum Symptoms

Here are some postpartum symptoms that no one expects.

HAIR LOSS: The hair changes that you saw in pregnancy were only temporary. Once you are no longer pregnant, you will be subjected to hair falling out. This does not mean that you are going bald; simply that you are losing hair that didn't fall out during pregnancy, according to your normal hair schedule.

SWEATING: As your body regulates its hormones and rids itself of excessive fluids, you will find yourself sweating, particularly the first week postpartum. This is true even if it is freezing outside. Try applying cool cloths and a change of night clothes if it becomes bothersome.

SWELLING: You thought that once the baby was born you would get your ankles back. Think again! Many women are given fluids in labor, particularly with an epidural or Cesarean birth. These fluids have to go somewhere in your body, and after birth you may feel like your whole body is slightly swollen, or you may notice that your legs and ankles are particularly puffy. Keep them elevated and be patient. You will get your slim ankles back.

Never hesitate to call your practitioner with any questions. This is especially true if any of the following occur:

- You have a fever higher than 101 degrees Fahrenheit.
- You have no bleeding.
- You are soaking a pad every hour.
- You have hot, swollen breasts.
- You have a foul smell or discharge from your vagina or incision.
- You are having painful urination or difficulty in urinating.

## Swaddle Your Baby

A baby emerges from a very cozy environment where he or she felt safely snuggled in mother's uterus without much room to move. Once out, they can move freely except they don't have any control over or understanding of what is going on.

Swaddling is a technique of wrapping your baby in a blanket snugly but safely. The topic may have been covered in your childbirth class and should definitely be discussed at new parenting classes. You can purchase special blankets to help you swaddle, as a way to calm your baby, or you can simply use a regular blanket.

Swaddling can help reduce how much your baby cries in the first weeks of life. Some babies respond very positively to this technique, while others merely tolerate it. Experiment with different ways to swaddle as well as different times to see what your baby likes best. For example, a baby may love being swaddled at naptime but not at other times.

## Understand Why Babies Cry

Everyone knows that babies cry. You knew it before you got pregnant. You probably also knew that a crying baby can rattle your nerves, give you a headache, or sap you of energy. What you didn't know before giving birth is the effect of a crying baby on the parent—when you are the parent in question. In addition to the usual responses, you must factor in sleep deprivation, and postpartum stress and strain.

To help provide some perspective, it is important to understand the range of reasons that a newborn can and will cry, including the following:

- Hunger
- Tiredness
- Over stimulated
- Under stimulated
- Pain
- Wet/dirty diaper
- Lonely
- Scared

This means that over time, you need to figure out your baby's code. Some parents insist they know exactly which cry means what, but not every baby has distinct cries you can read right away. If you know it's been a long time between feedings, then hunger is the likely culprit. Sometimes you will figure out the source of your baby's distress right away (such as a wet diaper), and sometimes you will not.

Feeling confused about why your baby is crying does not mean that you are a bad parent. It does mean that your baby is trying to communicate with you, so run through the basics, which should include a change of scenery when appropriate. If that doesn't stop the crying, try more comfort. When nothing works, and you're running out of ideas and patience, let someone else have a turn if possible. You may not realize it, but your baby can pick up on your stress and may even be crying because of it.

Eventually you and baby will hit your stride and be in tune. The crying will dissipate, and your confidence will grow. In the mean time, be kind to yourself, take breaks when you can, and never hesitate to ask for help!

## Return to Your Normal Bowel Movements

Something few women talk about is their first post-baby bowel movement. Many women dread this first bowel movement, particularly if they have had stitches in their perineum or rectum. It is perfectly normal to feel apprehensive or frightened.

After you have a baby, you should try to stick to a diet that is varied in fruits and vegetables and high in fiber to give your stools a normal consistency without resorting to medications. Some mothers choose to eat high-fiber foods, including some foods such as prunes, while others take fiber supplements.

If you have been taking certain pain medication, constipation can be a side effect, and your doctor or midwife may prescribe stool softeners or laxatives to treat it.

Do not allow your fear to delay your first bowel movement; you should go to the bathroom at your first urge. And try not to stress or strain. If you develop hemorrhoids, this is fairly common and while they may be painful, they will heal as your body heals from birth.

## Head Out for the First Time

Leaving the house for the first time after giving birth may seem like a big production, particularly if you were used to grabbing your coat and heading out. The following are some tips for getting out the door on time and with your mind intact:

- Plan ahead.
- Leave plenty of time to get ready.
- Dress yourself first, adding an extra layer like a T-shirt in case baby spits up. (You could also pack a change of clothes.)
- Pack a diaper bag.
- Gather all of your gear.
- Change and dress the baby.
- Head out!

Try to plan your trips when you know that your baby will be well fed and rested. Start with short trips with just a few stops. This will prevent you and baby from getting irritable or frustrated. Once you have a successful trip or two under your belt, you can try longer trips with more stops. Eventually traveling around town with baby will become second nature.

## Manage the Baby Blues

The baby blues is a fairly common phenomenon that shows up a couple of days after birth. The hormonal fluctuations that accompany birth and postpartum, along with the stress and strain of a new baby, add up and can leave you feeling overwhelmed.

When experiencing the baby blues, you may find that you cry more easily, seemingly about nothing. Your moods shift suddenly, and you may feel tense or restless.

As many as 80 percent of new mothers will experience some form of the baby blues, which can last anywhere from a few days to a few weeks. If you think you are suffering from the baby blues, be sure to talk to your practitioner, your partner, friends, and others. Reaching out for help can be a big boost and offer relief and comfort when you need it most.

## Get Help for Postpartum Depression

Postpartum depression (PPD) happens in about 10 percent of new mothers. It may start as a case of the baby blues that never goes away, or it may not show up for weeks or months after the birth of your baby. The symptoms can be similar to the baby blues, only they last longer or are more severe, or they can include the following other symptoms:

- Obsessive compulsive disorders (OCD)
- Mania
- Paranoia
- Loss of interest in baby, self, and food

Postpartum depression can be very frightening for everyone involved. It is important that the people around you understand what PPD looks like in case you need professional help and support. Women with any of the following risk factors have a greater chance of developing postpartum depression:

- Hormonal imbalance prior to pregnancy
- Single parent
- History of depression or mental illness
- Conflict in the marriage or other significant relationship
- Super woman syndrome (trying to do it all alone)
- Other issues causing stress or strain

Treatment can include therapy, medications, and even hospitalization in extreme cases. In rare cases, postpartum depression can turn into postpartum psychosis, which is a more extreme form of mental illness in which the mother loses touch with reality and can become a threat to herself and her children. For this reason, it is critically important to seek help for a mother exhibiting the early signs of depression.

## Go to Your Six-Week Postpartum Visit

Six weeks after the birth of your baby, you will go in for a postpartum checkup. This is a physical exam during which your practitioner checks your body to make sure that you are healing properly. This is also a time for you to ask questions about your birth, postpartum, body, birth control, future births, and anything else.

This visit typically includes the following:

- Pap smear and vaginal exam, even following a Cesarean birth

- Incision check

- Breast exam

- Discussion about postpartum birth control

- Weight check

- Blood pressure check

This is also your chance to show off your new baby to the office staff. They have helped you prepare for this baby since you found out that you were pregnant. Many practices have a board for displaying birth announcements, so don't forget to bring along a copy of yours.

## Select Postpartum Birth Control

Sex may be the furthest thing from your mind, and many practitioners ask that new mothers refrain from having sex for six weeks after giving birth (or at least until they stop bleeding). Even so, unless you were using condoms before getting pregnant, you will need to discuss birth control with your practitioner. A diaphragm needs to be refitted after giving birth because of changes to your body. The same is true with hormonal methods that require prescriptions. Plus, having a baby provides you with more options, including an IUD.

Consider the following when choosing a birth control method:

- How often you have sex (or plan to)

- Previous experience with birth control

- Milk supply, which can be affected by hormones

- Comfort level with touching your body (This relates to use of diaphragms and IUDs.)

- Commitment level to taking data for basal body temperatures (Will you avoid sex or use another method as backup during fertile times?)

- Child spacing issues (Don't choose a five-year or permanent plan if you want another baby in two to three years.)

Your practitioner can help guide you. You can choose one method of birth control and switch later. Some practitioners recommend that breast-feeding mothers use nonhormonal methods of birth control such as condoms, diaphragms, and certain IUDS, or low hormonal methods (progesterone only) such as the mini-pill and injectables. You also have the choice of using basal body temperatures (BBT) and the lactation amenorrhea methods (LAM) of birth control. These require specific classes to prevent pregnancy and cannot be taken lightly.

## Have Your First Period

It is common for mothers who feed their babies with breast milk only to have no periods until they either stop nursing or until their child begins eating other foods. For others, once you have stopped bleeding after the birth, possibly six or more weeks later, you may see your period return. Any bleeding after your postpartum bleeding has stopped is considered a period. It is also important to note that you can ovulate before you have a period.

When your period returns, it may be very erratic and it may last for fewer or more days than it used to. Some women also notice a change in the cramping or pain associated with their periods.

## Reconnect with Your Partner

Reconnecting with your partner is something that many women worry about prior to having a baby. It really does seem like in the first few weeks, you may have forgotten about it. This is harder for your partner to understand because he does not have the same physical demands as you, because he was not the one to give birth.

Reconnecting does not have to mean sex, although it certainly could. If you are both up for it, great, but if you're not, there are so many tender, meaningful ways to touch and connect that are nonsexual. Play footsie at dinner. Hold hands on the couch. Give each other back and neck massages. Kiss at least three times a day.

Communication is key, so talk to each other and be open about your feelings. Some days you may feel physically drained and don't want anyone else touching or making demands on you. You can be tender and loving without touching: Some couples exchange long glances, written notes, or even winks as a way to reconnect. And sometimes a smile says a lot.

Eventually you will get around to more physical and sexual touching. The following are some key suggestions for having a successful and pleasurable regrouping:

- A sense of humor
- Plenty of foreplay
- Avoid areas you say to steer clear of
- Lubrication
- Birth control
- Lots of understanding on both parts

You may need several attempts before you actually have sex again. This may be because you fall asleep or the baby wakes up. You may realize that cuddling and foreplay is all you are ready for right now.

When you do have intercourse, remember to go slowly. Talk to each other and be sure to tell your partner what feels good and what doesn't. Both of you are probably a tad nervous. Clear, calm communication can go a long way to making it a positive experience. Each sexual encounter will be better than the last if you follow these simple rules.

## Adjust Your Diet for Breastfeeding

Many mothers want to know what they should eat while nursing. There is no need to follow a restrictive diet as long as you make a point of eating well, and balanced, meals.

A few babies have food sensitivities to certain foods their mothers eat or drink, whether it's dairy, acidic foods such as tomatoes and citrus, caffeine, or alcohol. Try to pay attention to your diet in the early days and weeks of nursing to see what, if anything, your baby has trouble tolerating. If necessary, your practitioner or lactation consultant can help figure out what your baby is reacting to so you can avoid it in the future.

## Figure Out When and How to Sleep after Birth.

New mothers are told to "sleep when the baby sleeps." Good advice, but the problem is that we are accustomed to sleeping at night and breaking that mindset can be difficult. Not to mention that when the baby naps during the day, mothers are often eager to use the time for something other than sleep.

A new mother thinks, "Oh, I'll just throw in a load of laundry before I lie down..." The next thing you know, the one load of laundry has turned into doing the dishes, having a snack, writing a few thank you notes, and catching up on email. Just when you're ready to lie down, you hear your baby's familiar cry and there goes your nap.

Do your best to resist the call of stray chores. Most things can wait until you have had a nap, or even longer. Resting will help you feel sane and grounded. Doing random chores will not help in the same way. Think of sleep as your priority chore during the postpartum period.

## Get Everyone Fed

After your baby is born, you will not have the luxury of making complicated or time-consuming meals. Instead, you need dishes that can be prepared quickly and easily. Think twenty-minute meals that use five or fewer ingredients. If you don't already own a Crock-Pot, think about buying or borrowing one. They're great time savers because you throw all the ingredients in the night before or in the morning, and many hours later, you've got a hot meal. You can also enlist the help of anyone who has offered to drop by. When they ask if you need anything, skip the "Nothing, thanks," and ask if they wouldn't mind bringing over some prepared food so you have one less meal to worry about.

The hot meals—from friends, the freezer, or the Crock-Pot—usually take care of dinner, but what about the other meals? Stock up on cereal, instant oatmeal, and fruit bars to help get you through breakfast. For lunch, buy lots of soup and fixings for sandwiches. In addition, pick up some healthy options from the frozen food aisle. These products cook quickly, leave little or nothing to clean up, and provide well-balanced nutrition if you choose wisely.

Remember to have a ready stock of healthy snacks as well. Fresh fruits, nuts, dried fruits, crackers, popcorn, and other yummy treats will help maintain your energy levels throughout the day. Stash a few wherever you and the baby tend to hang out, so when hunger pangs strike, you have something close at hand.

### BREASTFEEDING AND SEX

Those old wives have plenty to say when it comes to breastfeeding and sex: You can't breastfeed if you have sex. Orgasm spoils your milk. Men won't want sex if you breastfeed. Ignore these myths, the truth is that breastfeeding and sex are perfectly compatible.

If the feeling is pleasurable, you can certainly tolerate breast stimulation during sex or foreplay. You should know that your breasts may leak, or they may not. If the leaking bothers you or your partner, you should skip this type of breast play or wear a bra with breast pads during sex.

Your breasts may be more sensitive than before, which can be a good thing or it may be painful. Talk to your partner about what feels good and what doesn't. Good communication is always the key to a great relationship, particularly sexual relations.

## Set Realistic Expectations for Yourself

Giving birth and being a parent is hard work and yet the tasks that you do as a parent are quite different from what we traditionally think of as work. This can lead mothers to think that their days are spent doing "nothing." This couldn't be further from the truth.

In reality, you are learning to care for and read another human being. And you are doing it while being sleep deprived and undergoing great shifts in your hormones.

The key to successfully handling the postpartum period is to go easy on yourself. Tell yourself every day that you are doing a great job, even when you don't feel like it. The affirmations that

you used in pregnancy are just as beneficial now; you just need to use postpartum variations. You might even
hang them over the changing table or your nursing station.

The following are some quick tips to help you feel good about yourself:

- Shower often—and alone.
- Buy a new outfit.
- Read a book—having nothing to do with babies—just for fun.
- Eat well, even when you are not hungry.
- Get outside regularly—for a stroll or even to take a walk at the mall.
- Remember that this phase is temporary.

A new kind of normal begins to set in more quickly than you might imagine. You may not even notice, and then one day you wake up and realize it's happened. You feel in control and more like you again. It's a great feeling.

## Get Back to Exercise

Exercise may not be the first thing on your mind after you have a baby, but it's a good idea to start doing some form of exercise almost immediately.

The first kind of exercise after a vaginal birth should be Kegels, just as you did during your pregnancy. These exercises are beneficial for many reasons. They help you tone the muscle and help blood flow return to that area, which speeds the healing process. Plus they may help you to avoid urinary incontinence down the road.

If you had a Cesarean, you can start doing deep breathing exercises in the first days after giving birth. If you do these a few times a day, you will help keep your lungs clear and support the healing process for your abdominal muscles. Place a hand on your lower abdomen, above your incision and inhale deeply enough that you feel your hand

move. Slowly exhale and repeat. You can also contract your stomach muscles and hold them for a count of five. Repeat four or five times.

Walking is something you can do as soon as you feel up to it. Go easily at first, walking for only a few minutes at a time. You should not be carrying anything at the beginning, even your baby, and pushing a stroller is not recommended.

More vigorous exercise can begin after four to six weeks for those who have had vaginal births. Let your bleeding and body be your guide. If you are still bleeding or don't feel well, wait until after your postpartum visit to the doctor or midwife to determine if you are ready. If you had a Cesarean, you will need to wait for this visit anyway; otherwise, you run the risk of damage because your abdominal muscles have been cut and need adequate time to fully heal.

The following are some tips for working out postpartum:

- Remember to start slowly.
- Do not jump back in to your prepregnancy routine.
- Your body may be very different when it comes to working out: Are you anemic? Do you have shortness of breath? Do you have a hernia? Do you have abdominal separation?
- You may need a new exercise bra to prevent you from straining your breasts.
- Consider trying something new that suits your changed lifestyle, such as taking a class that includes baby, such as Stroller Strides or baby yoga, or switching to a new fitness center that offers babysitting while you work out.
- Fitness DVDs and television shows are great for new moms.
- You can swim once you have stopped bleeding.
- Yoga and gentle stretching can feel great.

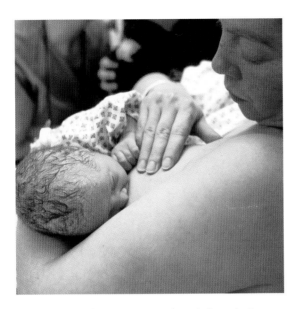

*As soon after birth as possible, put your baby to the breast. Even if they don't nurse, simply being at the breast is helpful.*

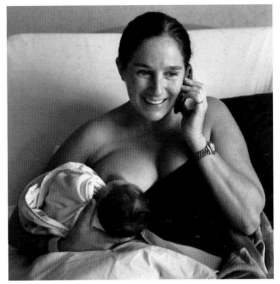

*Soon you'll be able to use a variety of positions while breastfeeding and go about normal activities.*

## Experiment with Positions for Breastfeeding

There are many positions that work for breast feeding. Sometimes a new mother adopts one position and sticks with it, while another woman may need to try them all before finding the best for her and her baby.

CRADLE HOLD: The cradle hold is the classic nursing position. If the baby's head is at your right breast, the head is resting in the crook of your right arm, and the length of his or her body is facing you. Your left hand can be used to stabilize or position the breast or the baby.

CROSS CRADLE HOLD: If the baby is at the right breast, the left hand is on the back of the baby's neck and the right hand is used to stabilize or position the breast or baby.

FOOTBALL HOLD: This is a good position for brand new babies, mothers who have had Cesareans, and those who need a good view of the baby's latch. If the baby is nursing on the left breast, he or she is lying on the mother's left side. The left hand is cradling the back of the baby's head while the right hand is assisting the baby. Use pillows or bolsters to raise the baby's body to be level with his or her head. If the baby is very long, bend the legs upward along the couch or bed where you are sitting.

SIDE LYING: You lie on either side and feed the baby from the bottom breast. Baby lies on his or her side facing you. You can either prop yourself up with your elbow and use the opposite hand for positioning, or lie down and have the bottom arm over your head for comfort.

Experiment to figure out which is comfortable and works best for you and your baby. Don't hesitate to ask a lactation consultant for help.

## Set Up a Breastfeeding Station

A breastfeeding station is simply the spot where you spend most of your time nursing. It can be a favorite chair, in your bed, or on the couch. Whichever spot you choose, you should equip it with all the necessary supplies for the time you are there.

Consider filling a basket or bin with the following:

- A book or magazine for pleasure
- A breastfeeding book
- A water bottle
- Snacks
- The TV remote control
- A phone
- Blank cards or birth announcements and a pen

These items will help you stay busy while nursing. It can also be a sanity saver not to have to get up and fetch something every few minutes while trying to nurse.

## Ensure That Your Baby Is Getting Enough to Eat

One of the biggest concerns a new mom has is whether or not the baby is eating enough. Here are some quick and easy ways to answer that question.

Your baby should eat eight to twelve times a day for the first four to six weeks or until he or she is steadily gaining weight. Most of these feedings should be two to three hours apart.

If your baby is two days old or younger, look for two wet and two dirty diapers per day. Starting when your baby is a week old, look for six to eight wet diapers and about three to five dirty diapers a day.

Some babies do what is called cluster feeding. This means that they pick a time of day and seem to eat nearly every hour. This is perfectly normal, assuming that the baby is going for longer stretches without eating during the rest of the day. Stretches between feedings can be as long as four hours—hopefully at night to allow you to sleep.

When babies have a growth spurt, they require more breast milk. In order to tell your body they need additional milk, they will nurse more frequently. This usually lasts for only a day or two. You may be surprised at how often they nurse during this period, but you should not assume there is a problem.

You cannot rely on how your breasts feel to determine if your baby is eating enough. You should also avoid looking at breast size, which has nothing to do with the amount of milk your baby is getting.

## Know When to Call a Lactation Consultant

A lactation consultant is a specialist at breastfeeding. You should call for help if the following occasions:

- You are having nipple soreness.
- You want advice.
- Your baby is not gaining sufficient weight.
- Your baby has special needs, such as poor suck, improper latch, or cleft lip

A lactation consultant can help by watching you feed your baby and offering supportive suggestions to improve what you are doing. She can also help you decide if assistive feeding devices such as a supplemental nursing system or specialty feeding cups could be beneficial. Lactation consultants also offer services such as baby weight checks and more, so be sure to ask what they provide and how they are covered by insurance.

## Deal with Engorgement

Engorgement is when your breasts are filled with milk, and it usually happens in the first few days after a baby is born. Engorged breasts feel hard and hot to the touch. This can be rather painful, and the best advice is to enlist the baby's help in relieving the swelling and pain by nursing.

Sometimes, especially with a very new baby, it is challenging to latch on to a swollen nipple. By applying a warm compress to the breast and expressing a bit of milk with your hand, you can usually get the baby to latch.

You might also try using cabbage leaves to relieve the swelling, but use caution because this method can also dry up your milk supply. There

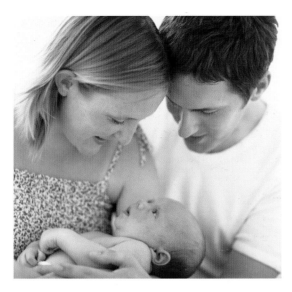

*The support that you get from dad is very important to the overall success of breastfeeding. Be sure to enlist his help!*

are other remedies, but the key is prevention. Nursing your baby on demand will help you avoid the discomfort of engorgement.

If the engorgement continues for a while, you can develop clogged milk ducts. This happens when the milk fails to drain properly from the ducts, and they become backed up. The condition can result from pressure on the breast from an ill-fitting bra or from the way you're holding the breast while nursing. You'll notice a lump or hard spot. Apply hot compresses or take a hot shower and gently massage the area to get the flow going again.

## Use a Breast Pump

A breast pump is designed to express breast milk for your baby. You will want to follow the instructions on your breast pump as far as putting it together and using it properly.

If you want to pump to save milk for later use (maybe for a date night out or because Dad wants to feed the baby), you will want to build up to it. The most important rule is to feed the baby first. Once you and baby have that down pat, it's fine to start building a stash of breast milk. During the early

morning, when your hormones levels are highest, it is a good time to add a pump session. You can also pump on one side while feeding the baby on the other side, once you have established your milk supply. Another trick is to pump your breasts after a feeding. This ensures that your baby gets the milk he or she need and within a few days, your body adjusts to supply extra milk at this feeding.

If you will be pumping on a regular schedule, such as at work, these pump times will replace the times when baby would be nursing, and an extra milk supply is therefore not needed. If you want more milk, try adding an extra pump session, though preferably not at work, where it can be difficult to stick to regular feeding times.

## Return to Work after Maternity Leave

One you are nearing the end of your maternity leave, you may begin to feel anxious about returning to work. These feelings are not at all unusual and should not be cause for concern.

The goal is to ease your transition back to work as much as possible. To do this takes a bit of planning. First, you should consider returning to work on a Wednesday or Thursday so your first week back is a partial week. Or you might consider starting with a half day on Wednesday or Thursday and then a full day or two after that. You may also decide to do two weeks of half time, rather than jumping right in to a full-time schedule.

Many mothers feel that this eases them and their family back into the workplace. If you find that you have issues to deal with, from child care to separation anxiety, then you have some breathing room in which to work it out. Going back to work can also be a tiring endeavor in the beginning. Starting slowly will help you ease into your work routine and gradually build stamina.

Once you are at work, pull out the binder that you made for maternity leave. It will help get you

## MEDICATIONS AND BREASTFEEDING

You may need to take medication while breastfeeding, but you should inform your practitioner or internist that you are nursing. Ideally, you already discussed all medication that you take on a regular basis before your birth.

Ask if the medications are compatible with breastfeeding. If they are, you are good to go but remember to raise the question again whenever he or she prescribes something for you. If the medications are not compatible, ask if there are similar medications that you can substitute.

Also tell your pharmacist that you are breastfeeding. This will help your efforts to nurse successfully without medication-related problems. You may run into a pharmacist or even practitioners who do not know a lot about the interaction between medications and breastfeeding. This can result in your being given incorrect information, or your being told to wean. First of all, make sure you are informed. There is a book on the topic called *Medications and Mother's Milk* by Dr. Thomas Hale. Then be sure that your practitioner and pharmacist are consulting this or a similar book for reliable, up-to-date information.

off to a fresh start and save your brain the strain of figuring things out in a vacuum. Hopefully, whoever has been keeping up with your projects has left you a progress report so you know what's up and what's ahead.

Remember to be kind to yourself. Do not panic if you feel lost or swamped for the first few days or weeks. Pack healthy snacks and lunch for maximum energy. Pump when you need to and do not feel guilty or self-conscious for taking mandated breaks. These tips—together with time and patience—should help make your return to work a positive and relatively stress-free experience.

### HOT MAMA

Stretchy pants are great the first couple of weeks after birth. But remember, you need to ditch them relatively quickly. Keeping your stretchy pants doesn't give you a sense of where your body is physically after having a baby and has a tendency to encourage you to keep some of the extra pounds. This may mean you buy a new pair of jeans or two until you finish losing the weight, which can take awhile. But the goal is to shed the weight and feel good about your body so you can be healthy for your baby.

# APPENDIX 1

## QUESTIONS TO ASK YOUR BIRTH PLACE

Take this list along when you tour your birth facility. As the tour director responds to your questions, do not hesitate to ask new questions that their answers raise. You should also have someone accompany you on the tour to help remember the answers and write notes when possible.

## Questions about Labor and Birth

- Do you offer classes for expectant parents?
- Who teaches the classes?
- How much do the classes cost?
- Do you have specialty classes, such as breastfeeding, VBAC, Cesarean, and Lamaze?
- Where do I go when it's time for labor: Labor and Delivery, the emergency room, or admitting?
- Is there a different place to go at night?
- Do I need to fill out any paperwork before being admitted in labor?
- Where can I find that paperwork?
- What will I need to bring with me when I'm in labor?
- Will my chart be sent over or will I need to hand carry it?
- Will I have to go to a triage area during labor or will I be shown directly to a private room?
- How long do mothers typically stay in triage?
- What types of rooms are available to give birth in?
- Can I labor, give birth, and recover in one room?

- What types of comfort measures do you encourage or practice?
- Is there a tub or shower in the birth room?
- Will I have access to birth balls, music, squat bar, etc.?
- Is there a kitchen area for me or my family?
- Am I allowed to bring food or drink from home?
- Do you provide clear liquids such as popsicles, broth, and Jell-O?
- Do you allow eating in labor? Is this true if you do not intend to receive anesthesia?
- Are IVs required of all laboring women or only those who are high risk or could I have a saline lock to provide access to my veins instead?
- Who would make this provision if it's not a standard policy? Can my doctor or midwife write a different order?
- What type of medications are available should I choose medication?
- What IV medications are used?
- Do you offer epidural anesthesia?
- Is there a special class to take for the epidural or other medications in labor?
- Do you have anesthesiologists who only do obstetrical anesthesia?
- Do you have 24-hour anesthesia available on site?
- Can I have a prelabor consult with the anesthesia group if I have special concerns?
- Under what circumstances can I not have anesthesia?

- Do you have visitor policies in labor?
- Do you have policies about siblings? Is there an age limit?
- How many people can be in the room when I am giving birth?
- Are cameras and film equipment allowed?
- Are there any periods during which we should turn off the cameras and film equipment?
- Can I use a camera stand?
- Do you allow professional photographers?
- What type of fetal monitoring do you offer: external, internal, or Doppler/fetoscope?
- What are the hospital policies on monitoring in labor?
- Do you offer telemetry (wireless) monitoring?
- How often do you experience an overflow of patients?
- What happens if all of your birthing rooms are taken?
- Do you ever send patients to other hospitals?
- Do you use students or residents in any way?
- Do I have the ability to refuse them or ask them to leave?
- What is your hospital's induction rate?
- How many patients receive augmentation in labor?
- What is your episiotomy rate?
- What is your epidural rate?
- What are your forceps and vacuum birth rates?
- What is your Cesarean rate?
- What is your VBAC rate? (If they do not provide these statistics, ask at the department of health or vital statistics.)
- Do you have doulas on staff?
- Do you have a listing of doulas?
- Are there requirements of doulas, such as certification, and if so, which ones?

- Does the facility offer a birth planning form?
- To whom should I send my birth plan?
- Does my birth plan need to be signed by my doctor or midwife and my pediatrician?
- Who is your facility certified through?
- Which accreditations do you have?
- Do you have a patient advocate on staff and if so, are they on call?

## Questions about Cesarean Birth

- Can my partner and my doula both stay with me for a Cesarean birth?
- Can we have photos of the birth and if so, who will take them?
- Will I be able to watch the surgery via mirror?
- Could the drapes be lowered?
- What is the policy about preoperative medications?
- What is the policy about postoperative pain relief?
- Do you do Duramorph or patient controlled analgesia (PCA)?
- Will the baby be available to me during the surgery time or in the recovery room?
- When can I begin nursing?
- If the Cesarean is planned, what is the admission procedure?
- Will my partner be able to go with the baby should he or she need to leave the room?

## Questions about Postpartum

- What is the average length of stay for a vaginal birth?
- What is the average length of stay for a Cesarean birth?
- Does insurance typically cover this stay?
- Will I have the same room postpartum that I did for labor and birth?
- Are all your postpartum rooms private and if not, when would my room not be private?
- Will I ever be moved from my room?
- Can my family stay with me in my room?
- Do the rooms have showers or tubs?
- Will I get a sitz baths?
- Do you offer portable sitz baths to take home?
- What pain relief options are available postpartum?
- Do the pain relief options differ following Cesarean births?
- Do the pain relief options differ for nursing moms?
- Is there a policy for early discharge?
- Who would I talk to about getting an early discharge?
- What are the meal policies?
- Whom do I talk to if I have special concerns about my diet?
- When can I eat after giving birth?
- Is food available 24/7?
- Are there places for my family to eat?

## Questions about Baby Care

- What is your policy on rooming in?
- Are there times that the baby cannot be in our room? What are these and can they be altered?
- If the baby must go to the nursery, can dad go along?
- Do pediatricians do their visits at the bedside or in the nursery? When would this not be appropriate?
- Do you have a lactation consultant?
- What are the lactation consultants hours?
- Does the lactation consultant see every nursing mom?
- Is the lactation consultant certified?
- Can I talk to someone about early vaccination schedules?
- What can you tell me about the mandatory metabolic testing of newborns?
- What are the policies about breastfeeding babies and bottles/pacifiers?
- Are you a designated baby friendly hospital? *(www.babyfriendly.org)*
- Are there sibling visitation policies?
- How many private rooms are available for postpartum and how are they assigned?
- When are circumcisions performed?
- Who performs circumcisions?
- What anesthesia is available for circumcisions?
- Do you allow ritual circumcisions?
- Do you provide a big enough room for social functions with ritual circumcisions?
- What if we do not want a circumcision?

# APPENDIX 2

## RESOURCES

### ABOUT PREGNANCY

*pregnancy.about.com*

This website offers information on pregnancy from conception to after birth. With the pregnancy week by week calendar, belly and ultrasound galleries, and lots of useful information, you're sure to find something here to enjoy throughout your entire pregnancy.

### AMERICAN ACADEMY OF HUSBAND COACHED CHILDBIRTH

*www.bradleybirth.com*

Based on the teachings of Dr. Robert Bradley, an obstetrician, the Bradley Method teaches natural childbirth and views birth as a natural process. It is a system of natural labor techniques in which a woman and her partner/coach play an active part.

### AMERICAN ACADEMY OF PEDIATRICS (AAP)

*www.aap.org*

This is the political body of pediatricians practicing in the United States. This group drafts policies based on research for pediatricians to use as guidelines in their practice. They also have many publications geared toward parents from baby safety and infant feeding to caring for your teen.

### AMERICAN ASSOCIATION OF BIRTH CENTERS (AABC)

*www.birthcenters.org*

Providing training and certification for birth centers, the AABC also maintains public information and a database of birth centers.

### AMERICAN COLLEGE OF NURSE MIDWIVES

*www.mymidwife.org*

This group creates the policy statements for certified nurse midwives as well as certified midwives around the United States.

### AMERICAN COLLEGE OF OBSTETRICIANS AND GYNECOLOGISTS (ACOG)

*www.acog.org*

Providing guidance in practice for obstetricians and gynecologists in the United States, ACOG holds conferences and generates research for doctors in the obstetrics and gynecologic field.

### AMERICAN PREGNANCY ASSOCIATION

*www.americanpregnancy.org*

The American Pregnancy Association is a national health organization committed to promoting reproductive and pregnancy wellness through education, research, advocacy, and community awareness.

### BABY FRIENDLY HOSPITAL INITIATIVE

*www.babyfriendly.org*

By choosing a hospital or birth center that has been certified as "baby friendly," parents can be assured that they will get the best start possible for their baby in terms of assistance and breastfeeding support. This group runs the certification program throughout the world.

## THE BIRTH ACTIVIST

*www.birthactivist.com*

This blog covers hot topics in pregnancy and childbirth, asking the hard questions and providing many points of view. It is premised on the belief that with all the information available, and not just the subset one person or organization wants you to have, you will be able to make the safest and best decisions for your family.

## BIRTH NETWORK NATIONAL

*www.birthnetwork.org*

This grassroots organization has chapters in many states. Each chapter focuses on the special needs of its particular community when it comes to pregnancy and birth support. There are educational meetings of various topics held.

## THE BIRTH SURVEY

*www.thebirthsurvey.com*

Ever wanted to share your birth experience and let everyone know how birth was for you? This survey allows you to do that, but it also lets you explore other practitioners and places of birth in your community and read what other mothers had to say about the care they received.

## CHILDBIRTH CONNECTION

*www.childbirthconnection.com*

Celebrating more than ninety years of helping mothers and families with educational needs in pregnancy, this group provides patient education to birthing families on a variety of topics, including Cesarean section and vaginal birth after Cesarean (VBAC).

## COALITION FOR IMPROVING MATERNITY SERVICES (CIMS)

*www.motherfriendly.org*

The mission of CIMS is to "promote a wellness model of maternity care that will improve birth outcomes and substantially reduce costs." With more than 90,000 members, they are moving forward in maternity care.

## DONA INTERNATIONAL (FORMERLY DOULAS OF NORTH AMERICA)

*www.dona.org*

The premiere doula organization in the world trains and certifies people to become professional supporters of laboring women and their families. This organization offers both birth doula and postpartum doula trainings as well as a vast referral network around the world.

## FIRST CANDLE

*www.firstcandle.org*

Formerly the SIDS Alliance (sudden infant death syndrome), First Candle is a nonprofit organization designed to help educate parents about infant health and safety as well as to provide a place for information if your baby has died.

## INTERNATIONAL CESAREAN AWARENESS NETWORK

*www.ican-online.org*

ICAN's goal is to help promote education surrounding Cesarean section and vaginal birth after Cesarean (VBAC) throughout the world. They provide consumer information on Cesareans, VBAC, and emotional and physical recovery as well as advocacy for families.

## INTERNATIONAL CHILDBIRTH EDUCATION ASSOCIATION (ICEA)

*www.icea.org*

ICEA trains and certifies childbirth educators, labor doulas, prenatal fitness teachers, and postpartum educators. This international organization holds trainings all over the country.

## INTERNATIONAL LACTATION CONSULTANT ASSOCIATION (ILCA)

*www.ilca.org*

ILCA provides the mechanism for testing to certify International Board Certified Lactation Consultants (IBCLCs), while offering professional conferences and a public database for IBCLCs.

## LA LECHE LEAGUE INTERNATIONAL

*www.llli.org*

This nonprofit organization is dedicated to supporting breastfeeding families through educational meetings, phone support, and in-person support from trained mothers who have been there with breastfeeding. They support a family's right to choose to breastfeed for any length of time from one day to one year or more.

## LAMAZE INTERNATIONAL

*www.lamaze.org*

The most recognized name in childbirth education, Lamaze trains and certifies childbirth educators throughout the world. They also provide information for families through their magazine and website as well as trainings for professionals such as the Labor Support for Nurses program, Breastfeeding Specialist, and other trainings. You will find an easy directory of childbirth educators around the world at their website.

## MIDWIVES ALLIANCE OF NORTH AMERICAN

*www.mana.org*

MANA is the midwifery organization for certified professional midwives and direct entry midwives. Here you can find information about home birth, birth centers, and choosing the right midwife for your pregnancy to support you in the midwives model of care.

## MOTHERING MAGAZINE

*www.mothering.com*

This magazine offers an online collection of articles and stories on pregnancy, birth and parenting, in addition to an online forum for women to discuss issues related to motherhood.

## NATIONAL ORGANIZATION FOR MOTHERS OF TWINS CLUBS

*www.nomotc.org*

Expecting more than one baby? NOMOTC offers a directory of twins and multiples clubs all over the United States.

## POSTPARTUM SUPPORT INTERNATIONAL

*www.postpartum.net*

Designed to provide support and education about postpartum emotional disorders such as the baby blues, postpartum depression, and more, this group offers the latest research and help lines available for families in the postpartum time frame.

## SOLACE FOR MOTHERS

*www.solaceformothers.org*

A place for mothers to talk about their recovery after a traumatic birth.

## VAGINAL BIRTH AFTER CESAREAN (VBAC)

*www.vbac.com*

This research-based website offers information about vaginal birth after Cesarean including the success rates, risks, benefits, and more— all presented in an easy-to-understand format.

## Acknowledgments

Writing a book takes more than simply sitting down and putting words to paper. There are so many steps involved. I'd like to thank the following people for hand-holding, cheerleading, word counting, and general support: Ashley Benz, Teri Shilling, Pat Predmore, Juliet Dietsch, Jana Pedowitz, Paula Pepperstone, Dr. Marcello Pietrantoni, Ann Grauer, Barb Doyen, Jill Alexander, Nancy King, and Jennifer Reich. There are also some people who put up with a very grouchy mother who spent too much time hunched over a computer some days, and yet they still love me: Hilary, Benjamin, Isaac, Lilah, Owen, Clara, Ada, and Noa. And a special thanks to my husband, Kevin, for all of the driving, meals, cleanup, foot massages, and pep talks.

## About the Authors

**Robin Elise Weiss, L.C.C.E., C.D. (DONA)** is a childbirth and postpartum educator, certified doula, and lactation counselor as well as the pregnancy/birth expert for About.com. She is the author of seven books on pregnancy and childbirth and she and her work have been featured in *Newsweek*, *Working Mother*, and *American Baby*. She lives in Louisville, Kentucky.

**Dr. Marcello Pietrantoni, M.D., F.A.C.O.G.,** is a perinatologist—a physician specializing in maternal and fetal health and complicated pregnancies. Dr. Pietrantoni is certified by the American Academy of Obstetrics and Gynecology. He is a member of American Medical Association, and the Society of Maternal Fetal Medicine. He has been a practicing perinatologist for more than seventeen years. He is currently in private practice in Louisville, Kentucky, where he lives with his family.

# INDEX